ALLE ZEIT WACH 1842

Spinal Angiomas

Advances in Diagnosis and Therapy

Edited by H. W. Pia and R. Djindjian

With 134 Figures

Springer-Verlag
Berlin Heidelberg New York 1978

Professor Dr. Dr. h.c. Hans Werner Pia
Direktor der Neurochirurgischen Universitäts-Klinik
Klinikstraße 29, D-6300 Giessen

René Djindjian †
Professeur de Neuroradiologie
à la Faculté de Médecine de Paris

ISBN-13: 978-3-642-66722-0 e-ISBN-13: 978-3-642-66720-6
DOI: 10.1007/978-3-642-66720-6

Library of Congress Catalog Card Number: Main entry under title: Spinal angiomas. Bibliography: p. Includes index. 1. Spinal cord-Tumors. 2. Angioma. I. Pia, Hans-Werner. II. Djindjian, René. [DNLM: 1. Hemangioma-Diagnosis. 2. Hemangioma-Therapy. 3. Spinal cord neoplasms-Diagnosis. 4. Spinal cord neoplasms-Therapy. WL400 S757] RC280.S7S64 616.9'92'82 77-15055

Softcover reprint of the hardcover 1st edition 1978

Printing: Beltz, Offsetdruck, Hemsbach/Bergstraße
Bookbinding: J. Schäffer OHG, Grünstadt

2127/3140-543210

In Memory of
RENE DJINDJIAN

Preface

The rapid development of diagnostic and therapeutic procedures in the management of spinal angiomas has opened up new possibilities and provided better chances for the patients concerned. The greatest impetus to this progress was given by the introduction of selective and superselective spinal angiography, microsurgical technique, and embolization. These sophisticated techniques and the skill required for their use are far from being routine in the neurosurgical and neuroradiologic departments. In spite of the rarity of spinal angiomas, the application of the above-mentioned procedures is the prerequisite for improving early diagnosis and giving timely adequate treatment. Delay in diagnosis and treatment are still the main cause of unsatisfactory results.

In the last 10 - 20 years, several groups in Europe and the USA have done important and fundamental work in introducing and developing the diganostic and therapeutic armamentarium. Based on the pioneering work of their teachers and the classic contribution of Wyburn – Mason in 1943, they simultaneously improved the morphologic, physiologic, and clinical basis of our knowledge.

Although progress is going on and many problems have to be solved, the general principles of clinical diagnosis, operative treatment, and embolization have been laid down and are to be published in a special monograph on this topic.

Several meetings in which most of the contributors participated led to the idea of combining the experiences of the experts in a single, factual, and frank discussion. We feel that it is precisely the diverse and controversial aspects and the personal character of this book which portray the existing situation in certain fields. We hope that this may stimulate neurologists, neurosurgeons, and neuroradiologists to join our efforts to improve the fate of patients suffering from spinal angiomas.

We are very grateful to the Springer Company, for their acceptance and realization of our idea and also their indulgence in allowing several proposals for additional contributors, occasioned by new developments during the preparation and production of this book.

Our thanks are also extended to our friends who have participated in this book and to all those who have helped in its preparation, especially our neurosurgical friend Charles Langmaid for translation and correction.

Giessen and Paris, December 1976

Hans Werner Pia
René Djindjian

On behalf of the contributors I deeply regret that René Djindjian could not witness the completion of our book. He died before it was published.

Giessen, January 1978

Hans Werner Pia

Contents

Embolization

List of Contributors

Dr. Agnolo Lino Agnoli, Neuroradiolog. Abteilung, Zentrum für Radiologie, Röntgenabteilung Chirurgie der Justus Liebig–Universität, Klinikstr. 29, D–6300 Giessen

Dr. Michel Djindjian. Service de Neurochirurgie, Hôpital Lariboisière, 2, Rue A. Paré, F–75010 Paris

Prof. Dr. René Djindjian †, Département de Neuroradiologie à la Faculté de Médecine de Paris

Dr. John L. Doppman, Department of Radiology, Clinical Center, National Institute of Health, Bethesda MD 20014/USA

Dr. R.W. Fiedeler, Neurochirurgische Klinik, Rämistraße 100, CH–8091 Zürich

Prof. Dr. Hermann Hager, Abteilung Neuropathologie, Zentrum für Neurologie der Justus Liebig-Universität Giessen, Am Steg 22, D–6300 Giessen

Prof. Dr. R. Houdart, Service de Neurochirurgie, Hôpital Lariboisière, 2, Rue A. Paré, F–75010 Paris

Prof. Dr. Kurt Jellinger, Ludwig Boltzmann-Institut für klinische Neurobiologie, Wolkersbergenstr. 1, A–1130 Wien

Dr. Albrecht Laun, Zentrum für Neurochirurgie der Justus Liebig-Universität Giessen, Klinkstr. 29, D–6300 Giessen

Prof. Dr. Guy Lazorthes, Clinique de Neurochirurgie, Hôpital de Rangueil, F–31054 Toulouse

Prof. Dr. Dr. h.c. Hans Werner Pia, Zentrum für Neurochirurgie der Justus Liebig-Universität Giessen, Klinikstr. 19, D–6300 Giessen

Dr. Th. P. Rankin, Neurochirurgische Universitätsklinik, Kantonspital Zürich, Rämistraße 100, CH–8091 Zürich

Prof. Dr. A. Rey, Service de Neurochirurgie, Hôpital Lariboisière,
2, Rue A. Paré, F–75010 Paris

Prof. Dr. Heinzgeorg Vogelsang, Department Radiologie, Abteilung II-Neuroradiologie der Medizinischen Hochschule Hannover, Karl-Wiechert-Allee 9, D–3000 Hannover 61

Prof. Dr. Mahmut Gazy Yasargil, Neurochirurgische Universitätsklinik, Kantonspital Zürich, Rämistraße 100, CH–8091 Zürich

Morphologic Aspects

Blood Supply and Vascular Pathology of the Spinal Cord

Guy Lazorthes

The pathology of the spinal cord has for a long time been dominated by myelitis. Nowadays it is thought that many of the previously described "syndromes" are, in fact, vascular myelopathies. Three events have shed new light on spinal pathology:

1. Research into the blood supply and circulation of the central nervous system has not only recalled some long-standing and often neglected developments by Adamkiewicz (1882), Kadyi (1889), and Tanon (1910) but has also provided new details (Lazorthes, 1957, 1958, 1964; Corbin, 1961).
2. More systematic anatomic and clinical investigations of the pathologic spinal cord have also produced some very interesting observations (Ullman and Alajouanine, 1938; Zülch, 1954-1955; Lhermitte and Corbin, 1960; Garcin et al., 1963; Jellinger, 1966; Neumayer, 1967; Fazio, 1970).
3. New techniques of exploration and examination, especially angiography of the vessels of the spinal cord by selective injection, have placed the anatomic contributions in an appropriate clinical and surgical framework (Houdart et al., 1965; Di Chiro, 1967).

A final analysis shows quite clearly that in spite of the complexity and fragility of the central nervous system (brain, brain stem, or spinal cord) and the susceptibility of the neurone to ischemia and anoxemia, there is fortunately a correspondingly very particular blood supply and circulation which has no analogy with that of other internal organs. In actual fact, the central nervous system is provided:

1. on the arterial side, with safety systems which are capable of becoming pathways of supply, and these systems are unlike those met within any other part of the human body,
2. on the venous side, with multiple drainage channels, and
3. with regulating and protective mechanisms.

I. Arterial Blood Supply and the Afferent Channels

In the case of the spinal cord, as with all other parts of the central nervous system, there exist anastomotic safety systems arranged on several levels (Lazorthes, 1962). They are called into play in cases of physiologic or pathologic circulatory insufficiency.

The first system, which is extraspinal, connects the entering vessels. The other two systems, which are intraspinal, can be called respectively periaxial and intraaxial, according to their position. We will consider: 1. the circulation on the entering vessels, 2. the circulation in the perimedullary region, and 3. the intramedullary circulation.

1. The Circulation in the Vessels of the Arterial Inflow

The afferent arterial vessels of the spinal cord are more numerous and more extensive than those of the brain, and their details are less well-known than those of the brain and brain stem.

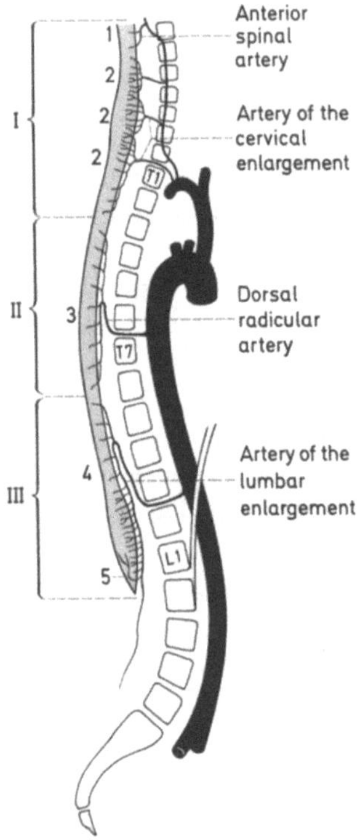

Fig. 1. The three vascular territories of the spinal cord (Lazorthes, 1957)

The division of the spinal cord into three distinct territories (Fig. 1) according to their unequal blood supply, which we proposed in 1957, and which has been adopted by every author since, must be retained for the study of the circulation. Each of these three territories, i.e., each of these three vascular areas, represents not only an anatomic unity but also a functional unity. Hence, this division has a morphologic and even more so a physiologic significance.

The Upper or Cervicothoracic Region

The Upper Cervical Spinal Cord

The first four cervical segments (C 1 - C 4) have generally little or no radicular inflow. They are supplied by the anterior spinal artery. This vessel originates from the convergence of two branches coming from the vertebral arteries. The arterial supply is represented by the "suboccipital anastomotic confluence" formed by the anastomosis of the vertebral, occipital, and the ascending and deep cervical arteries (Lazorthes and Gouazé, 1968). It is capable of taking over from the terminal segment of the vertebral artery and thus protecting the circulation of the brain stem and the cerebrum, but even more so that of the upper cervical spinal cord which depends on it. In thromboses of the vertebral artery, the distal segment of this artery can obtain a collateral supply from the occipital or deep cervical or ascending cervical arteries.

Cervical Enlargement

The last four cervical segments and the first two thoracic segments (C5 – D 2) constitute the functional unit of the upper limb and possess an independent blood supply. They are, indeed, supplied by two to four large radicular arteries, originating from the vertebral arteries and the ascending and deep cervical arteries; the lowest one (Fig. 2) arrives with the seventh or eighth cervical root, is the most important and has been designated the artery of the cervical enlargement (Lazorthes, 1962). We have investigated the part played by various arteries of the neck in the blood supply of the cervical spinal cord, by the injection of colloidal barium into each of them (Lazorthes and Gouazé, 1966).

The functional value of the anatomic contributions can only be verified in vivo by experiments on animals, or as a result of fortuitous clinical observations. We have, in the

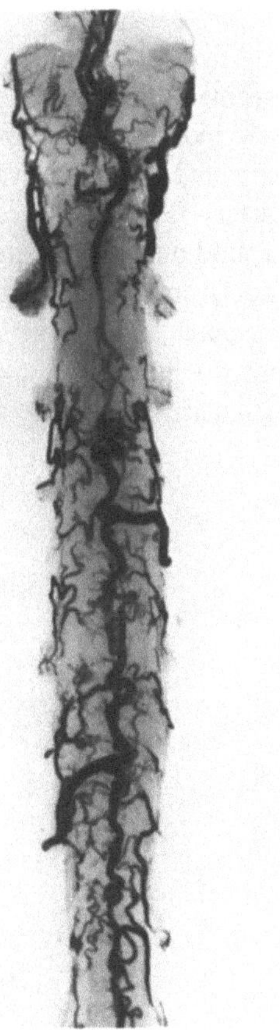

Fig. 2. Arteries of the cervical enlargement. The lowest is called "the artery of the cervical enlargement." It is generally the most important (Lazorthes, 1962)

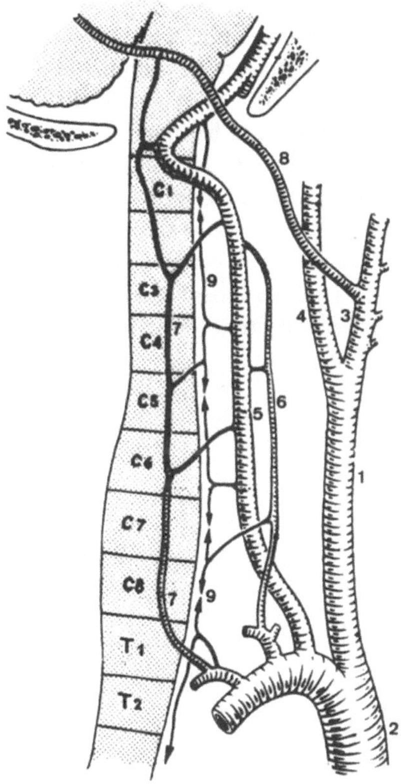

Fig. 3. Blood supply of the cervicothoracic region and the collateral pathways: 1. common carotid, 2. innominate artery, 3. external carotid, 4. internal carotid, 5. vertebral artery, 6. ascending cervical artery, 7. deep cervical artery, 8. occipital artery, 9. anterior spinal artery

case of the monkey, the dog, the cat, and the rabbit, been able to obtain information about the functional areas of the cervical spinal cord by the injection of biologic fluorescents. We have been able to show that the subclavian and external carotid systems are capable, in these animals, of taking over the blood supply to the cervical spinal cord in the event of ligation of both vertebral arteries (Fig. 3).

The anastomotic collaterals of the external carotid are responsible for the upper two-thirds of the cervical spinal cord; the subclavians ensure the blood supply of the cervical enlargement. Finally, if one vertebral artery is tied, the supply to all of the cervical spinal cord is taken over by the other vertebral artery (Lazorthes et al., 1968).

The second thoracic spinal segment represents a border zone situated between the upper area, which is supplied by the collaterals of the subclavian artery, and the two areas, intermediate and lower, whose blood supply depends directly on the thoracic and abdominal aorta. Obviously this dividing line is subject to wide individual variations which means that it may be higher or, more often lower, e.g., at D 3. The zone without arterial afferents corresponds in general to the second and third thoracic segments.

The Intermediate or Midthoracic Region

The third, fourth, fifth, sixth, seventh, and eighth thoracic segments usually receive a single artery which arrives with the fifth, sixth or seventh thoracic root. It must, however, be remembered that when any of the dorsal spinal arteries is injected where it leaves the aorta – where it can be more properly called the intercostal artery (Fig. 4) – it can be seen that the greatest portion of the injection is very quickly found on the opposite side as well as in the more superficial and in the deeper layers. The dorsal spinal arteries are, in fact, connected by their various collaterals in the vertebral, intraspinal, and retrovertebral planes. Selective aortic angiography can display them, but from the point of view of the cord, there are few possible supplies at this level, which is particularly vulnerable and is the site of predilection for ischemic lesions.

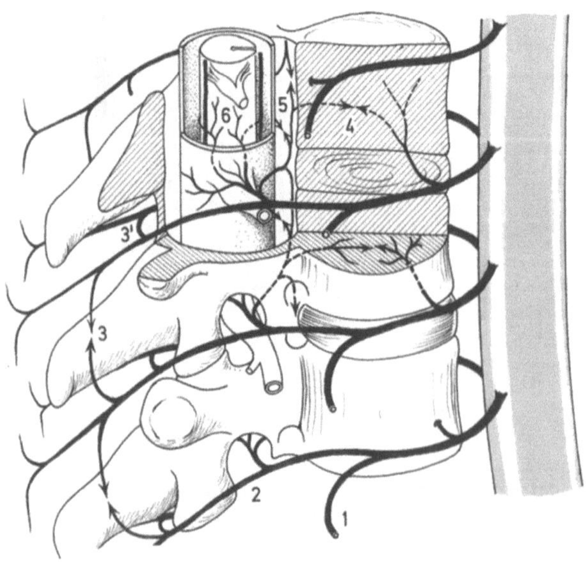

Fig. 4. Arteries of the midthoracic region: 1. intercostal artery, 2. dorsal spinal branch, 3. retrovertebral anastomosis, 4. intravertebral anastomosis, 5. extradural anastomosis, 6. medullary artery

We have attempted to demonstrate this by the following experiment (Fig. 5): after ligation of the thoracic aorta, below the origin of the subclavian artery from which the highest intercostal artery comes (this provides the last radicular artery vascularizing the upper or cervicothoracic region), and above the intercostal or lumbar artery from which the artery of the lumbar enlargement (Adamkiewcz artery) which vascularizes the lower region comes, an injection of the aortic segment thus isolated allows us to determine the small contribution from the aorta to the midthoracic spinal cord, the scanty supply available, and the precariousness of the blood supply of the spinal cord in this intermediate region.

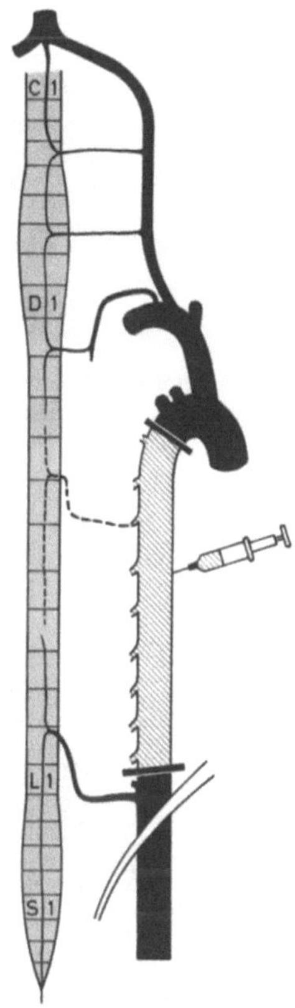

Fig. 5. Experiment to show the poor blood supply of the midthoracic spinal cord

The Lower or Thoracolumbosacral Region

At the level of the lower thoracic, lumbar, and sacral spinal cord segments, the available blood supply usually depends essentially on one artery, the large anterior radicular artery of Adamkiewicz, which we decided to call the artery of the lumbar enlargement (Lazorthes, 1957) (Fig. 6). It is usually the only arterial contribution in this area, which represents approximately the lower third of the spinal cord; when it is very high up and arrives with the seventh, eighth, ninth, or tenth thoracic roots, a second anterior radicular artery may be found lower down. The posterior radicular arteries are more numerous (Fig. 7).

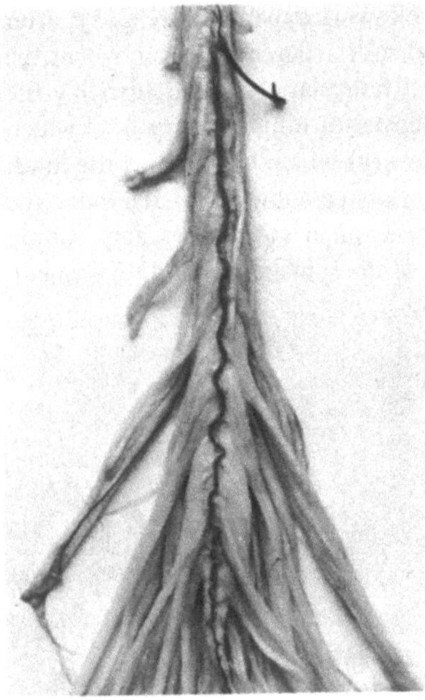

Fig. 6. Artery of Adamkiewicz or "of the lumbar enlargement" of Lazorthes

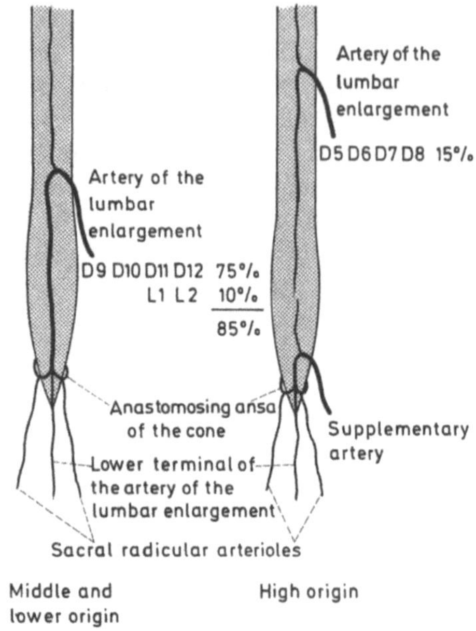

Fig. 7. Artery of the lumbar enlargement and its variations (Lazorthes, 1957)

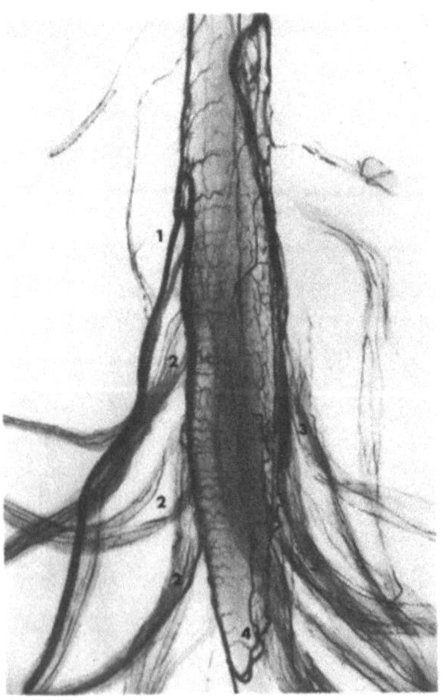

Fig. 8. Arterial supply of the lumbar enlargement: 1. artery of Adamkiewicz or "of the lumbar enlargement," 2. and 3. arteries of the sacral roots, 4. anastomotic loop of the conus (Lazorthes, 1957)

The system is essentially composed of the "lower radicular inputs" which we described in 1962 (Lazorthes et al., 1968) (Fig.8). On each root of the cauda equina, below the artery of the lumbar enlargement, there exist one or more arteries, thin, but nevertheless real, which converge on the anterior spinal artery for the anterior ones, and on the posterior spinal arteries for the posterior ones. We have shown in the case of animals (monkey and dog), by injecting fluorescent neurotropic markers (Lazorthes et al., 1967),

Fig. 9. Ligature of the lumbar artery. One of them gives off the artery of Adamkiewicz. The injection of biologic fluorescents shows the importance of the inferior supply.
(a) Diagrammatic sketch.
(b) Spinal cord of monkey, dorsal view

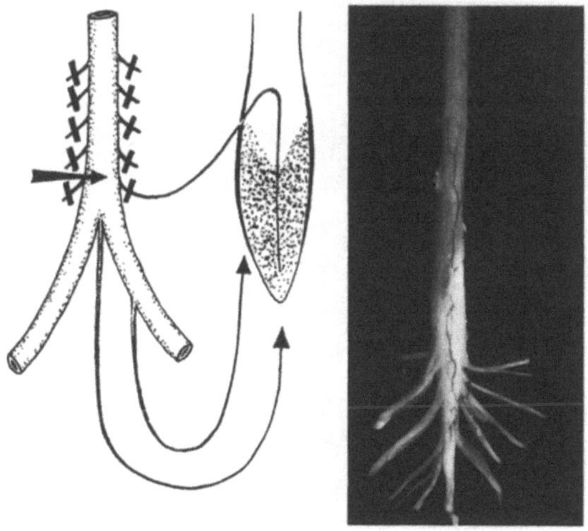

(a) (b)

that these radicular inputs are capable of opening up in the event of a deficiency in the main inflow and that they can take over the supply of the lumbar enlargement (Fig. 9).

In the case of man, if a solution of colloidal barium is injected into the abdominal aorta, below the origin of the artery of the lumbar enlargement, the contrast material is found at the level of the whole lumbar enlargement. It undoubtedly gets there through the arteries which accompany the roots of the cauda equina, coming from the lumbar, iliolumbar, middle sacral, and lateral sacral arteries and then through the anastomotic loop of the conus (Lazorthes, 1957).

2. The Circulation in the Perimedullary Arterial Network

In the case of the brain, two levels can be distinguished in the periaxial arterial blood supply: on the one hand, the basal anastomotic circle (circle of Willis) which represents a theoretically ideal safety device and has no equivalent in any other part of the human body; on the other hand, there is the cortical network composed of the three cerebral arteries and their anastomoses.

In the case of the spinal cord, there is nothing comparable: the periaxial network is composed of an important anterior, median longitudinal channel which extends the vertebrobasilar trunk along the spinal cord, of other longitudinal channels of lesser importance, and lastly, of the transverse anastomoses which connect these.

The Longitudinal Spinal Channels

There are two questions which arise viz., the continuity of these longitudinal channels and the direction of the circulation in the anterior spinal artery. What should be thought about *the anterior spinal complex?* Suh and Alexander (1939) stated that, if an injection is made into the arteries of the first cervical segments, the material does not go beyond the cervical spinal cord; that if it is made into the arteries of the lumbar region, it rises into the lower and middle thoracic segments. This finding suggested to the authors the theory that the flow in the anterior spinal trunk goes in opposite directions, descend-

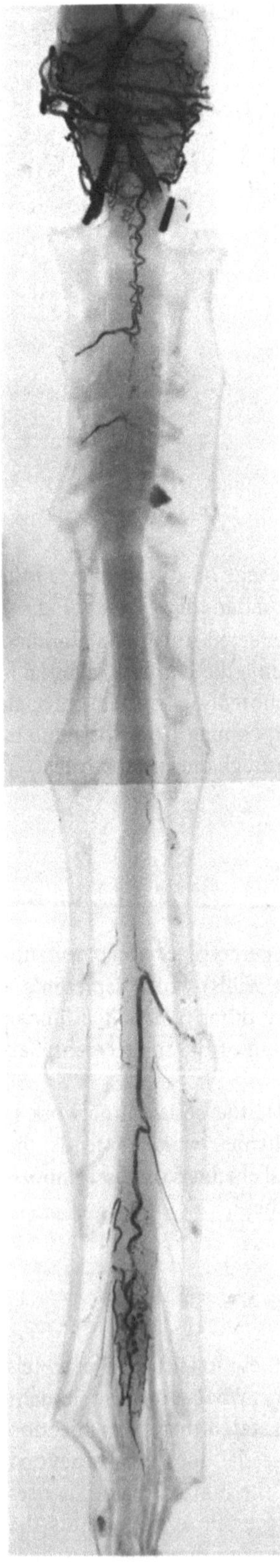

Fig. 10. Injection into the basilar artery goes into the anterior spinal artery , but when it reaches the middle cervical segments it leaves the vertebral canal by means of a radicular artery and passes into the general circulation. The material appears again in the artery of Adamkiewicz

ing in the upper cervical part and ascending in the lower (lumbosacral and lower thoracic) part. The perimedullary arteries of the upper thoracic region, the point of convergence of the two flows, would thus represent an anastomotic channel too inadequate to allow any connection between the upper and lower vascular territories.

Zülch (1954, 1962) points out, moreover, that the flow makes its way upward in the ascending branch of a radicular artery and downward in the descending branch. Along the cervical spinal cord, the flow would descend to approximately D 4. Lower down, along the thoracic spinal cord, it would be ascending from D 9 / D 10 to D 4, and descending as far as the start of the lumbar spinal cord. Along the lumbosacral cord, the flow is ascending for a very short distance above the point of entry of the large radicular artery (approximately L 2) and descending below that. There would be a vulnerable point at D 4 between the cervical and thoracic flow and another at L 1 between the lower thoracic and upper lumbar inflow (Fig. 10).

With the aim of investigating the circulation in the anterior spinal artery, we have carried out a certain number of experiments (1958), one of which seems to us to be conclusive. In a fetus, we tied the two vertebral arteries after their entry into the skull, then by injection of the basilar trunk under pressure, we injected the anterior spinal complex from top to bottom. On the x-ray photographs, we could establish that the opaque material did not descend beyond the cervical enlargement; no injection was visible in the perimedullary thoracic arterial network. On the other hand, the material was found much lower down in the artery of the lumbar enlargement; it had not reached there through the perimedullary channels, but had come out of the spine through one of the cervical radicular arteries, and afterward had filled the arterial system, the aorta and the artery giving rise to the artery of the lumbar enlargement (Fig. 10). This experiment proves that, even in the case of the fetus, not to mention of the adult, neither the anterior spinal artery nor the perimedullary arterial network constitutes a longitudinal anastomotic channel capable of playing an adequate part in the event of an obstruction of one of the supplying vessels. It is logical to suppose that in the adult, one can count even less on the functioning of this channel. This impossibility of injection beyond C 4 or C 5 was also found by Corbin (1961) and by Taylor (1964).

In a second series of experiments in 1962, we initially confirmed the fact that the injection of one of the vertebral arteries in its intracranial portion rarely allows the material to be pushed below C 4; only once did it reach D 6, but this injection was rather artificial and far removed from physiologic conditions. We then injected the artery of the lumbar enlargement four times and saw the injection fill the anterior spinal trunk from the bottom to the top. Furthermore, it should be pointed out that this injection was only effective superficially, as from the midthoracic region onward it was always incomplete in the deeper layers. In conclusion, the continuity of the anterior spinal trunk does not seem to us to be guaranteed, and even less so that of the posterior spinal vessels.

As far as the direction of flow is concerned, in the anterior spinal artery, it can be agreed that at the level of the first cervical segments the blood flow goes in a craniocaudal direction, that along the lumbosacral spinal cord it also makes its way downward, below the entry of the artery of the lumbar enlargement (large radicular artery of Adamkiewicz), and that in the intermediate region the flow is not in one specific direction, but in opposite directions in each of these branches. The descending flow appears, in general, to be the more important.

The Perimedullary Network

The value of *the perimedullary network* (Fig. 11) has been much discussed. Charpy (1921) and Testut (1928) admit that it represents a sort of reservoir which receives the blood from the radicular arteries and distributes it along the whole length of the spinal cord. Its physiologic homogenity should cancel out the inequality of the original segmental distribution and it would make the flow in the spinal cord uniform. This view is certainly too optimistic; the perimedullary network is not a faultless anastomotic supply system and it certainly does not protect the whole spinal cord. The small diameter of the vessels leads one to think that the supplies ensured by the perimedullary network cannot go beyond the adjoining spinal segments, and thus, they protect only the peripheral or superficial compartment, that is, only the white matter.

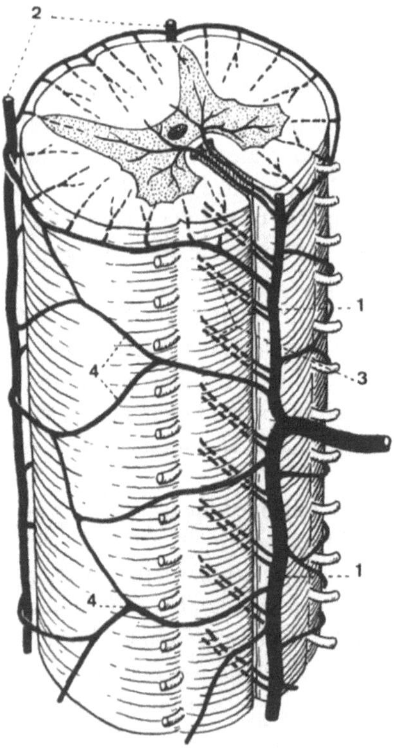

Fig. 11. The perimedullary network: 1. anterior spinal artery, 2. posterior spinal arteries, 3. central arteries, 4. perimedullary arteries

There is no need to distinguish in this perimedullary network separate anterior and posterior arterial territories as certain authors have proposed (Lhermitte and Corbin, 1961). This schematization seems excessive to us. The distinction between the two perimedullary arterial territories is not clearly defined. Even more so, it is difficult to envisage the selective involvement of one or the other and the possibility of the appearance of distinctive syndromes.

3. The Intramedullary Arterial Circulation

In the interior of the whole central nervous system, spinal cord, brain stem, and cerebrum, there exist two vascular systems which can be called anterior or central, and posterior or peripheral, according to whether one is referring to their position or to their territories of supply.

As far as the spinal cord is concerned, in contrast to that which supplies the brain stem and cerebrum, the two systems are not very distinct superficially. However, it must be admitted that the anterior radicular arteries supply the anterior spinal trunk and go essentially to the central area, whereas the posterior radicular arteries go to the posterior spinal vessels and distribute themselves principally in the peripheral area. Actually they are joined together quite closely by the perimedullary network.

The essential question remains of knowing whether or not the arteries of the central nervous system are end arteries. Different authors do not agree on this subject. Several have supported the existence of real anastomoses between the various vascular territories of the central nervous system. On the other hand, most maintain that the intra-axial arteries behave like end arteries as in the description given by Conheim (1872); that is to say, that they only communicate from one to another by a network of capillaries measur-

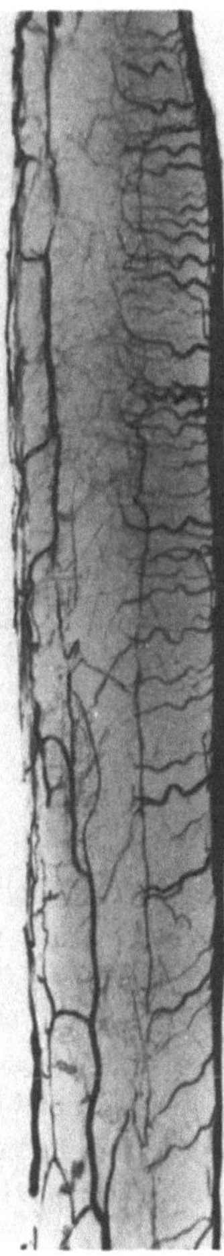

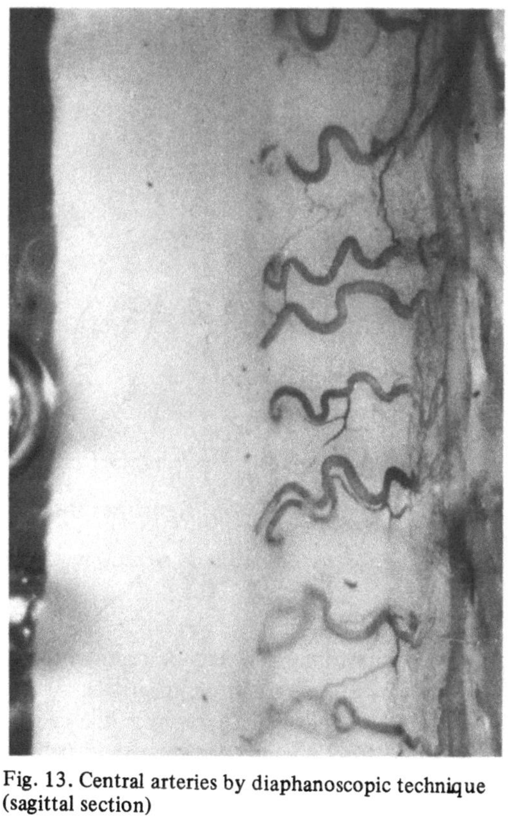

Fig. 13. Central arteries by diaphanoscopic technique (sagittal section)

◀ Fig. 12. Central arteries shown by angiography (sagittal section)

ing 7 – 13 μ, which is not functional. Injections of colored or radiopaque substances do not pass through this microscopic anastomotic network. This seems to be true as far as the brain is concerned, where the central and peripheral regions are separate and independent, without any possible communication.

A central artery or a peripheral artery only ensures a sufficient blood supply in the limited area of its terminal capillary network. Is it the same as far as the spinal cord is concerned?

1. *The peripheral arteries* are interconnected by a network of such a caliber that it cannot be functional. Their anastomoses, if there are any, seem unimportant and without function.
2. *The central arteries* (Figs. 12, 13) on the other hand would appear to anastomose.

It must first of all be conceded that each one spreads out its terminal branches to a distance varying from 2 to 3 cm. According to Jellinger (1966), each central artery supplies a zone 15 – 20 mm high, which can be as much as 50 – 60 mm. As it is already known that the number of central arteries per cm varies from one to eight (Lazorthes, 1957) (Fig. 14), this means that there exists an important overlapping of the areas irrigated by the central arteries, especially at the level of the enlargements, where the density of the central arteries is greater. Each central artery supplies several cellular groups and each cellular group is irrigated by several arteries. In addition, the central arteries anastomose one with the other.

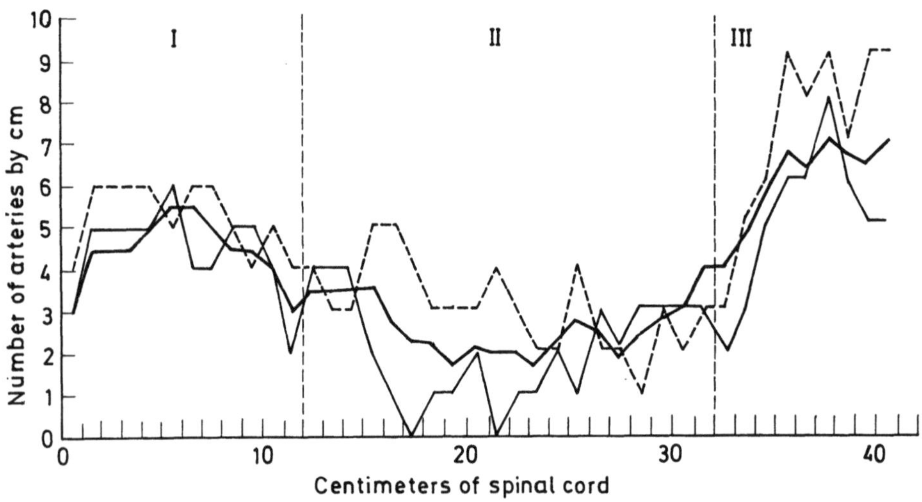

Fig. 14. Study of the central arteries to show number of arteries per cm (Lazorthes, 1957)

a) A first anastomosis would be represented by the ascending and descending ramifications which separate from the trunk of the central arteries at the level of the grey commissure and which join up in the center of the cord with the corresponding ramifications from the arteries above and below so as to form a paramedian vascular channel running along the sides of the central canal, as already noted by Adamkiewicz (Fig. 15). This anastomotic system, which is developed principally in the dorsal region of the spinal cord (Fig. 16) would compensate to some extent for the precarious hemodynamic situation of this region, which results from the smallness and the frequent discontinuity of the anterior spinal artery and the lack of central vessels.

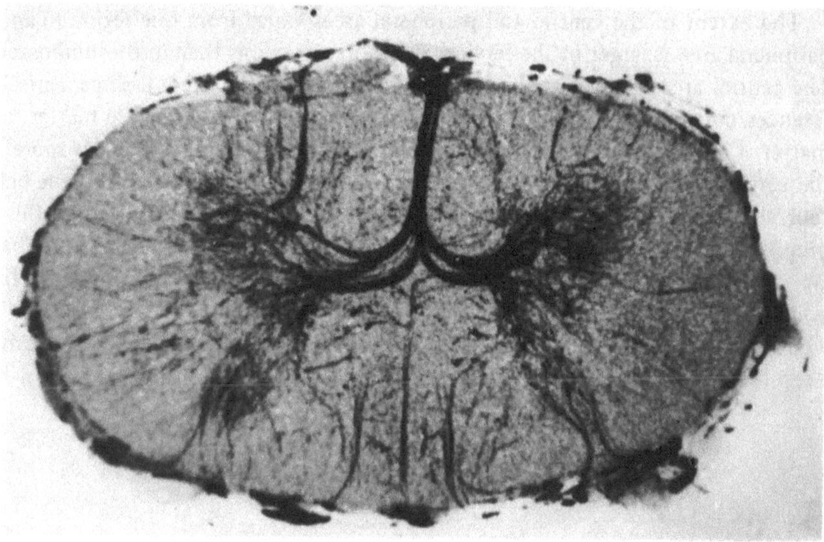

Fig. 15. Arteries of the cervical enlargement shown by angiographic injection (horizontal section)

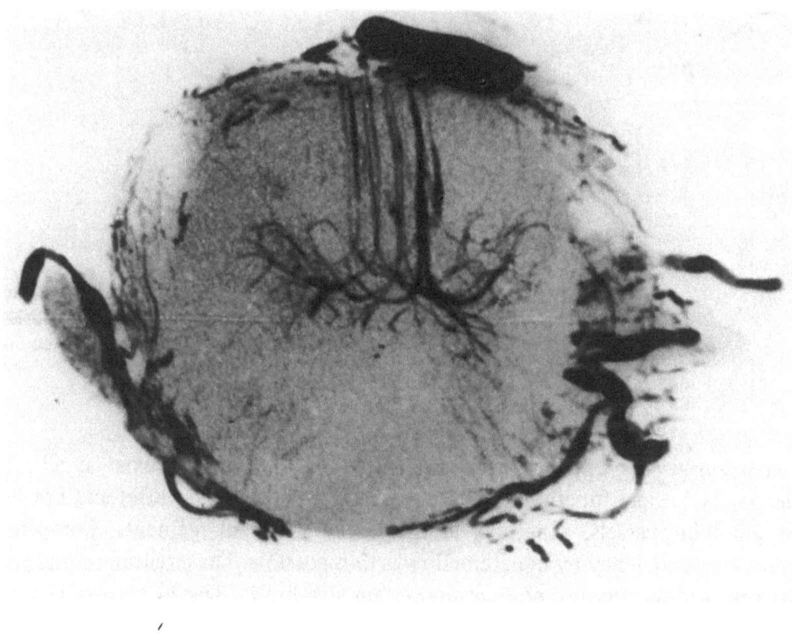

Fig. 16. Arteries of the lumbar portion of the spinal cord shown by angiography (horizontal section)

b) Transverse anastomoses may exist between the central arteries at the same level and could connect the arteries of one side with those of the opposite side, by passing either in front of or behind the central canal (Pitzorns).

c) *The central arteries and the peripheral arteries* only communicate through the capillary network. It would seem that in vivo a peripheral artery or a central artery can only provide for the circulation of its own capillary network. The intramedullary arteries can be considered as end arteries, in the sense suggested by Conheim (1872).

The extent of the central and peripheral areas varies from one region to another. The peripheral area is larger in the cervical and thoracic regions than in the lumbosacral region. The central area is larger at the level of the cervical and lumbar enlargements. These differences correspond to the greater or lesser importance of the white matter or the grey matter. Can it be concluded that a lesion in the anterior spinal trunk is more serious in the cervical and lumbosacral regions than in the thoracic region? Is the zone between the central and peripheral areas clearly defined? Some writers have suggested this and have proposed some very precise demarcations. Others have, on the contrary, described an overlapping of the areas (Fig. 17). In particular, Turnbull et al. (1966) have defined these points of overlapping which are found at the meeting point of the two areas. This zone would no longer be vulnerable, as had been thought, but on the contrary is privileged, as a result of its possessing a double blood supply.

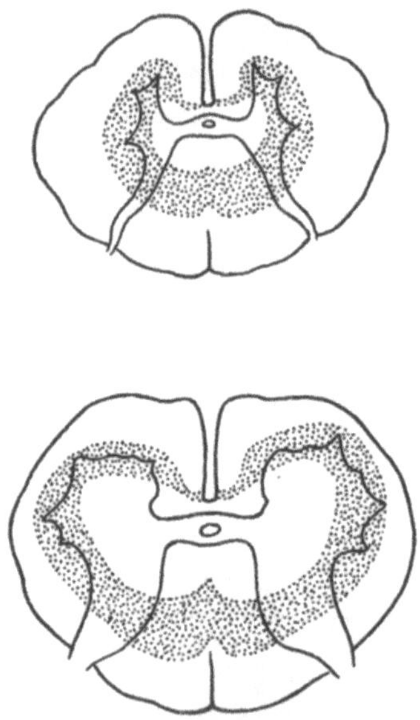

Fig. 17. Central and peripheral territories. Dorsal and lumbar spinal cord. This shows the "common areas" as described by Turnbull et al. (1966)

Conclusions: The supply channels of the arterial circulation exist at all levels but are unequal and their functional capacity is not infallible. The afferents are numerous on the supplying vessels, expecially at the level of the enlargements. Compensation for a circulatory deficiency by collateral flow is thus possible. The circumferential perimedullary network is only anastomotic within certain size limits. The intramedullary anastomoses between the central arteries and the peripheral arteries also have a functional value only for a narrow frontier zone.

II. Vascular Physiology and Pathology of the Spinal Cord

All these investigations have led neurologists and neurosurgeons to think about the possible involvement of a vascular factor in a certain number of misclassed spinal syndromes. Circulatory insufficiency of the spinal cord can be the result of either the narrowing or obstruction of one of the arterial channels, or a general circulatory failure with or without any arterial lesion, or often a combination of both the anatomic and hemodynamic factors.

1. The General or Hemodynamic Factor

A simple pressure drop in a patient whose arteries are normal seldom produces, by itself, lesions or ischemic disorders, unless the very low figure of 40 – 50 mm Hg is reached. The cerebral blood flow is dangerously impaired at an earlier stage, viz., from 70 mm Hg downward.

If an increase in vascular resistance due to diffuse arterial disease is combined with a pressure drop, the safety threshold rises and the decrease of the blood flow intervenes earlier. A sudden fall in arterial pressure due to cardiovascular collapse or traumatic shock, or during a coronary thrombosis, produces an ischemia in the poorly vascularized zones. In the case of the elderly patient, the association of diffuse arteriosclerosis with low blood pressure plays a very important part.

2. The Local Factor – The Vascular Resistance

The arterial channels irrigating the spinal cord can be narrowed or obstructed at various points along their course. As with cerebral circulatory insufficiency, it has been learnt during recent years that the cause of the circulatory deficiency is situated not only along the periaxial or intra-axial ramifications, but often in the larger, main arterial trunks as well.

Causes

The pathologic lesion is either *parietal intrinsic:* obliterating arteritis, dissecting aneurysm of the aorta, or due to some act of vascular surgery, i.e., section, ligature, clamping, puncture for aortography (if the supply is not adequate, the results are serious), or *parietal extrinsic:* arterial compression (tumor, extradural inflammation, disk), or *circulatory:* hyperviscosity of the blood.

Site

A Lesion of One of the Arterial Channels of Supply to the Spinal Cord
One of the main supplying arteries – vertebral, aorta, intercostal arteries, lumbar arteries – can be stenosed or thrombosed. In the case of unilateral thrombosis of the vertebral artery and if the other artery is itself reduced in caliber, it is seen that the supply can come from the collaterals of the subclavian and external carotid arteries. In vertebral thromboses, the distal segment of this artery can receive an anastomotic supply from the occipital, deep cervical, and ascending cervical arteries. One of the anterior radicular arteries can be involved, compressed, or obstructed.

A Lesion of the Juxtamedullary and Intramedullary Arteries
The perimedullary arteries, in particular the anterior spinal, can be involved either by arteritis or by compression (cervical arthrosis, herniated disk, cervical disk herniation, hyperextension, or hyperflexion of the cervical spine, vertebral manipulations of the cervical spine).
Obstruction of the anterior spinal artery generally induces a multisegmental softening whose extent is variable. This softening is central; the peripheral area is protected by the

peripheral network. Softening in the central area (the lesion *"en crayon"* of Zülch) seems to be the result of obstruction of the anterior spinal channel without compensation. Obstruction of a single central artery (sulcocommissural artery) ought, as a rule, to give rise to a central segmental softening often unilateral. In actual fact, if one admits, on the one hand, the overlapping of the area of the overlapping central arteries whose ramifications intermingle like the branches of adjacent trees, and on the other hand, the existence of periependymal vertical anastomoses, the obstruction of a single central artery ought to be of no consequence; only the obstruction of several adjacent central arteries ought to be able to cause an ischemic focus.

Obstruction of the peripheral network which is seldom complete and circular shows itself as a rule by a softening of the white matter of the head of the posterior horn. This obstruction, limited to the posterior spinal arteries and to the posterior arterial territory, would give rise to what Perier et al. (1960) called the posterior spinal syndrome.

3. The Cellular Factor

Reduction of the arterial supply of a given area does not necessarily imply that the amount of blood which flows into it is either sufficient or inadequate for its metabolic requirements. In the central nervous system, the blood supply is probably directly proportional to the number of neurons as well as to the density of the synaptic endings; in the midthoracic spinal cord, the grey matter and, therefore, the neurons and the synaptic endings are less numerous than in the cervical and lumbar spinal cords.

4. The Site of Lesions

Certain critical zones, where the vascularization is not so rich, are more liable than others to circulatory deficiency. In general, as with the cerebral circulation, it is the regions which are farthest from the main vessels of supply and situated in the border zones between two areas which are the most vulnerable and the first ones to be affected. The "last meadows" are the first to lack water and the most vulnerable to decreases in the flow from the spring (Schneider).

Vertically

1. Softenings resulting from acute circulatory failure are frequent in the midthoracic region of the spinal cord as can be ascertained by the reading of treatises of neurology and published observations. In the same way, anatomic reports very often point out that progressive stenosis or thrombosis in spinal arteriosclerosis, neuroanemic syndromes, necrotic myelitis of Foix and Alajouanine, periarteritis nodosa, myelopathies provoked by radiotherapy and other radiation, are maximal at the level of the midthoracic spinal cord. This elective localization probably also explains why, from their investigation of the spinal cord in the elderly, Graux et al. (1962) established the concept of an inconspicuous neurologic involvement of the upper limbs and upper half of the trunk, and a more obvious one of the lower limbs and lower half of the trunk.
2. Softening which follows the obstruction of one of the arterial channels is multisegmental; each radiculomedullary artery divides on its arrival at the spinal cord into an ascending and a descending branch; the ischemic area will, therefore, generally extend above

and below the entry of the artery. In depth, the softening is more widespread in the central area, than in the peripheral area. In the central area, indeed, the supply is poor although anastomoses connecting the central arteries have been described, whereas in the peripheral system anastomoses can develop more definitely through the perimedullary network, which includes several radicular arteries. Complete transverse softening probably corresponds to an involvement of the central and peripheral areas, i.e., it arises from a complete interruption of the superficial and deep circulation in several segments.
The obstruction of the radicular artery which goes to the lumbar enlargement (large anterior radicular artery of Adamkiewicz) can be responsible for a flaccid paraplegia with sensory disorders more or less extensive according to the level of this artery (Cossa's "syndrome of the artery of the lumbar enlargement"). Stenosis or spasm of the artery of the lumbar enlargement can be the origin of a spinal intermittent claudication syndrome.

Transversely

Transversely, at the level of each segment, there also exists a boundary zone between the limits of the two arterial flows, central and peripheral. The two flows are, according to classic descriptions, almost independent and anastomose very little. Many authors describe them as being juxtaposed, which leads to admitting that the circular border zone which is at the junction of the two areas ought to be the first affected by ischemia. This is the concept of Zülch (1954, 1966) who has, nervertheless, described the central softening (*"en crayon"*) which is frequently seen. On the other hand, the description of Turnbull et al. (1962) admits the existence of a circular intermediate zone between the two areas where the endings of the central and peripheral arteries overlap and in this way explains the central location of ischemic necrosis.

Conclusion

1. Circulatory insufficiency of the spinal cord is the result of anatomic and hemodynamic causes. Narrowing of the arterial channels of the spinal cord and functional circulatory disorders have shared responsibilities. In addition, as with cerebral circulatory insufficiency, there is a cellular metabolic factor.

2. Circulatory insufficiency of the spinal cord is all the more serious when it attacks an artery situated far from the heart. In fact, the possibilities of supply through anastomoses are that much greater when the obstruction is situated far from the spinal cord.

3. The more rapidly medullary circulatory insufficiency establishes itself, the less chance there is that the compensatory and anastomotic mechanisms can intervene effectively, because they are "caught unawares."

4. Clinical examination gives an inaccurate idea of the site of the arterial involvement; only selective arteriographic examination (Djindjian's technique) is capable of demonstrating the lesion.

Pathology of Spinal Vascular Malformations and Vascular Tumors

Kurt Jellinger

While vascular malformations of the brain have been well-known for many years, similar disorders of the spinal cord have been largely disregarded, and there has been no uniformity of opinion concerning the nature and origin of these rather uncommon lesions. Although recent refinements in neuroradiology and neurosurgery have focussed attention on spinal vascular anomalies and have encouraged a rational surgical approach to their treatment, there is still limited understanding of the functional morphology, origin, and pathology of spinal angiomas and the pathogenesis of associated lesions which are closely related to the natural history of these malformations. The essential distinction between vascular (angiomatous) malformations and vascular tumors dating from the study by Cushing and Bailey (1918) is now generally agreed upon, although the relationship of the two groups is still less than completely clear. Recent comprehensive reviews on spinal angiomas were given by Djindjian *et al.* (1969) and Aminoff (1976), while spinal hemangioblastomas were reviewed by Hurth *et al.* (1975), and Browne *et al.* (1976).

Terminology and Classification

Ever since Virchow's (1863) first anatomic description and classification of angiomas, there has been great confusion in the nomenclature of these vascular lesions which are known to occur in all parts of the CNS, though with varying frequency. The earliest report of an angioma of the spinal cord was given in 1885 by Hebold and Gaupp (1888) who referred to "hemorrhoids of the pia mater" and recognized them as a source of spinal subarachnoid hemorrhage. Later authors used various terms. e.g., cirsoid angiomas, spinal varicosis, hemangioma, arteriovenous aneurysm, etc. (f.rev. Béraud, 1972). Spinal hemangioblastomas were initially described in 1912 by Schultze and later recognized to be identical with those in the cerebellum (Cushing and Bailey, 1928; Wyburn – Mason, (1943).

If one uses the classification proposed by Russell and Rubinstein (1972) and Rubinstein (1972), one can reasonably distinguish the following groups of vascular malformations and tumors of the CNS, including the spinal cord (Table 1):

1. *Congenital vascular anomalies* consisting of a) *saccular aneurysms* of the arteries resulting from developmental defects of the vessel wall (aplasia or hypoplasia of the muscle coat) and b) *vascular malformations* or *angiomas* (blood vessel hamartomas) caused by

Table 1. Classification of vascular malformations and tumors

Virchow (1863
1. Angioma cavernosum
2. Angioma racemosum
   a) Teleangiectatic or capillary
   b) Venous
   c) Arterial
   d) Arteriovenous

Cushing and Bailey (1928)
1. Vascular malformations
   a) Teleangiectasias
   b) Venous angiomas
   c) Arterial (arteriovenous) a.
2. Hemangioblastoma

Bergstrand et al. (1937)
1. Cavernous angioma
2. Racemose angiomas
   a) Teleangiectasias
   b) Sturge – Webeı disease
   c) Racemose arterial angioma
   d) Racemose venous angioma
   e) Arteriovenous angioma
3. Hemangioblastoma (-reticuloma)
4. Angioglioma

Turner and Kernohan (1941)
1. Vascular malformations
   a) Teleangiectasias
   b) Angiomas (hamartomas)
      Venous
      Arterial
      Arteriovenous
2. Vascular neoplasms
   a) Capillary
      Capillary angioma
      Hemangioendothelioma
      Capillary hemangioblastoma
   b) Cavernous
      Cavernous hemangioma
      Cavernous hemangioblastoma
   c) Sarcomatous

Wyburn - Mason (1943)
1. Anomalies
   a) Venous – secondary
      Angioma racemosum venosum
   b) Arteriovenous
   c) Arterial – isolated
      associated with cardiopathy
   d) Syphilitic aneurysms
   e) Teleangiectasias

Zülch (1956)
1. Angiomas and aneurysms
   a) *Angioma cavernosum*
   b) *A. capillare ectaticum*
      (teleangiectasia)
   c) *Angioma arteriovenosum aneurysmaticum*
   d) *Angioma capillare et venosum calcificans* (Sturge–Weber)
2. Angioblastoma (Lindau tumor)

McCormick (1966)
1. Teleangiectasias including Sturge–Weber syndrome
2. Varix including vein of Galen malformations
3. Cavernous malformation ("angioma")
4. Arteriovenous malformation ("angioma")
5. Venous malformation ("angioma")

Rubinstein (1972) – modified
1. Vascular malformations (hamartoma)
   a) Capillary teleangiectasis
   b) Cavernous angioma (cavernoma)
   c) Arteriovenous malformation
      (AV angioma, cirsoid angioma)
   d) Venous malformation (angioma)
   e) Capillary venous angioma
      (Sturge–Weber)
2. Vascular tumors
   a) Capillary hemangioblastoma
3. Vascular tumors of the meninges
   ("angioblastic meningiomas")
   a) Hemangioblastoma
   b) Hemangiopericytoma

faulty embryonic development. Although some angiomas are growing and thus can form a tumor-like mass, they lack evidence of any cellular proliferation which is the criterion of any true neoplasm.

2. *Vascular tumors* resulting from autonomous growth of vasoformative cells. According to their presumed cellular derivation, two major types are distinguished: a) capillary

hemangioblastomas or hemangioendotheliomas ("angioreticulomas") and b) *hemangio-pericytomas,* previously considered to be a subgroup of angioblastic meningiomas (Rubinstein, 1972).

It should be recognized, however, that the distinction between vascular malformations and vascular neoplasms is not always easy to make, since the two groups may coexist (Krishnan and Smith, 1961; Raynor and Kingman, 1965; Pia, 1973).

In the spinal region only vascular malformations (angiomas) are of practical interest, while vascular tumors and saccular aneurysms are very rare, though occasionally coexisting with angiomas. Although most authors agree that both these latter types of lesion are to be distinguished from angiomas, they will be briefly considered in view of their significance in clinical and angiographic differential diagnosis.

Congenital Saccular Aneurysms

Isolated berry aneurysms of the spinal vasculature, i.e., congenital saccular dilatations of a spinal cord artery comparable to intracranial aneurysms, are extremely rare, only seven *bona fide* cases being reported in the literature. They may arise from the posterior spinal artery (Baló, 1925; Bräutigam, 1960; Henson and Croft, 1956; Ledinsky et al., 1963), the anterior spinal artery (Mares et al., 1967; Leech et al., 1976), or the central spinal artery (Guizzetti and Cordero, 1903). All of these instances presented subarachnoid bleedings, some with hematomyelia (Bräutigam, 1960; Guizzetti and Cordero 1903). A mycotic aneurysm on a lumbar vessel producing subarachnoid hemorrhage has also been described (Henson and Croft, 1956). The combined occurrence of arterial aneurysm with AV angiomas in the spinal cord has been reported in about 6% of the latter anomaly (Herdt et al., 1971). A calcified intramedullary aneurysm in spinal angioma was reported (Deeb et al. 1977).

Spinal Vascular Malformations (Angiomas)

Definition

Angiomas are localized collections of blood vessels, abnormal in structure and in number, representing a developmental anomaly of the spinal circulatory system showing persistence of a primitive pattern of vascular pathways with altered hemodynamics.

Embryology

Early in embryologic development, primitive vessels spread from the walls of the yolk sac and digestive tube and reach the neural plate as it closes to form the neural tube. The blood vessels have their origin in solid cords of angioblasts, differentiating from mesoderm which, through dissolution of their inner portion form tubular structures. In the development of the CNS vascular system, five stages are distinguished (Padget, 1948; Streeter, 1918). In the first stage (3 – 4 weeks = 5 – 9 mm CRL), there is a primitive extraneural vascular plexus; in the second stage (3–5 weeks = 10–12 mm), arteries, veins,

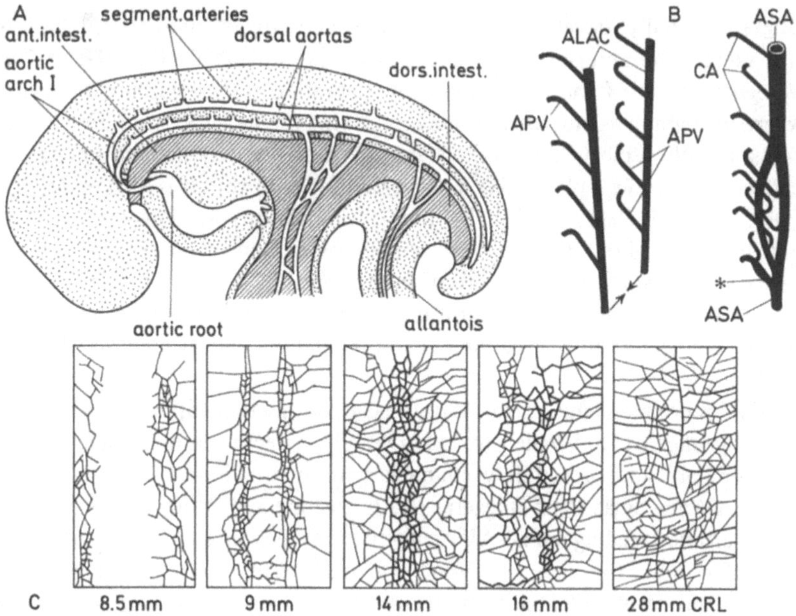

Fig. 1. Development of spinal cord blood vessels. (A) Arterial system in 3-week-old embryo, (B) Primitive arterial longitudinal anastomotic channels (ALAC) migrate medially and fuse to form anterior spinal artery (ASA). Anterior perforating vessels (APV) become the central arteries (Turnbull, 1972), (C) Development of anterior spinal arteries at different stages 8.5 - 28 mm CRL (Corbin, 1961)

and capillaries with communications between them appear, and the vessel wall develops by differentiation of mesenchymal cells; in the third stage (7–8 weeks = 12–24 mm) three layers of vessels develop, forming independent systems for the integument, dura, and the pia and CNS; in the fourth stage (2nd month), the adult pattern of vascular trunks becomes apparent; and in the fifth stage mature vessels.

The development of the *spinal vascular system* follows four stages (Turnbull, 1972):

1. *Primitive Segmental Stage* (2–3 weeks): 31 pairs of segmental vessels originating from the dorsal aortas grow toward the neural tube along developing nerve roots (Fig. 1A). Upon gaining the neural tube, each vessel divides into anterior and posterior branches, the latter supplying the spine, meninges, and cord. The terminal branches of the segmental vessels which accompany the nerve roots ramify to form capillary networks on the lateral surface of the neural tube. Longitudinal anastomotic channels form in the lateral capillary networks, the first to appear being the primitive anterior arterial tracts, representing the paired primordia of the anterior spinal artery (Fig. 1C).

2. *Initial Stage* (3rd–6th week): Later, arterial anastomoses develop on the posterior aspect of the cord forming a capillary network on the surface of the entire cord, the anterior and posterior systems being separated. At this stage, longitudinal venous channels evolve on both surfaces. The first vessels expand and become connected forming paired longitudinal endoneural channels. These sinuses sprout vessels and change into a capillary network which extends in all directions and interconnects with capillaries growing inward from the surface. The primitive anterior *tracts* give rise to the anterior penetrating vessels which become the central arteries (Fig. 1B).

3. *Transitional Stage* (6th week–4th month): Formation of the adult pattern of vascularization progresses in craniocaudal direction. a) The two anterior longitudinal tracts

migrate medially, develop interconnections and largely fuse (Torr, 1957). Where they do not merge, the anterior spinal artery remains duplicated (Fig. 1C). b) *Summation and desegmentation* of the cord supply by reduction in the number of segmental arteries. Microangiography demonstrates adult patterns of the superficial cord vessels in 10-week fetuses, with typical "hair-pin" arrangement of the thoracic and lumbar radiculomedullary arteries, while a plexus-like arrangement of cord vessels is seen up to 12 and 14 weeks (Di Chiro and Wener, 1973). By the 4th month of gestation, capillaries are distributed equally throughout the gray and white matter, and in the following months there is a relative increase in the vascularity of the former.

4. *Terminal Stage* (after 4 months): The anterior spinal artery shows a straight course in the younger fetuses becoming tortuous in the cervical area and later in the lumbar portion.

Maldevelopment during the second stage of vascular formation, around 6 weeks, leads to persistence of thin-walled tortuous vessels, defective in media and elastica, with primitive capillary and precapillary channels and abnormal arteriovenous shunts, characteristic of AV angiomas (Van Bogaert, 1950; Cushing and Bailey, 1928; Kaplan et al., 1961). Some arteries feeding spinal AV malformations may be supernumerary segmental arteries persisting from the rich embryonic vascular system. Similar changes are suggested to occur from developmental disorders during the early third stage which may lead to segmental neurocutaneous vascular malformations of the skin, the dura, and CNS, or all three. The earlier differentiation of the ventral and rostral parts of the spinal vasculature would explain the preferential occurrence of angiomas on the dorsal surface and in the caudal region.

Etiology

Several hypotheses have been advanced concerning the origin of spinal vascular malformations. Previous authors held that they were caused by some toxic or infective agent (Foix and Alajouanine, 1926; Mair and Folkerts, 1953). Although exacerbation has sometimes occurred during pregnancy (Aminoff, 1976; Brion et al., 1952; Newman, 1959) or following a spinal injury (Sargent, 1925), traumatic factors do not play a significant role in the pathogenesis of the disorder (Béraud, 1972). According to another theory, these vascular anomalies are mechanical in origin and, similar to varicosities of the lower extremities, are due to the upright position of man and interference with the free return of venous blood from the spinal canal (Lindemann, 1912; Stochdorph, 1969; Suter—Lochmatter, 1950). This suggestion is *refuted* by the angiographic demonstration of arterial feeders (Di Chiro et al., 1967; Di Chiro and Wener, 1973; Djindjian, 1970; Doppman et al., 1969) and the close morphologic resemblance of spinal angiomas to those found intracranially. Most authors accept the notion of a *congenital* etiology which is strongly supported by the frequent coexistence of spinal vascular malformations with other congenital anomalies and dysplasias (Table 2).

Incidence

In large series of autopsy material, vertebral hemangiomas were found in 10—12% of spines (Odom et al., 1957; Schmorl and Junghanns, 1932; Töpfer, 1928; Yasargil, 1971), while they account for 4. 4% of neurosurgically treated tumors of the spine (Arseni and Simionescu, 1958). In neurosurgical series, the incidence of spinal angiomas ranges from

3. 3% (Krayenbühl and Yasargil, 1963) to 12. 5% (Nittner and Tönnis, 1950; Vanderkelen et al., 1975) of spinal space-occupying lesions with an average of 8 – 10% (Di Chiro et al., 1967; Pia and Vogelsang, 1965). In Pia's (1973) material spinal angiomas accounted for more than 40% of all vascular malformations of the CNS. In our own series of 290 post-mortem and biopsy cases of CNS vascular anomalies, spinal angiomas represented 16.5% of the total and accounted for 31% of the neurosurgically treated cases.

Location and Major Sites

The location and extent of angiomas varies according to 1) the different layers involved, 2) the site within the vertebral canal, and 3) the spinal level. Within the different layers, the following sites may be involved: vertebral extradural, intradural, subpial arachnoidal, and intramedullary. In addition to isolated vascular anomalies, frequently there are *combined* or complex and *multiple* angiomas with simultaneous involvement of all the contiguous layers from the skin to the dura and subarachnoid space (Pia, 1973; Seze et al., 1966). In 15 – 20% there are concomitant cutaneous and/or vertebral angiomas at the same level (Djindjian et al., 1971; Doppman et al., 1969).

Vertebral angiomas may be isolated, most commonly affecting the middle and lower thoracic spine and less often the cervical and lumbar region (Arseni and Simionescu, 1958; McAllister et al., 1975; Seiler, 1971), but may extend into the extradural space (McAllister et al., 1975).

Extradural angiomas, accounting for 15 – 20% of all spinal vascular anomalies (Bischof and Schettler, 1967; Pia, 1973) and for about 4. 7% of all spinal space-occupying lesions (Rasmussen et al., 1940), are rarely isolated (Papo et al., 1973; Vanderkelen et al., 1975). Their feeding vessels usually exhibit no communication with the spinal cord arteries and, thus, these malformations play no part in the vascular supply of the cord. A spinal epidural angioma draining into intrathecal veins was reported by Kendall and Logue (1977). The functional anatomic separation of the extradural angiomas, the majority of which are exclusively extradural, and those in the subdural space and spinal cord (Globus and Doshay, 1929) has to be considered in both angiographic diagnosis and treatment (Di Chiro and Wener, 1973; Djindjian et al., 1969; Vogelsang, 1970).

Intradural angiomas may be isolated, and quite often penetrate the spinal cord to a variable extent, but they almost never extend to the epidural space (Djindjian et al., 1969).

Subpial angiomas represent the most frequent and classic intradural type of vascular malformation showing one or more pedicles. Many intradural angiomas are confined to the cord surface and probably exhibit no communication with the intramedullary vascular system (Bailey and Sperl, 1969; Brion et al., 1952; Kaufmann et al; 1970; Ommaya et al., 1969; Shephard, 1963), and it has been rare to demonstrate by arteriography a common vascular supply to the cord and the malformed vessels (Di Chiro and Wener, 1973; Djindjian, 1970; Djindjian, 1966, 1969, 1971; Doppman et al., 1969; Kaufmann et al., 1970). In other cases, a collateral system may exist with the anomaly and may be capable, under certain circumstances, of furnishing a more or less adequate blood supply to the cord tissue (Béraud, 1972; Luessenhop and Dela Cruz, 1969). On the other hand, the association of the vascularization of the angioma and the spinal cord may produce cord ischemia by "steal" phenomena (*see* chronic progressive radiculomyelopathy, p.35).

Isolated *intramedullary* vascular malformations are rare (Aminoff, 1976; Antoni, 1962; Bergstrand et al., 1964; Garcin and Lapresle, 1968; Odom et al., 1957; Schröder

Table 2. Dysplasias associated with spinal angiomas

1. *Cutaneous lesions:*	Hemangiomas Nevi (usually metameric) Angiolipomas
2. *Vertebral anomalies:*	Scoliosis, Kyphoscoliosis Vertebral angiomas
3. *Vascular dysplasias:*	Soft tissue hemangiomas Angiomas and AV fistulas of extremities Vascular deformities (variectasias) Disseminated hemangiomas Klippel-Trenauney-Weber syndrome Hemangiomas in viscera (liver) Osler-Rendu syndrome Lymphatic dysplasias (angioelephantiasis)
4. *Vascular anomalies of CNS:*	Intracranial angiomas Cerebrospinal angiomatosis Saccular aneurysms (cerebral or spinal arteries)
5. *Vascular tumors:*	Hemangioblastomas – cerebellum, spinal cord Retinocerebellar angiomatosis Hippel-Lindau disease, etc.
6. *CNS dysplasias:*	Syringomyelia Spina bifida, etc.

and Brunngraber, 1964), while association of extramedullary and intramedullary angiomas is seen in about one-fifth of the cases (Djindjian et al., 1966, 1969; Shephard, 1963). Within the spinal canal, both the epidural and intradural vascular anomalies are mainly located on the *dorsal* aspect, although the latter not infrequently extend over the ventral surface or may invade the cord. In the Paris material, 44% of intradural AV angiomas were on the dorsal surface alone, 48% were retromedullary with invasion of the cord, while 8% were intramedullary malformations (Djindjian, 1969; Houdart et al., 1968).

Regional localization allows the identification of three major varieties (Djindjian et al., 1969; Béraud, 1972):

1. *Cervical angiomas,* accounting for 10 – 15% of all spinal vascular malformations, are usually of medium size, extending over one to three or more segments. Their afferents are usually bilateral and obtain their hypertrophied branches from the subclavian artery, vertebral artery, ascending cervical artery, cervico-intercostal and thyreo-cervical trunks, or from aberrant supplementary feeders arising from intercostal branches (Bailey and Sperl, 1969; Djindjian, 1970; Djindjian et al., 1966, 1969). Rare angiomas in the upper cervical region and lower medulla receive their afferents from the vertebrobasilar system (Bailey and Sperl, 1969; Djindjian, 1969; Pouyanne et al., 1950). Unilateral or bilateral feeders may arise either from the anterior spinal artery of from both the anterior and posterior spinal arteries and may penetrate the spinal cord. These anomalies usually drain into the intracranial sinuses.

2. *Cervicothoracic* and *thoracic* forms (20 – 30%), located over the lower cervical and upper thoracic cord, tend to be voluminous and cover three to four segments or more (Djindjian et al., 1966, 1969, 1971). Their feeders are less numerous (two to three) and, as a rule, unilateral. They come from the aortic intercostal vessels. The hypertrophic veins drain via the extradural plexuses into the intracranial sinuses and the azygos and caval systems.

3. *Thoracolumbar, lumbar,* and *lumbosacral* angiomas account for 50–70% of all spinal vascular anomalies, the majority being located below T 8 to T 10 (Bischof and

Schettler, 1967; Djindjian et al., 1969; Krayenbühl and Yasargil, 1963; Pia, 1973; Pia and Volgelsang, 1965; Vogelsang, 1973; Wyburn – Mason, 1943; Yasargil, 1971). They are usually smaller and contain only one large feeding artery originating from caudal intercostal and lumbar branches, the iliolumbar and internal iliac arteries or the artery of Adamkiewicz, while others are nourished from the posterolateral or posterior spinal arteries. They drain into the azygos and caval systems. At other sites, extensive malformations covering large parts or even the whole length of the cord are rare (Bérand, 1972; Djindjian et al., 1969; Pia, 1973).

Morphologic Types

The major anatomic types of spinal vascular malformations and their preferential sites are summarized in Table 3.

Teleangiectasias (capillary angiomas) are small, mostly solitary groups of abnormally dilated capillaries separated by interstitial or nervous tissue. They account for about 20% of all spinal vascular anomalies (Wyburn – Mason, 1943) and occur in both the extradural and intradural spaces. The latter often lie subpially, communicating with the medullary arteries or emerging from them, which does not imply any intramedullary involvement. Subpial teleangiectasias may cause spinal subarachnoid hemorrhage (Gaupp, 1888; Odom, 1962). Rare intramedullary teleangiectasias are isolated, with a preference for the posterior columns, or can be rather diffuse (Goulon et al., 1971). They may cause hematomyelia (Garcin et al., 1951; Hiecke, 1949; Koos and Böck, 1970; van Reeth, 1952; Russell, 1932), myelomalacia, or diffuse progressive myelopathy (Garcin and Lapresle, 1968). The intramedullary location of teleangiectasias is often associated with intradural AV angiomas. Mixed angiomas in which capillary proliferation coexists with cavernous changes may occur, and occasionally no differentiation between teleangiectasias and cavernoma can be made (Bergstrand et al., 1964; Voigt and Yasargil, 1976). Therefore, the evolution of

Table 3. Location of major types of spinal angiomas

Location and Extension	Isolated	Combined	Morphologic Type
1. Vertebral	Frequent	1+2, 1+2+3	*Cavernous* angioma
		1+3	*Capillary* angioma
		1+2+3 (+5)	Venous angioma
2. Extradural	Rare	1+2; 1+2+3	*Cavernous* angioma
		(2+)	Capillary + cavernous a.
			Capillary angioma
			Arteriovenous angioma
3. Subdural	Frequent	3+4+5; 3+5	*Arteriovenous* a.
			Capillary angioma
			Venous angioma (varix?)
			Arterial angioma
4. Leptomeningeal (subarachnoid)	Rare	4+5	*Capillary* angioma
			Arteriovenous a.
			Cavernous a.
			Venous a. (?)
5. Intramedullary	Rare	5+3, 5+4	*Arteriovenous* a.
		5+1	*Capillary* angioma
		5+3+2+1	*Cavernous* angioma
			Capillary + venous a. (?)

cavernoma from teleangiectasia has been suggested (van Reeth, 1952; Russell and Rubinstein, 1972; Wyburn – Mason, 1943).

Cavernomas which account for 5 – 16 % of spinal vascular anomalies (Bergstrand et al., 1964; pers. mat.) range in size from pinpoint to mulberry-sized lesions and have no extra development of supplying arteries or veins. Grossly, they appear as solitary well-circumscribed lesions, dark brown or blue in color. They are composed of closely clustered, sinusoidal thin-walled channels, lined by a single endothelial layer, with little or no intervening parenchymatous tissue (Fig. 2C). Their usual sites are the vertebral bodies and, less frequently, the extradural and intradural space, while intramedullary cavernomas are rare (Bergstrand et al., 1964; Hadlich, 1930; Losacco, 1966; Moyer and Köhler, 1917; Artner et al., 1973; Schröder and Brunngraber, 1964; Wyburn – Mason, 1943). While multiple cavernomas are found in the brain (Voigt and Yasargil, 1976) and in parenchymatous organs (Rubinstein, 1972; Russell and Rubinstein, 1972), they usually appear as a solitary lesion in the spinal cord. They may cause progressive myelopathy (Schröder and Brunngraber, 1964) or hemorrhage which may be subarachnoid or intramedullary (Fig. 2A). We observed a cherry-sized intramedullary cavernoma at C 3 to C 5 which was successfully removed from a female aged 62 who suffered from progressive paraplegia (Figs. 2B, C). In addition, typical AV angiomas may contain cavernous areas.

Venous malformations, also referred to as cirsoid or racemose varices, are entirely composed of veins. They consist either of an enlarged tortuous single vein with one or many draining pedicles or of a compact group of such distended veins. The histologic appearance is that of many veins, varying greatly in caliber and often showing marked hyalin or collagenous thickening, thrombosis, or secondary inflammation. Racemose venous angiomas are located extradurally in vertebral bodies and within the cord. However, for the majority of intradural vascular anomalies previously classified as spinal varices (Globus and Doshay, 1929; Hebold, 1885; Lindemann, 1912; Osterland, 1960), spinal varicosis (Bischof and Schettler, 1967; Krayenbühl and Yasargil, 1963; Suterlochmatter, 1950; Wyburn – Mason, 1943) or racemose venous angioma (David et al., 1962; Koeppen et al., 1974; Resche et al., 1974; Scholz and Manuelidis 1951; Scholz and Wechsler, 1959), spinal angiography, by demonstrating arterial feeders offered the definite proof that they are actually AV angiomas (Di Chiro et al., 1967; Di Chiro and Wener, 1973; Djindjian, 1970; Djindjian, 1966, 1969, 1971; Doppman et al., 1969). Slowing of circulation, darker-colored vessels, and partial thrombosis giving the impression of a venous origin may cause difficulties in the *in vivo* separation of arteries and veins during surgery. The histologic distinction between arterial and venous channels may be virtually impossible because of the severe structural abnormalities of the vessel walls (Adotti et al., 1971; Jellinger et al., 1968).

Admittedly, some degree of varicosity is often observed over the lower segments of the cord (Fig. 3A), and morphometric studies in a large post-mortem material of aged humans revealed increased caliber and tortuousity of intradural veins over the posterior surface of the lumbosacral cord (Jellinger, 1966). It may be difficult to draw a sharp distinction between these and the true hamartomas. The extensive and multiform anastomoses of the vertebral venous plexus with almost all other venous systems may cause a "varicose-like" dilatation of the spinal veins in cases with cor pulmonale or drainage disorders in the caval veins (Lorenz, 1901; Stochdorph, 1969), although the backflow of the venous blood into the spinal cord is apparently limited by various anatomic peculiarities including valves located at the intradural entry of the radicular veins. The identification of this type of venous disorder requires a careful and complete autopsy with a particular search throughout the venous drainage of the body. The problem is complicated in that venous

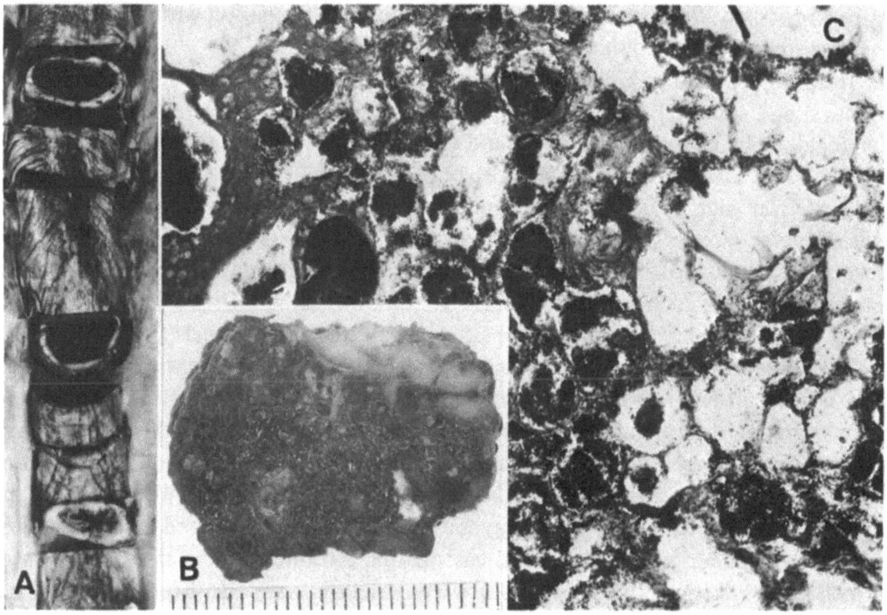

Fig. 2. (A) Hematomyelia resulting from ruptured intramedullary angioma, (B, C) Biopsy specimen of intramedullary cavernous angioma of the cervical cord. C-H. & E. x 45

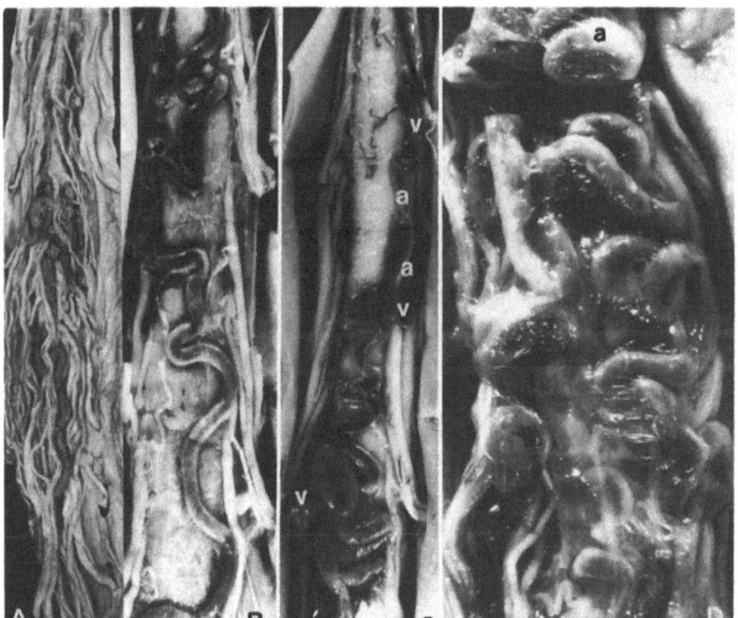

Fig. 3. (A) Marked "varicose" tortuosity of intradural veins over posterior surface of caudal spinal cord in aged female, (B) Plain arteriovenous fistula composed of one or two tightly coiled continuous vessels spread along a large longitudinal section of the cord, (C) Glomus-type of AV angioma presenting a localized plexus of vessels with single arterial feeder (a) and several draining veins (v) over thoracolumbar spinal cord, (D) "Juvenile" type of AV angioma over posterior surface of thoracolumbar cord. Voluminous malformation with "aneurysmal" dilatation (a) and thickened arachnoid

thrombosis may supervene in a congenital vascular malformation with resultant confusion between spinal thrombophlebitis and AVM (Hughes, 1966).

Definite proof of *arterial* racemose angiomas previously suggested to occur in the extradural and subdural spaces (Brasch, 1900; Epstein et al., 1949) has never been obtained by angiography or histology (Bergstrand et al., 1964; Di Chiro and Wener, 1973; Djindjian et al., 1969; Houdart et al., 1968; Wyburn – Mason, 1943). This type is to be distinguished from significant dilatation and/or coiling of the spinal arteries, the *"hypertrophied spinal arteries syndrome,"* which may occur in two conditions, resulting in a reversal of blood flow. One consists of "hemodynamically active" lesions involving a low pressure run off, such as a highly vascular tumor or an AV fistula located in the spinal cord, outside the cord, or paravertebrally outside the spinal canal (Di Chiro and Wener, 1973). The other condition that causes a reversal of blood flow within the spinal cord arteries is stenotic or obstructive vascular disease located either in the spinal cord arteries themselves or in the major extraspinal arterial channels, such as the vertebral arteries (Dorndorf and Gänshirt, 1972; Labauge et al., 1969) or the aorta, e.g., in cases of coarctation of the aorta (Christian and Noder, 1954; Haberer, 1903; Weenink and Smilde, 1964). Compression of the cord may result from markedly dilated and tortuous spinal arteries, and aneurysms of the spinal vasculature, attributed to increased arterial pressure in collateral systems bypassing the aortic constriction, have also been reported (Mares et al., 1967; Sargent, 1925).

Arteriovenous malformations (AVM) constitute the commonest type of vascular anomaly in both the brain (Bergstrand et al., 1936; McCormick, 1966; Pool, 1972) and spinal cord. Their incidence is 1. 5 – 7 % (average 4%) of intracranial (Jellinger, 1975; Krayenbühl and Yasargil, 1972; Perret and Nishioka, 1966; Rubinstein, 1972; Russell and Rubinstein, 1972; Sahs et al., 1969) and 3. 4 – 11% of spinal space-occupying lesions with a suggested ratio of brain to cord AVMs of about 8:1 (Di Chiro et al., 1971) to 4:1 (Lombardi and Migliavacca 1959). The arteries and veins composing these anomalies are abnormally developed; arteriovenous shunting is common. As a result, a tortuous vascular mass occupies the surface of the spinal cord, usually on its posterior aspect, although similar anomalies do occur in front of the cord (Fig. 6A). In most cases in intradural AVMs, the convoluted vessels are situated in the leptomeninges which are opaque due to fibrous thickening and iron pigmentation resulting from earlier spontaneous hemorrhage.

The *gross appearance* of the AVM is highly variable. There is a slightly enlarged but otherwise normal arterial system with a normal course and transdural penetration of the radicular tributaries. It is difficult at necropsy, but easy during life with arteriography, to determine the arteries feeding the malformation. These may come from one or several pedicles and may be unilateral or bilateral. Most spinal AVMs are supplied by one or more of the radiculo-pial arteries and only a minority are supplied either partly or completely by radiculo-medullary vessels. These arteries, often of large size, and abnormal in appearance or pattern, lead to the malformation which comprises a cluster of dilated vessels or sinuses. The venous drainage is enlarged, with one or more dilated pedicles, but it is often possible to make out a completely arranged venous system abnormal only because of dilatation. Superimposed on the normal vessels is a large dilated vein with impressive tributaries which seem to form one continuous venous channel or a more localized vascular plexus. In others still, the malformation is more extensive and consists of a highly tortuous conglomeration of grossly dilated blood vessels; aneurysmal sacs of various size may be seen resembling grossly those of berry aneurysms, which are rarely associated with an AVM. The veins may travel a long way from the AV shunt, upward and downward, and can assume a size much larger than the malformation itself. As post-mortem specimens, the AVMs are less impressive than when demonstrated by angiography or when exposed at operation, when the tangled vessels are engorged and pulsating. Although the extent of the malformation is better appreciated by angiography than by anatomic examination, there may be considerable discrepancy between the anomaly at arteriography and the larger size at surgery or morphologic examination, which is the result mainly of thrombosis of most of the lesions (Pia and Vogelsang, 1965; Vogelsang, 1973; Wirth et al., 1970). However, the angiographic classification of AVMs of the spinal cord, based on functional anatomic characteristics can quite often be confirmed by gross morphologic examination. Three patterns are distinguished (Di Chiro et al., 1971; Di Chiro and Wener, 1973; Ommaya et al., 1969), the first two types being found only in adults:

1. Simple *A V fistulas,* the single coiled vessel AVM or angiographic type I, are characterized by one or two tightly coiled continuous vessels along a large extent of the cord. The fistulas are direct, but the recognition of the change from arterial to venous character is difficult, even by histologic examination of the specimen. This difficulty is often due to grossly disturbed structures and reactive changes of the vessels (Adotti et al., 1971; Jellinger et al., 1968). This type of a simple AV fistulous communication probably represents the large majority of spinal vascular anomalies previously referred to as "spinal varicosis" (Rubinstein, 1972).

2. A frequent pattern, corresponding to the *"glomus type"* or angiographic type II, the cirsoid AV angiomas or type III of the AV fistulas (Vollmar et al., 1964), morphologically presents as a small localized vascular plexus or a conglomeration of vessels into which single or multiple arterial feeders converge and from which one or several draining veins depart. While the arterial feeders usually show only slight enlargement or originate from normal radicular tributaries, the tortuous veins form an abnormal group of large varicosities or one large continuous venous channel.

3. The third pattern or "*juvenile*" type is reminiscent of large cerebral AVMs. Multiple large feeding arteries supply voluminous conglomerations of greatly dilated vascular masses that often appear to fill the spinal canal or may penetrate the cord (Figs. 6 A-D). This type, most frequent in children, may also occur in adults, as seen in two of our cases.

The *histologic picture* of spinal AVMs, although similar to cerebral angiomas, may present considerable problems in recognizing the true nature of the constituent vessels, readily demonstrated by angiography. Histologic distinction between arteries and veins was reported by Adotti et al. (1971) in 14 of their 25 biopsies, and was possible in 18 of 23 intradural AVMs in our material, while identification of an arterial feeder was possible in only four cases each of both series. Disorganization in the structure of the vascular wall is common, including reduplication, interruption, or distortion of the internal elastic lamina of arteries (Fig. 5B), variation in the thickness of the media or muscularis, aneurysmal thinning and dilatation of the vessels, or focal thickening and hyperplasia of the lumen (Fig. 5C). These muscular sphincters, seen in four of 25 histologically examined spinal AVMs (Adotti et al., 1971) may play some role in blood flow regulation. True atheromatous plaques are rare, while thrombosis or organization and endothelialisation (Fig. 4E), and finally, calcification of the vessel walls (Fig. 5A), or metaplastic bone formation may occur. The veins are dilated and thin-walled (Figs. 4B,C, 7E, F), or considerably thickened due to mural connective tissue proliferation, and severe fibrous of hyalin transformation, with usually lack of any muscular coat (Figs. 4A,5C,7A, C). Although these vessels do not show elastic lamellae (Ansari, 1965), they were called "arterialized" veins (Cushing and Bailey, 1928) or "fistulous veins" (Antoni, 1962). The same vascular space may show a wall suggestive of any artery along one segment and a venous structure along another, probably representing an AV fistulous communication

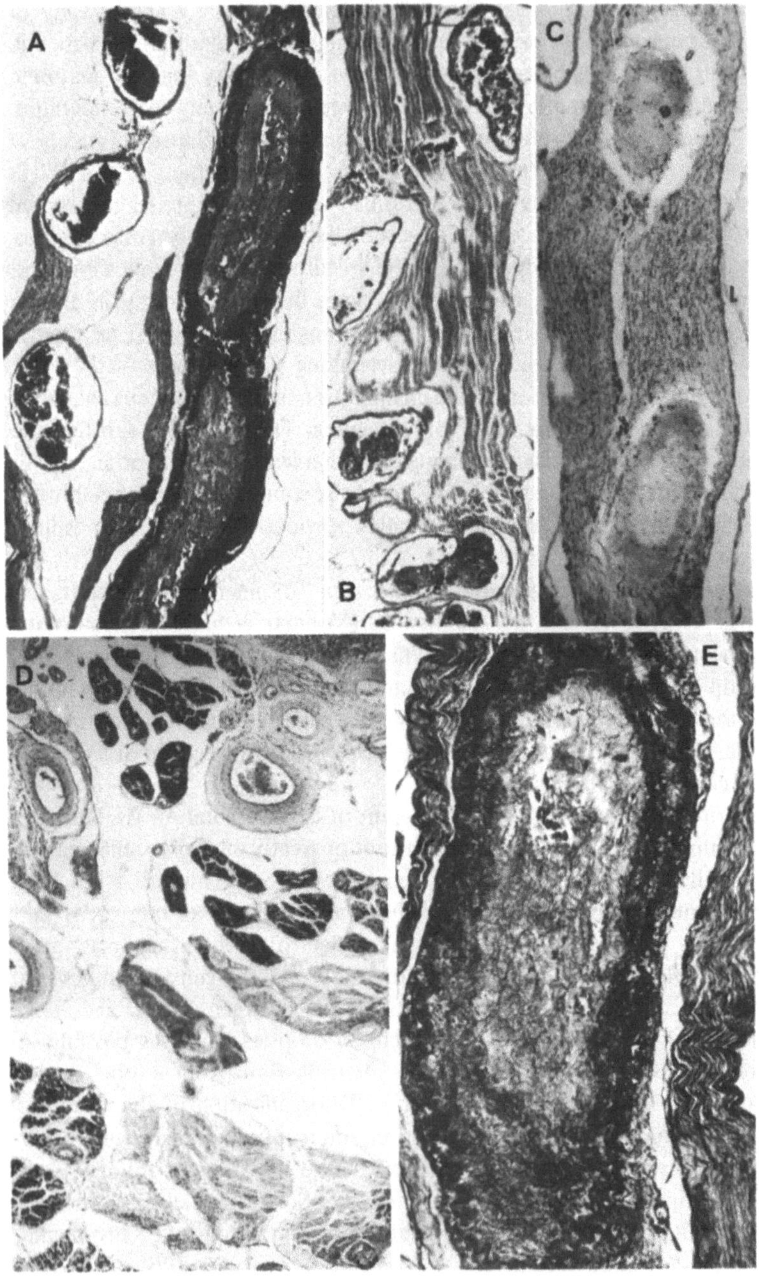

Fig. 4. Radicular vessels (A) Dilated veins and obliterated artery in intradural part of L 5 root. van Gieson x 40, (B) Dilated and tortuous veins in L 3 root. El.v.G. x 40, (C) Complete demyelination of L 3 root with obliterated veins and deposits of hemosiderin. L.F.B. x 50, (D) Demyelination of posterior roots at S 4 with dilated, thick-walled meningeal vessels. L.F.B. x 40, (E) Obliterated vessels in intradural part of T 3 root. Biopsy specimen of AV angioma in female aged 38 years presenting with recurrent paraparesis and negative spinal angiography. v.G. x 100

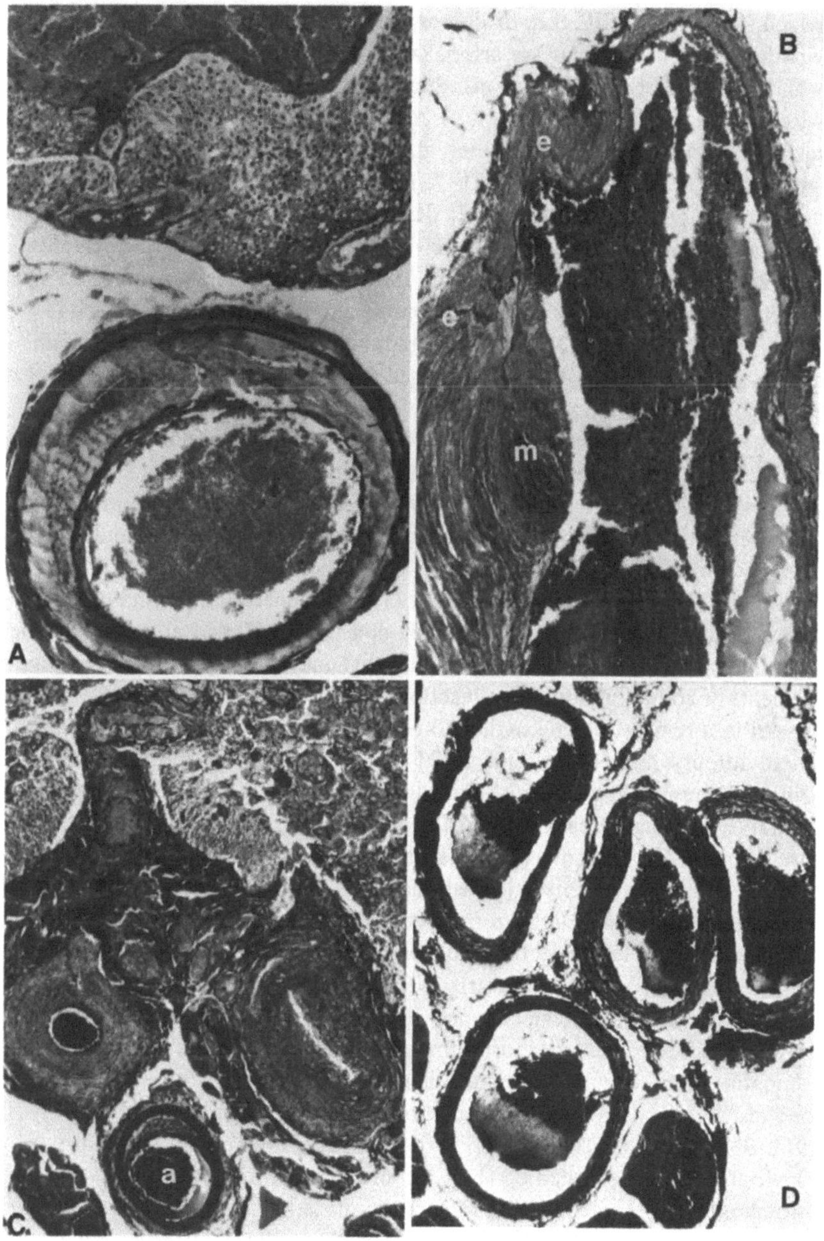

Fig. 5. Radicular and spinal cord vessels. (A) Calcified vessel and dilated vein (v) in anterior L 5 root. H & E. x 100, (B) Radicular artery at L 3 showing subintimal fibrosis, destruction of internal elastic lamina (e) and cushion-like hyperplasia of media (m). v.G. x 65, (C) Thick walled fibrotic veins on anterior surface of sacral cord extending into necrotic cord tissue (arrow), subintimal fibrosis of anterior spinal artery (a). El.v.G. x 100, (D) Dilated and tortuous veins around T 9 posterior root, v.G. x 40

which, however, is difficult to demonstrate. In this connection, it has been questioned whether the AV angiomas are arterialized from the earliest stage of their development or whether they start as venous lesions which subsequently acquire a fistulous communication with an artery. The identification of AVMs in young children, usually showing the complex "juvenile" type (Di Chiro et al., 1971; Di Chiro and Wener, 1973; Reichmann and Sorenson, 1971; Vogelsang, 1973), strongly suggests that no transition of this kind needs to be postulated although it does not exclude this possibility in older subjects. The proportion of intradural spinal angiomas demonstrated in children, previously considered to be rather rare (Béraud, 1972), has considerably increased since the introduction of angiography. They represented about 10% of Vogelsang's (1973) material, while in our series of 23 cases of intradural spinal AV angiomas examined by biopsy and/or autopsy, there were two girls aged 6 and 9 years, respectively, one of whom had a cervical AV malformation at the C 2 to C 5 level successfully removed.

In addition to the anomalies of the pial vessels, there is almost constant involvement of the *radicular tributaries,* mainly of the lumbosacral roots and cauda equina. These changes which are very similar to or even more severe than those in the pial vessels, are often restricted to the intradural portion of the radicular arteries and veins and are often associated with severe root lesions (Figs. 4, 5, 9E).

In 10 – 20% of the cases, the pial AVM may penetrate into the cord and extend over several segments (Figs. 6A, B, D). They consist of bulks of abnormal arteries and veins with interspaced nervous tissue (Fig. 6C) that may show gliosis, various amounts of iron pigment, or some inflammatory reaction. The AVM may replace large areas of the cord, as seen in a female aged 63 with a 30-year clinical history suggestive of multiple sclerosis, where autopsy disclosed a large AVM of the cervical and thoracic cord (Fig. 6D) with some areas resembling capillary hemangioblastoma (Fig. 6E) and a coexisting small right frontal cavernoma. Occasional hemangioblastomatous areas may be observed in an otherwise typical AV angioma (Engelhardt and Gruse, 1973; Pia, 1973), and association of AVM and capillary hemangioblastoma of the spinal cord does occur (Fig. 9).

There are sometimes large or many small abnormal vessels inside the spinal cord which resemble capillary teleangiectasias, or venous angiomas (Scholz, 1951; Scholz and Wechsler, 1959), and rarely, AVMs (Ansari, 1965; Flament et al., 1960; Jellinger et al., 1968). These thick-walled vascular channels have the size and position usually suggesting that they are altered capillaries or veins and, less often arteries which may show direct communication with the extramedullary AVM (Figs. 5C, 6A – C, 8A) or are seen at a long distance from the pial malformation suggesting a separate blood supply (David et al., 1962; Jellinger et al., 1968; Linoli 1958; Reinisch, 1963). They have fibrous hyaline walls which are sometimes calcified (Fig. 8), and recent thrombosis or organization of earlier thrombosis may be seen. Within necrotic areas, an increase in the number of ectatic vessels may be associated with fibrinoid necrosis, collagenous thickening, and mineralization (Figs. 8C, D); it may be difficult to draw a strict distinction between true vascular anomalies and reactive changes secondary to the extramedullary angioma (Jellinger et al., 1968; Koeppen et al., 1974).

Complications of Spinal Angiomas

There are several lesions secondary to spinal vascular malformations. Acute or recurrent *subarachnoid hemorrhage* has been reported in 10 – 30% of several series of spinal AVMs (Bergstrand et al., 1964; Houdart et al., 1968; Krayenbühl et al., 1969; Odom, 1962;

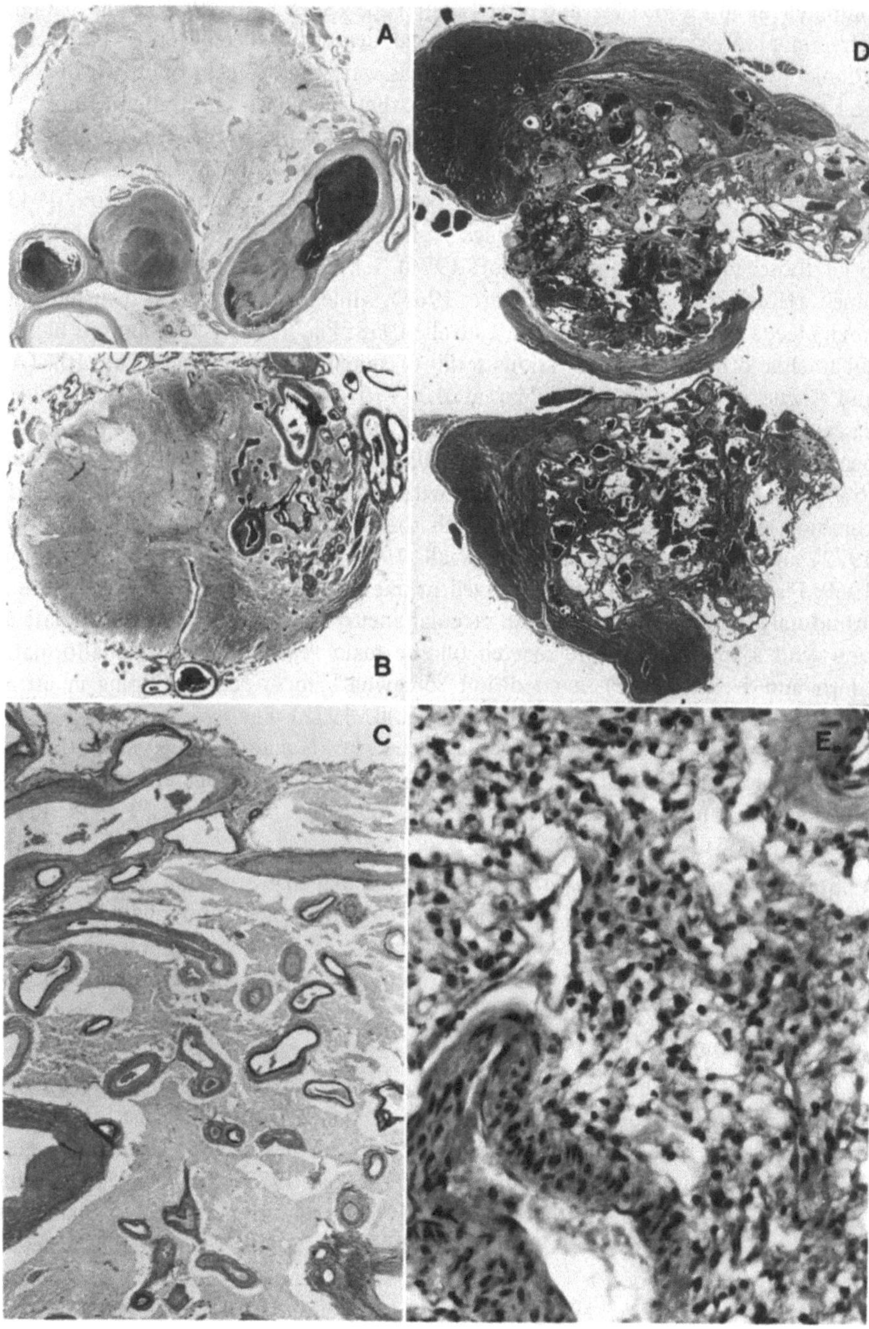

Fig. 6. (A-C) Arteriovenous malformation over anterior part of the cervical cord. (A) with large intramedullary portion in the thoracic cord, (B, C = H. & E. x 45), (D) AV angioma replacing large areas of cervical and upper thoracic spinal cord. L.F.B., (E) Hemangioblastoma area in intramedullary AV angioma. H. & E. x 250

Ommaya et al., 1969; Pia and Vogelsang, 1965; Shephard, 1963) while patients with intracranial AVM present with subarachnoid hemorrhage in 20–60% (Olivecrona and Tönnis, 1971; Pool, 1962). Whereas angiomas were the cause in only two of 6368 cerebral subarachnoid bleeds (Sahs et al., 1969), they have been said to be the most common cause of subarachnoid bleeding confined to the spinal theca (Black, 1900; Béraud, 1972; Gaupp, 1888; Henson and Croft, 1956; Höök and Lidvall, 1958; Lorenz, 1901; Losacco, 1966; Odom, 1961; Pia, 1973; Pia and Vogelsang, 1965; Wyburn–Mason, 1943). The incidence of subarachnoid hemorrhage from angiomas with a large shunt is higher than from those with small ones (Aminoff 1976). It often represents the earliest sign of the illness (Houdart et al., 1968; Shephard, 1963), while in some patients recurrent subarachnoid bleeds may occur (Höök and Lidvall, 1958; Pia, 1973). The reported incidence of subarachnoid hemorrhage in various series of spinal angiomas ranges from 10% (Aminoff and Logue 1974) to 30% (Djindjian et al., 1970) and averaged 12.6% in a series of 421 cases reviewed by Aminoff (1976). On the other hand, definite proof of subarachnoid hemorrhage was received in only three of 50 cases of angiographically proven spinal AVM (6%), all of which showed combination with arterial aneurysm (Herdt et al., 1971). This combination is well-documented in both the brain (Perret, 1966; Ule and Kolkmann, 1972) and spinal cord (Höök and Lidvall, 1958; Hopkins et al., 1966; Kunc and Bret, 1969; Pia, 1973) and has been observed in one among 23 morphologically proven spinal intradural AVMs of our series. The saccular aneurysms, always found in intimate association with a spinal AVM, are located on the main vessel feeding the malformation (Di Chiro and Wener, 1973), a condition somewhat similar to the finding in intracranial AVMs associated with aneurysm (Shenkin et al., 1971). The two lesions have been found to coexist in the same relative percentages, i.e., in 7% and 6% of AVMs in the brain and cord, respectively; and in 75% of the patients with both lesions either intracranially or intraspinally, subarachnoid hemorrhage was observed (Herdt et al., 1971; Perret and Nishioka, 1966).

Spinal *extradural hematoma* arising from vascular malformation with or without previous minor trauma is rare. The bleeding may originate from dilated epidural veins (Lougheed and Hoffmann, 1960), a venous angioma and dilated lumbar varicose plexus (Cube, 1962; Dawson, 1963), or other vascular anomaly not clearly identified as an angioma or varicosity (Herrmann et al., 1965). Spinal *subdural hematoma* associated with AVM is rare (Pia, 1973).

Hematomyelia, a large intramedullary hemorrhage spreading over several segments, represents a rather frequent complication of spinal vascular malformations, particularly AVMs and cavernous angiomas (Ansari, 1965; Buckley, 1936; Houdart et al., 1968; Marty, 1899; Odom, 1957; Ohlmacher, 1899; Pia, 1973; Reznik, 1965; Richardson, 1938; Vraa-Jensen, 1949; Wyburn–Mason, 1943), and intramedullary capillary angiomas or teleangiectasias (Hiecke, 1949; Koos and Böck, 1970; van Reeth, 1952; Russell, 1932). Hematomyelia may occur with or without subarachnoid hemorrhage but the two are often associated (Balck, 1900; Béraud, 1972; Blahd, 1923; Buckley, 1936; Koos and Böck, 1970).

Compression damage to the spinal cord and roots may result from large intradural vascular malformations acting as space-occupying lesions (Bailey and Sperl, 1969; Guillain and Alajouanine, 1925; Hopkins et al., 1966; Krayenbühl et al., 1970; Kunc and Bret, 1969; Ommaya et al., 1969; Sargent, 1925; Shephard, 1963; Steimle et al., 1971). The cord is usually compressed by bulky venous components of large AVMs (Guillain and Alajouanine, 1925), which also cause damage to the spinal roots (Figs. 6A, E).

Ischemic changes and infarction of the cord are common complications of vascular anomalies (Antoni, 1962; Brion et al., 1952; Cushing et al., 1928; Flament et al., 1960), which may cause transient attacks (Aminoff, 1976; Palmer, 1972), "apoplectiform" progression (Pia, 1973; Sargent, 1925; Wyburn–Mason, 1943), or chronic disease.

Chronic progressive radiculomyelopathy, with recurrent or progressive ascending flaccid paraparesis and anesthesia is a rather frequent complication of spinal vascular anomalies in middle or later life. This conditon, often referred to as Foix-Alajouanine disease (Bodechtel, 1957) or Foix-Alajouanine syndrome (FAS) (Koeppen et al., 1975), originally described as "subacute necrotizing myelopathy" (Foix and Alajouanine, 1926), and later renamed "angiohypertrophic necrotizing myelitis" (Bednar, 1970; Osterland, 1960), "angiodysgenetic myelomalacia" (Bodechtel, 1957; Flament et al., 1960; Reinisch, 1963), or "angiodysgenetic necrotizing myelopathy" (David et al., 1962; Jellinger et al., 1968; Scholz and Hanuelidis, 1951; Scholz and Wechsler, 1959) was previously attributed to "endomesovasculitis" of the spinal cord vessels (Foix and Alajouanine, 1926) or to spinal thrombophlebitis (Greenfield and Turner, 1959; Hair and Folkerts, 1953), although its relationship to spinal angiomas, mainly of venous type, was described earlier (Lhermitte et al., 1931; Lindemann, 1912). It is now agreed upon that the FAS is *not* a separate nosologic entity but represents a particular form of chronic radiculomyelopathy, the underlying pathology of which in most cases is an intradural AVM (Ansari, 1965; Antoni, 1962; Brion et al., 1952; Djindjian et al., 1969; Pia and Vogelsang, 1965; Wirth et al., 1970) or a variety of vascular anomalies, the true nature of which (venous, arteriovenous) is under discussion, as the complexity and secondary changes of these malformations make a definite morphologic assessment difficult (Berger et al., 1973; Jellinger et al., 1968). The numerous case reports of the condition have been reviewed by Jellinger et al. (1968) and Koeppen et al. (1974), the total estimated number of documented post-mortem cases being about 65, including ten personal observations. The majority of the patients are males over 50 years old; our series included nine males and one female aged 27–72 years (average 61 years) with a duration of illness ranging from 3–9 years (average 5.5 years).

Grossly, the spinal cord covered by coiled and convoluted vessels more on the dorsal than on the anterior surface (Fig. 3B–D), tends to be greatly shrunken, cystic in some parts, and discolored. No distinction between grey and white matter can be made. The microscopic picture, in addition to considerable thickening and redundancy of the vessels in the subarachnoid space and along the intradural parts of the spinal roots, shows extensive demyelination and necrosis of the cord, being more advanced in the lumbosacral areas (Fig. 7D, H.), but extending up to the midthoracic level (Fig. 7B, E–G). The necrosis may effect one half of the cord (Fig. 7C), the whole transverse section (Fig. 7D), or is limited to the central parts (Fig. 7E) and marginal areas (Fig. 7B). Areas of acute necrosis contain focal collection of plasmatic exudates akin to coagulation necrosis or "plasmatic infiltration necrosis" (Scholz and Manuelidis, 1951; Scholz and Wechsler, 1959), with lipid degradation and gliosis, later progressing to fibrous collagenous scarring which is very evident in the lumbosacral area (Fig. 7H). The upper parts of the cord show Wallerian degeneration of the dorsal columns (Fig. 7A), often associated with pial vascular anomalies. The lesions of the radicular tributaries are often associated with severe damage to the lumbosacral nerve roots ranging from flaky or segmental demyelination to complete nerve fibre depletion and fibrous scarring (Figs. 4C, D, 9C, D). These radicular changes apparently occur before damage to the cord and thus may explain the initial clinical signs and symptoms. About half of the patients have an acute onset of pain and dysesthesia (Aminoff, 1976; Bischoff and Schettler, 1967; Krayenbühl et al., 1969) or complain of intermittent sciatica (Jellinger et al., 1968; Pia, 1973; Wirth et al., 1970) and "dysbasia intermittens spinalis"

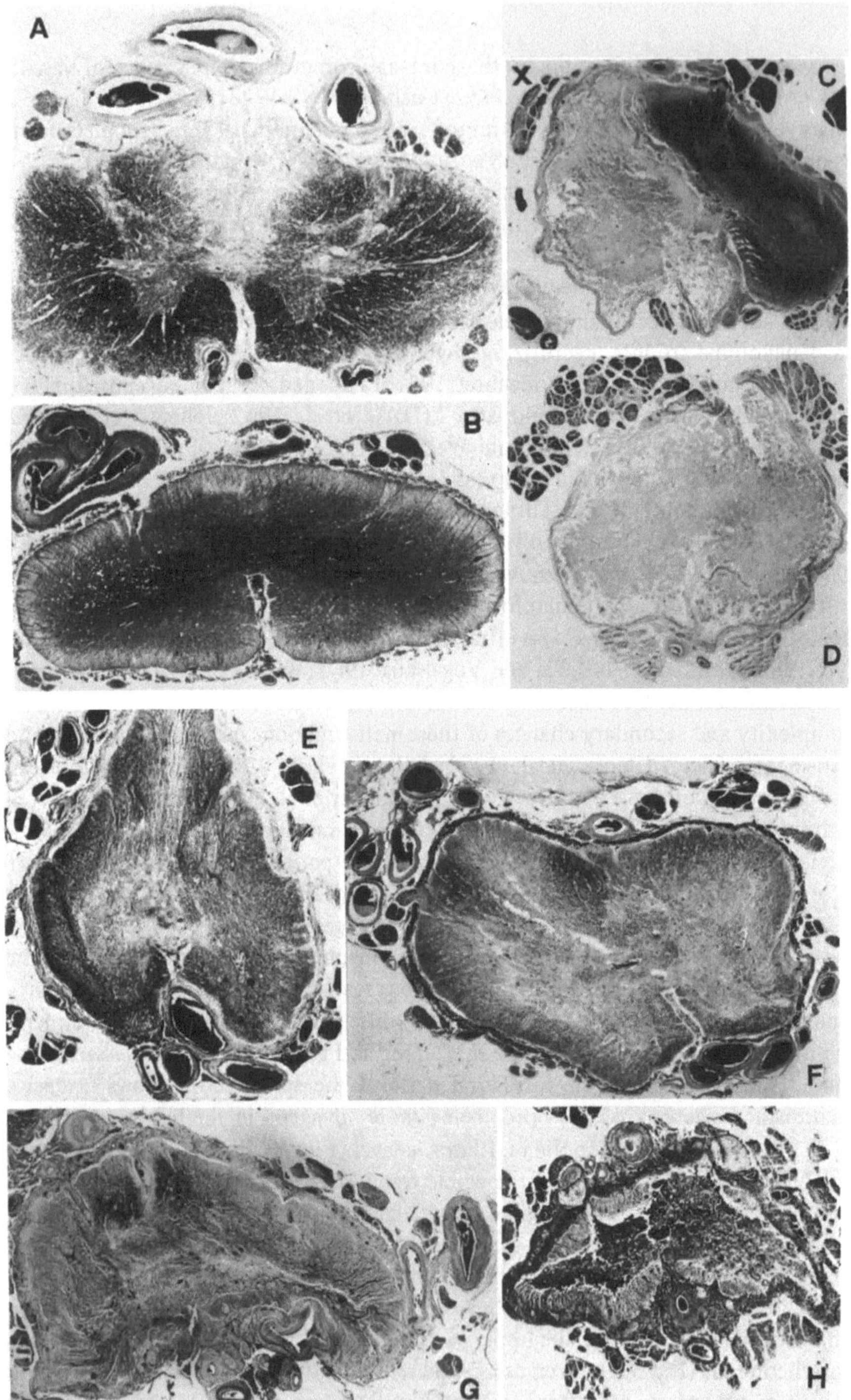

Fig. 7. "Angiodysgenetic" myelopathies. (A) Dilated thick-walled veins on dorsal surface of cervical cord with Wallerian degeneration of dorsal columns. L.F.B., (B) Convoluted pial veins and marginal demyelination of midthoracic cord, Heidenhain x 5, (C, D) Necrosis of right half of lumbar segment with demyelination of posterior roots (x) and complete transverse necrosis of sacral cord with demyelinated spinal roots. L.F.B., (E-H) Incomplete to complete transverse necrosis at different levels (E = T 4; F = T 7; G = T 8; H = L 5) with central collagenous scar at lumbar level (II)

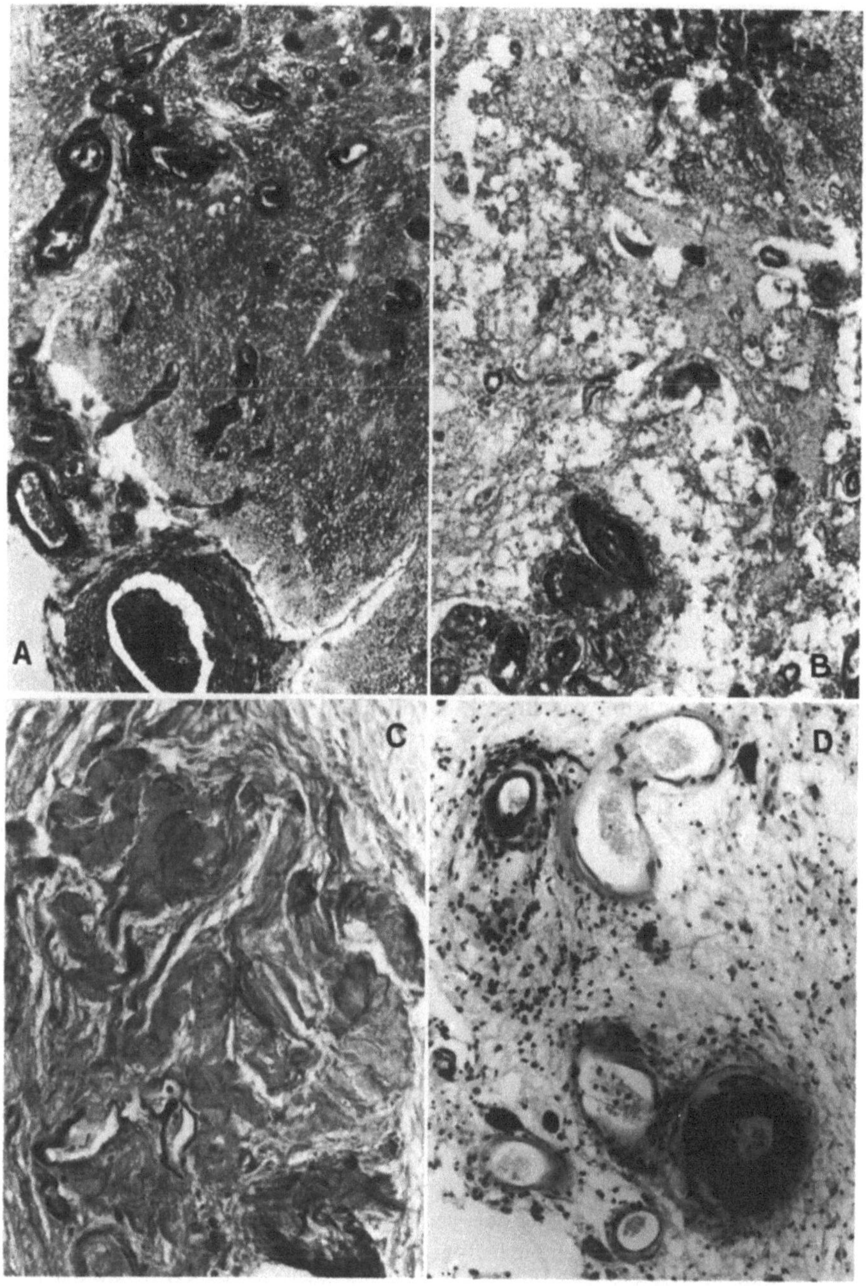

Fig. 8. Intramedullary vessels in "angiodysgenetic" myelopathy. (A) Proliferated vessels in demyelinated dorsal white matter of lumbar cord. L.F.B. x 15, (B) Accumulation of fibrotic intramedullar vessels, El.v.G. x 260, (C) Extravasation of fibrinoid and hyalin masses in necrotic grey matter of thoracic cord. v.G. x 100, (D) Fibrinoid necrosis and mineralization of teleangiectatic vessels in necrotic gray matter. C.V. x 100

(Foix and Alajouanine, 1926) with transient weakness and sensory disturbances (Wirth et al., 1970), followed by progressive radiculospinal symptoms. In a number of patients with surgically treated sciatica, similar lumbosacral extradural vascular anomalies have been demonstrated (Gümbel et al., 1969). There is a striking increase and proliferation of intramedullary blood vessels within and outside the necrotic areas (Fig. 8). These abundant vascular channels, the histology of which often does not allow their designation as veins or arteries, show fibrinoid necrosis (Fig. 8B, D), transformation into "collagen tubes" (Fig. 8C) and *mineralization* (Figs. 5A, 8D). Histochemical and scanning electron-microscopic studies identified an excess of calcium and abnormal distribution of phosphorus and sulfur (Koeppen et al., 1974). Although continuous penetration of pial vascular anomalies into the spinal cord has been observed (Jellinger et al., 1968; Kothe, 1953), the identity of vascular lesions within the necrotic foci of FAS and delayed radiation myelopathy (Jellinger and Sturm, 1971) allow the conclusion that the intramedullary vascular lesions are, at least in part, secondary phenomena. It is believed that the disease of the intramedullary vessels with the associated necrosis of the cord tissue and spinal roots, both considered the significant lesion in FAS, represent a reaction to the superficial vascular malformation, although the relationship between the two pathologic processes is not fully elucidated (Jellinger et al., 1968; Koeppen et al., 1974).

Several theories explaining the development of chronic radiculomyelopathy in AVM have been put forward. One hypothesis suggests that damage to the cord and roots is caused by pressure effects of the angioma (Guillain and Alajouanine, 1925; Krayenbühl and Yasargil, 1963; Kunc and Bret, 1969; Shephard, 1963) while others attribute myelomalacia to thrombosis of the abnormal vessels in the malformation (Flament et al., 1960; Pia and Vogelsang, 1965) although thrombosis is rarely demonstrated by angiography or surgery (Wirth et al., 1970; Aminoff and Logue, 1974). Other important factors are: 1) disturbances of the venous drainage of the cord due to slowing down of the flow in the discharging venous channels, confirmed by angiography (Di Chiro et al., 1967, 1971, 1973; Djindjian et al., 1966, 1969, 1970, 1971; Doppman et al., 1969) or blockage of the outflow in the greatly distendend convolutions and obstructed radicular tributaries (Jellinger et al., 1968; Losacco, 1966; Lorenz, 1901), and "steal phenomena" resulting from the fact that the venous sink of the AVM acting as a shunt siphons off important blood supply from the spinal cord (Chatterjee, 1969; Di Chiro and Wener, 1973; Kaufmann et al., 1970; Krayenbühl and Yasargil, 1972; Shephard, 1963). All or some of these factors are suggested to result, via a complex chain of action, in chronic ischemia and disturbances of the blood-brain barrier with extravasation of plasmatic substances and ensuing necrosis of the parenchyma. The intramedullary vascular lesions either primary or secondary in origin are believed to enhance the development of damage to the cord that obviously represents the final result of a long-standing pathologic process causally related to the vascular malformation, although its pathogenetic factors are not yet fully understood. Spinal angiography has not only succeeded in eliminating FAS as a clinicopathologic entity, but will it is hoped contribute further to eliminating this and other delayed sequelae of spinal angiomas by facilitating their early clinical diagnosis and providing the basis for successful surgical treatment.

Associated Lesions in Spinal Angiomas

A considerable proportion of spinal angiomas – up to 25% (Djindjian et al., 1971) – are associated with other neural or extraneural vascular lesions and various dysplasias which are in favor of a common dysembryogenetic basis of these changes and emphasize the hamartomatous character of the spinal vascular anomalies (Table 2).

Concomitant *cutaneous angiomas*, present in 8% - 26% of the cases of spinal vascular malformations (Adotti et al., 1971; Di Chiro et al., 1971; Djindjian et al., 1971; Doppman et al., 1969) due to their often metameric location may be valuable as a guide in detecting the location of the cord lesion. However, cutaneous angiomas may also occur in a non-segmental distribution in some patients with a spinal angioma (Doppman et al., 1969; Djindjian et al., 1970; Aminoff and Logue 1974), and may also be associated with other types of spinal vascular hamartoma, and with epidural and vertebral angioma (Aminoff 1976). Within this cutaneomedullary angiomatosis syndrome, nevi of "port wine" character may occur in the skin of the corresponding dermatome (Cobb, 1915; Giampalmo, 1943) or at other sites of the trunk and extremities (van Bogaert, 1950; Djindjian et al., 1971; Wyburn–Mason, 1943). Other cutaneous lesions include cavernomas (Foix and Alajouanine, 1926) and angiolipomas (Berenbruch, 1890; van Bogaert, 1950).

Vertebral anomalies accompanying spinal angiomas include kyphosis or kyphoscoliosis (Aminoff, 1976; Dalloz, 1963; Djindjian et al., 1971) and vertebral angiomas seen in about 10% of spinal cord angiomas (Djindjian et al., 1971) producing the syndrome of "vertebromedullary angiomatosis" (Newman, 1959). A metameric affection of all contiguous layers from the skin to the spinal cord may exist – "cutaneovertebromedullary angiomatosis" (Djindjian et al., 1971; Pia, 1973; Seze et al., 1966) – while Turner and Kernohan (1941) reported a patient with spinal, cutaneous, and intramedullary angiomas and segmental distribution.

Other *extramedullary vascular anomalies* accompanying spinal angiomas include a wide variety of dysplasias, e.g. multiple teleangiectasias and cavernomas in soft tissues (Gagel and Meszaros, 1948; Goulon et al., 1971) and visceral organs (Di Chiro, 1957; Djindjian et al., 1971), venous angiomas and AV fistulas in the extremities (Djindjian et al., 1971), or rare combinations with the Klippel-Trenaunay-Weber syndrome (Djindjian et al., 1971; Krayenbühl et al., 1970), and with hereditary hemorrhagic teleangiectasia or Osler-Rendu syndrome (Djindjian et al., 1971; Merry and Appleton, 1976), and hereditary cutaneous hemangioma (Kaplan et al., 1976). There may be combinations of spinal AVM with anomalies of the lymphatic system and other mesenchymal dysplasias (Djindjian et al., 1971).

Multiple vascular anomalies of the CNS include: 1) the association of an AVM of the spinal cord with one of the brain (Di Chiro, 1957; Di Chiro et al., 1971; Houdart et al., 1968; Wyburn–Mason, 1943) or cerebellum, and rare cases of cerebrospinal angiomatosis and 2) the association of an AVM of the spinal cord with single or multiple *"berry" aneurysms* on spinal arteries (Herdt et al., 1971) and intracranial arteries (Brion et al., 1952; Jellinger et al., 1968; Wyburn–Mason, 1943). One of our cases of FAS due to thoracolumbar AVM after a 6-year illness died from ruptured berry aneurysm of the left internal carotid artery.

The association is known of spinal AVMs with *hemangioblastomas* of the spinal cord (Djindjian et al., 1971; Guidetti and Fortuna, 1967; Guillain et al., 1932; Jellinger et al., 1968; Klug, 1948; Krishnan and Smith, 1961; Pia, 1973; Wyburn–Mason, 1943) and cerebellum (Dilenge et al.,1976) or retinocerebellar angiomatosis (Di Chiro, 1957) and with other *tumors* of the spinal cord and cauda, e.g., ependymoma (Krishnan and Smith, 1961; Urieger, 1974), neurofibroma (Hoffman and Bagan, 1967), and lipoma (Jellinger et al., 1968).

Interesting associations are that of spinal AVM with *CNS dysplasias,* e.g., syringomyelia (Russell, 1932), syringomyelia and syringobulbia (Hetzel, 1960), meningocele, (Mair and Folkerts, 1953) and spina bifida (Wyburn–Mason, 1943). An intramedullary hemangio-

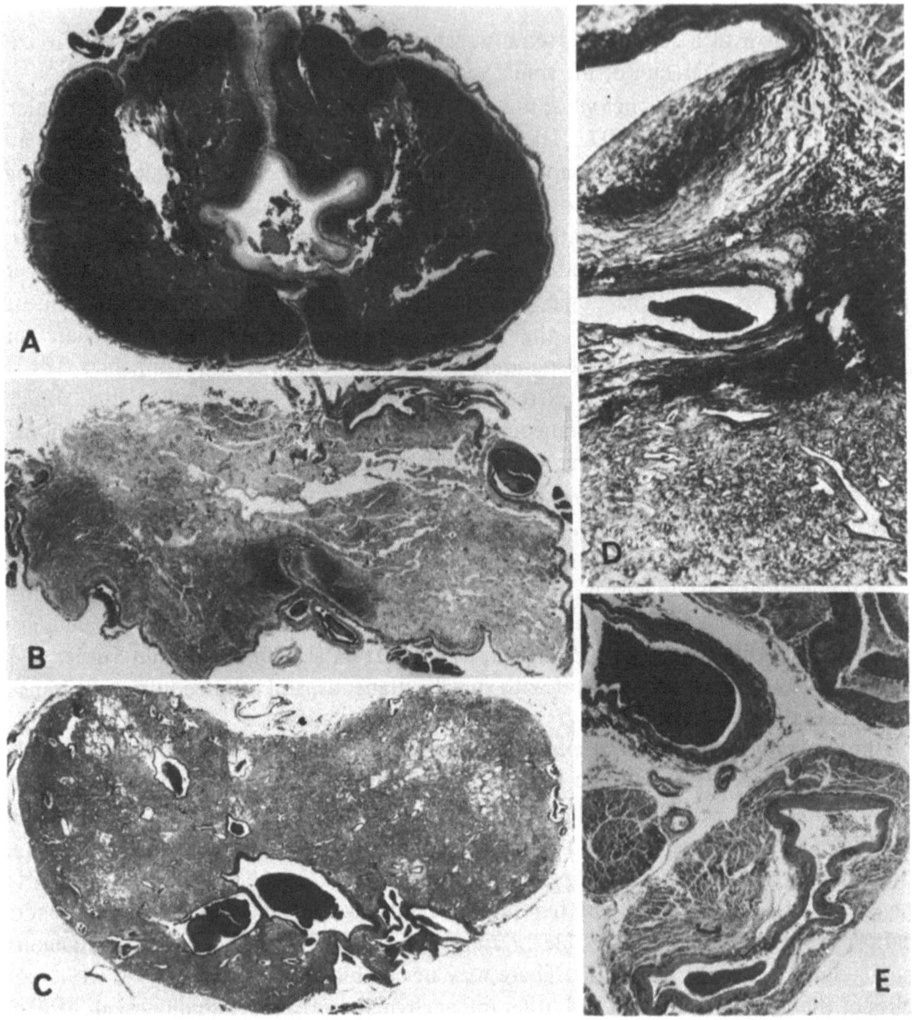

Fig. 9. Intramedullary hemangioblastoma of the lumbar cord (C = Gomori x 5) with angiomatous dorsal pial vessels (D = El.v.G. x 60) associated with AV angioma from low thoracic cord to cauda equina (E = El.v.G. x 40), necrotic myelopathy at the low thoracic and upper lumbar segments (B = L.F.B. x 6), and syringomyelia with degeneration of medial dorsal columns of the cervical cord (A = L.F.B. x 5)

blastoma of the cauda with intradural AVM and necrotizing myelopathy of the thoracic cord combined with cervical syringomyelia was seen in a male aged 25 years (Fig. 9). Although it has been argued that the syringomyelic cavity might be due to transudation of plasma from the tumor vessels, the separate occurrence of syringomyelia and AVM supports the view that they constitute separate congenital anomalies (Rubinstein, 1972; Wyburn–Mason, 1943), representing parts of dysgenetic syndromes (phacomatoses) that are closely allied to each other.

Spinal Vascular Tumors

Vascular neoplasms affecting the spinal cord are rather are. They include two major types – hemangioblastomas and hemangiopericytomas – both of which may cause diagnostic problems.

Capillary Hemangioblastoma (Hemangioendothelioma, Angioreticuloma)

The first spinal hemangioblastoma was reported in 1912 by Schultze. A recent review of 138 cases including 30 cases of their own was given by Hurth et al. (1975). These tumors constitute 1–2.5% of all intracranial neoplasms being mainly located in the posterior fossa with 10–12% supratentorial forms (Jeffreys, 1974; Leu and Rüttner, 1972; Rubinstein, 1972), while their incidence among the tumors of the spinal cord and cauda ranges from 1.3–14% with an average of 4–5% (Browne et al., 1976; Leu and Rüttner, 1972; Palmer, 1972; Resche et al., 1974; Sloof et al., 1964). Among 70 angioblastomas, we observed four spinal cord tumors. *Grossly,* the tumors are well-circumscribed and may be either solid or cystic (Fig. 10B, C), containing yellow areas and dilated blood spaces. The characteristic histologic feature consists in the presence of large numbers of thin-walled, closely packed blood vessels lined by plump endothelial cells and separated by large, polygonal interstitial or "stromal" cells with foamy cytoplasm often showing considerable lipid storage (Fig. 10D). There is a delicate connective tissue stroma. Recent electron-microscopic and organ culture studies demonstrated three cell types – endothelial cells, pericytes, and stromal cells – all of which are neoplastic (Spence and Rubinstein, 1975; Toga et al., 1976), suggesting that capillary hemangioblastomas originate from vasoformative elements showing variable angiogenic differentiation to form capillary walls. The stromal cells, the histogenesis of which has been a matter of discussion (Cushing and Bailey, 1928; Hurth et al., 1975; Russell and Rubinstein, 1972), are now regarded as an aberrant cell type of angiogenic mesenchymal lineage which does not interconvert into endothelial cells (Spence and Rubinstein, 1975).

Spinal angioblastomas which constitute 10–12% of all spinal vascular anomalies and vascular neoplasms may occur at all levels of the spinal cord. Among 138 tumors (Hurth et al., 1975), 17 were extradural and 121 subdural, ten of which showed an extramedullary location, 28 were on the posterior roots, and 83 within the cord. They are located mainly in the cervical (Fig. 10A) and thoracic cord. The lesions are most often single (Bergstrand et al., 1964; Browne et al., 1976; Guidetti and Fortuna, 1967; Hurth et al., 1975; Sloof et al., 1974; Wyburn–Mason, 1943), intramedullary (60%), and mainly located in the dorsal parts of the cord; 30% show purely intramedullary and 6% both intra- and extramedullary location, occasionally replacing the whole cord tissue (Fig. 10B). Cysts within or close to the tumor are present in about 50% of the cases. There is associated syringomyelia in 67% of intramedullary cases (Browne et al., 1976) and meningeal varicosity or AVM in 48% of all cases (Browne et al., 1976; Di Chiro and Wener, 1973; Djindjian et al., 1971; Guidetti and Fortuna, 1967; Guillian et al., 1932; Klug, 1948; Pia, 1973; Wyburn–Mason, 1943). This association was observed in almost 7% of spinal AVMs (Pia, 1973). Diagnostic problems may arise from the fact that AVMs occasionally contain hemangioblastomatous areas (Fig. 6E), while hemangioblastomas often show angioma-like sinusoid blood spaces and wide vascular channels (Figs. 9D, 10B). The tight clusters of sinusoidal thin-walled vessels may explain the angiographic picture of these tumors charac-

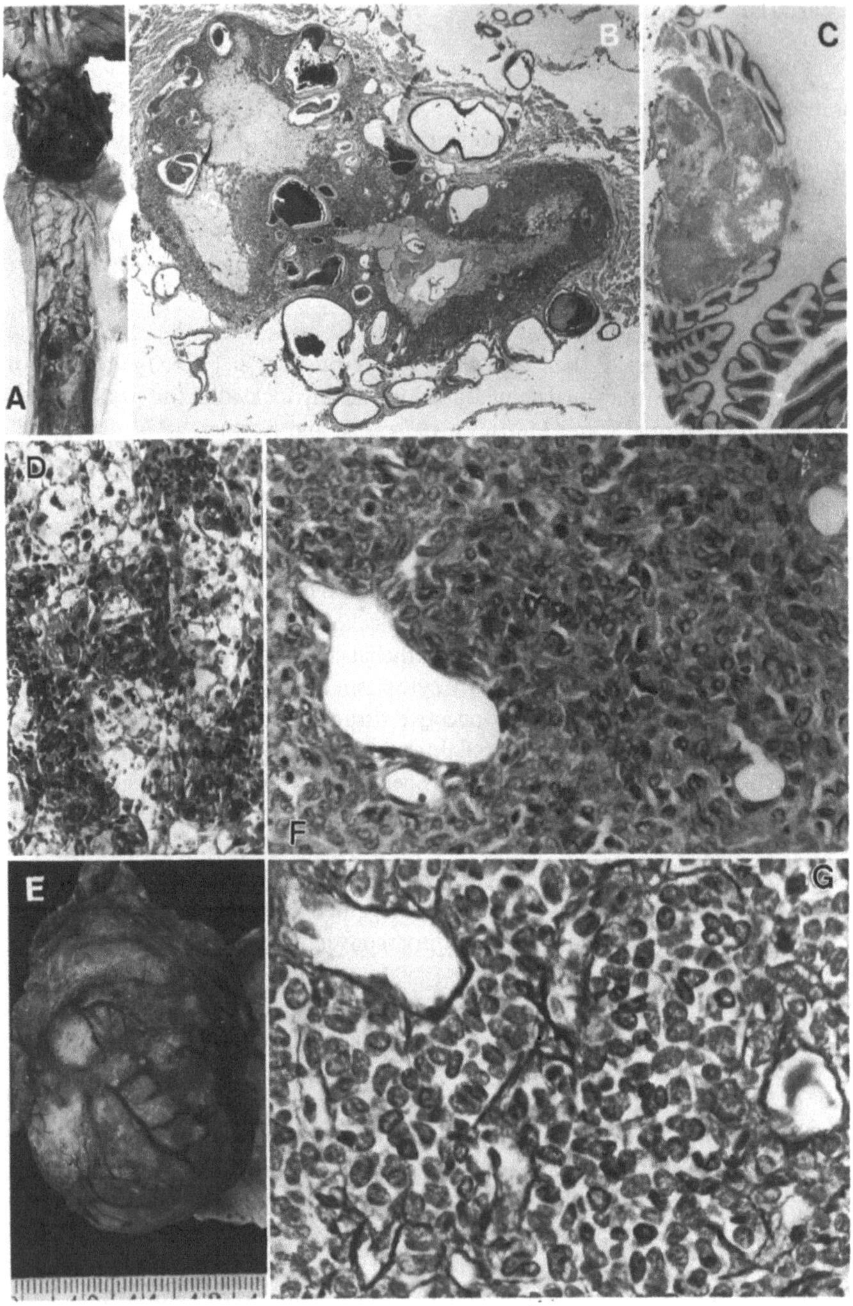

Fig. 10 (A–C). Hemangioblastomas of the upper cervical cord (A, B) and cerebellum, (C) in male aged 73 years with von Hippel-Lindau disease, (D) Low power shows stromal cells. (H. & E. x 100). (E–G) Meningeal hemangiopericytoma of the cauda equina. (E) Biopsy specimen of tumor attached to the dura, (F) Endothelial-lined vascular channels surrounded by densely arranged tumor cells (H. & E x 260), (G) Network of reticulin fibres outlining vascular architecture. (Gomori x 400)

terized by densely staining nodules with a vascular "blush" and rapid shunting into a distended vein (Browne et al., 1976; Di Chiro and Wener, 1973; Herdt et al., 1972; Hurth et al., 1975), which usually can be differentiated from an AVM, but occasionally may mimic the glomus type II of AVM (Di Chiro et al., 1971). The spinal hemangioblastomas are fed by the posterior system and less often by the anterior system (Hurth et al., 1975) or by different vessels, resulting in an angiographic "jigsaw puzzle" arrangement of the tumoral blush (Di Chiro and Wener, 1973). Hemangioblastomas in other CNS locations and retinocerebellar angiomatosis (von Hippel-Lindau disease) are present in 33% of the cases with spinal cord angioblastomas (Browne et al., 1976), often associated with syringomyelia (Hurth et al., 1975; Rubinstein, 1972) or with spinal AVM and syringomyelia (Fig. 9). In a male aged 73 years with a 16-year history of cervical tumor and glaucoma, autopsy disclosed multiple angioblastomas of the medulla, cervical cord, and cerebellum (Fig. 10A–D) with ossified angioblastoma of the retina, multiple cysts in the kidneys, and renal hypernephroma.

Hemangiopericytoma of the Meninges

Hemangiopericytoma is a vascular tumor in the soft tissues, predominantly arising from pericytes (Stout and Murray, 1942) which rarely occurs in the cranial vault and spinal canal. The frequent attachment of cerebrospinal hemangiopericytoma to meninges and the finding of meningiomatous whorls in tissue culture lent support to their inclusion with the "angioblastic" meningiomas (Muller and Mealey, 1971), but they have a unique biologic behavior and prognosis as they tend to recur and metastasize, which justifies their differentiation from the common group of angioblastic meningiomas (Jakesz, 1976; Jellinger and Slowik, 1975; Kastendieck and Klöppel, 1976; Olivecrona and Tönnis, 1971; Rubinstein, 1972). Grossly, these tumors are attached to meninges, encapsulated, occasionally lobulated, solid, and indistinguishable from other varieties of meningeal tumor (Fig. 10E). Histologically however, they show a distinct pattern unlike that seen in meningiomas. Numerous vessels, either slit-shaped or patent, lined with endothelium, are surrounded by densely packed, mostly spindle-shaped cells with round or elongated nuclei (Fig. 10F). Mitotic figures are frequent. The vascular network is particularly pronounced and well outlined by reticulin stains (Fig. 10G). The ultrastructure of these tumors conforming in all respects to hemangiopericytomas in other organ systems (Battifora, 1973) supports the concept of their pericytic origin, occasionally suggesting some leiomyoblastic differentiation (Pena, 1975; Popoff and Malinin, 1974), and opposes the presumed meningothelial derivation of the neoplasm (Kastendieck and Klöppel, 1976; Marc et al., 1975; Toga et al., 1976). It is postulated that all the "angioblastic meningiomas" share a common origin from polyblastic mesenchymal cells originating in or derived from the meninges (Horten et al., 1977).

Hemangiopericytomas account for 1–3% of intracranial "meningiomas" (Jellinger and Slowik, 1975; Pitkethley et al., 1970), but only a small number of these tumors has been observed in the spinal canal (Grode, 1972; Pitkethley et al., 1970; Schirger et al., 1958). Among 35 hemangiopericytomas found in a series of 1900 meningiomas in the files of the AFIP, there were only three spinal tumors, two at the upper cervical and one at the thoracic level (Pitkethley et al., 1970). Among 21 hemangiopericytomas in a series of 1300 meningiomas (including 200 spinal tumors), we found only two located in the spinal canal. One was a large tumor of the cauda equina (Fig. 10E–G) in a female aged 43 years who had several recurrences within 5 years and finally died with liver metastases. The angiographic findings common to these tumors include a myriad of tiny irregular feeding vessels springing from a main trunk, an intense fluffy type of stain, lack of early veins, and prolonged tumor circulation time. When located intracranially, they show a dual arterial supply from the internal carotid or vertebral circulation rather than from external (meningeal) vessels (Gullotta and Heller, 1974; Marc et al., 1975). Although angiographic demonstration of spinal hemangiopericytoma has not been reported to the best of our knowledge, differentiation from other vascular tumors particularly hemangioblastoma and highly vascularized endotheliomatous meningioma appears important from both the angiographic and histologic aspects.

Summary

Spinal vascular malformations, accounting for 3.3–12.5% of spinal space-occupying lesions, include vertebral angiomas, extradural, intradural, subpial, and intramedullary angiomas, which occur as isololated or complex vascular anomalies and may involve various layers at the same level. The preferential occurrence of angiomas on the dorsal surface of the cord and in the caudal regions is related to the embryologic development of the spinal vasculature. Frequent association of spinal angiomas (20-25%) with other vascular anomalies and dysplasias emphasizes their hamartomatous nature and developmental origin. Spinal angiomas include the following morphologic types: 1) capillary teleangiectasias with extra- and intradural and rare intramedullary location, 2) cavernomas, mainly arising in vertebral bodies and rarely within and outside the cord, 3) venous angiomas, mainly located in vertebral bodies and in the extradural space, intradural forms being rare, and 4) arteriovenous malformations (AVM) constituting the commonest type. They are composed of arteries and veins abnormal in appearance and pattern, with AV shunts, and present as simple AV fistulas, cirsoid angiomas with localized vascular plexuses and large complex convolutions ("juvenile" type). AVMs include the majority of vascular anomalies previously referred to as venous angiomas or spinal varicosis, although the histologic recognition of the true nature of the constituent vessels, readily demonstrated by angiography, is difficult due to severe structural abnormalities and secondary changes in the vessel walls. The AVM affects both the pial and radicular vessels and may penetrate into the cord, but the distinction between true intramedullary vascular anomalies and reactive changes is difficult. The complications of spinal angiomas include rare extradural hematoma, subarachnoid hemorrhage, hematomyelia, compression lesions of the cord and roots, and ischemic changes causing chronic progressive radiculomyelopathy, previously referred to as Foix-Alajouanine syndrome. Chronic damage to the cord and spinal roots results from pressure effects, thrombosis of the abnormal vessels, disorders of venous drainage, and "steal" phenomena related to the vascular anomaly. Vascular neoplasms affecting the spinal cord include capillary hemangioblastomas (average 4–5% of spinal cord tumors), occasionally combined with AVM, and rare hemangiopericytomas, the differentiation of which from vascular malformations appears important from angiographic and morphologic aspects.

Discussion

Operative Findings in Spinal Angiomas

Hermann Hager

The occurrence of vascular malformations within the spinal cord and its coverings is not unusual in our biopsy material . This demonstration comprises a number of representative cases from the neurosurgical clinic of the University of Giessen. The usual arteriovenous malformation of the spinal cord is a solitary tortuous vascular mass. Usually, the larger abnormal vessels are situated in the posterior leptomeninges. The malformation may be restricted to the subarachnoid space, but more commonly it invades and alters the dorsal segments of the cord. The feeding arteries become dilated and hypertrophic as a result of locally increased blood flow.

In the vessel walls, the normal lamination of elastic and muscle fibers is altered. Sclerosis of the intima and mural fibrosis occurs. Often the media is imperfectly developed or varies greatly in thickness (Fig. 1A). The veins constitute the bulk of the channels within the lobulated mass. The walls of the veins show irregular collagenous thickening. Thrombosis with varying degrees of organization is sometimes observed. In some vessels, a distinction between artery and vein is difficult.

The next case (Fig. 1B), an angioma from T 8 to L 2, shows severe thickening, degenerative changes of arterial walls, and old thrombus of the veins.

In the next case a sudden paraplegia was caused by a spinal angioma of T 11 to L 1. This angioma consisted chiefly of thin-walled convoluted veins. The arteries showed thickened fibrous walls. Occasionally *thrombotic* occlusions can be seen.

In the next example, the angioma was situated in the thoracic region, invading the spinal cord (Fig. 1C). The angiomatous complex shows a tortuous bundle of vessels, predominantly arteries with extremely thickened walls.

The next case had a long history with subarachnoid bleeding and paraparesis of the legs nine years before. The clinical diagnosis was an extensive spinal angioma. The biopsy shows extremely thickened arterial walls and remains of old thrombotic processes (Fig. 1D).

The next patient suffered from muscular atrophy, spastic paraparesis, and sensory disorders in the right leg. The angioma shows a complex arrangement of fibrous, thick-walled arteries and dilated veins.

The last patient showed increasing signs of a transverse lesion of the thoracic spinal cord. The clinical diagnosis was an extradural tumor (Fig. 1E). The biopsy shows a large cavernous hemangioma with small, unequal spaces separated by fine fibrous strands. One can see in the center a large area of thrombosis with reactive changes in the surrounding tissue. There is no cellular stroma beyond the limiting walls of the blood spaces.

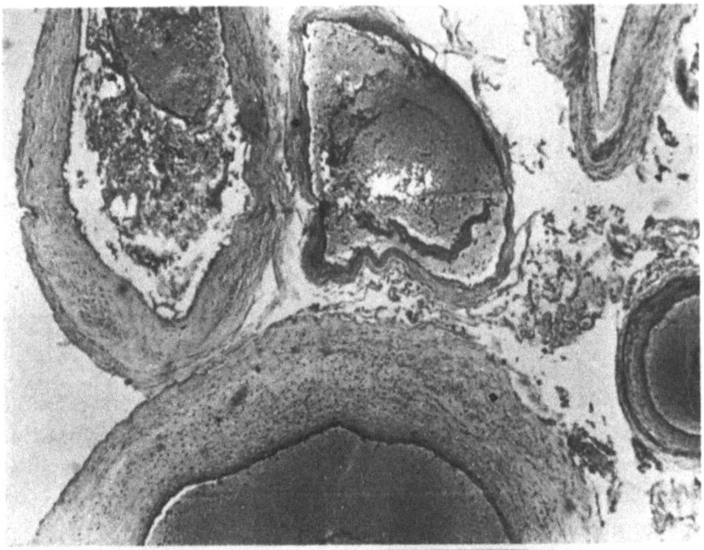

Fig. 1A

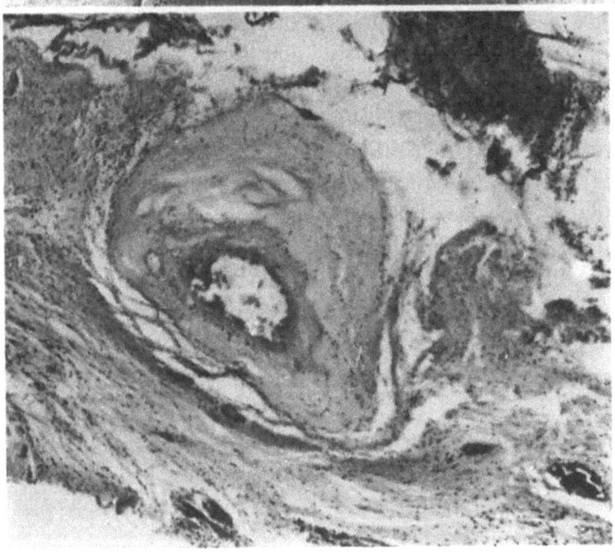

Fig. 1B

Fig. 1. (A) Patient with AV angioma T 10 – L 1 with incomplete cauda syndrome. The vessel walls show sclerosis of the intima and mural fibrosis. (B) Angioma from T 8 – L 2 with severe thickening and degenerative changes of arterial walls, (C) Angioma from the thoracic region, invading the spinal cord; tortuous bundle of vessels, predominantly arteries with thickened walls, (D) Extensive spinal angioma; subarachnoid bleeding and paraparesis nine years before; extremely thickened arterial walls, (E) Patient with transverse lesion of the thoracic spinal cord; cavernous hemangioma with small unequal spaces separated by fine fibrous strands. In the center, large area of thrombosis

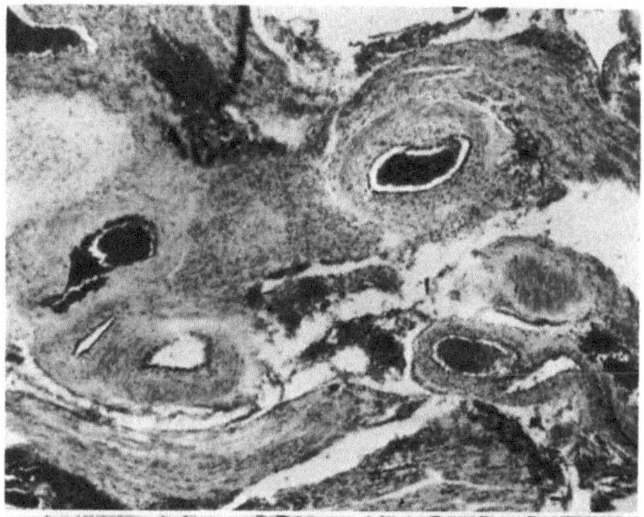
Fig. 1C

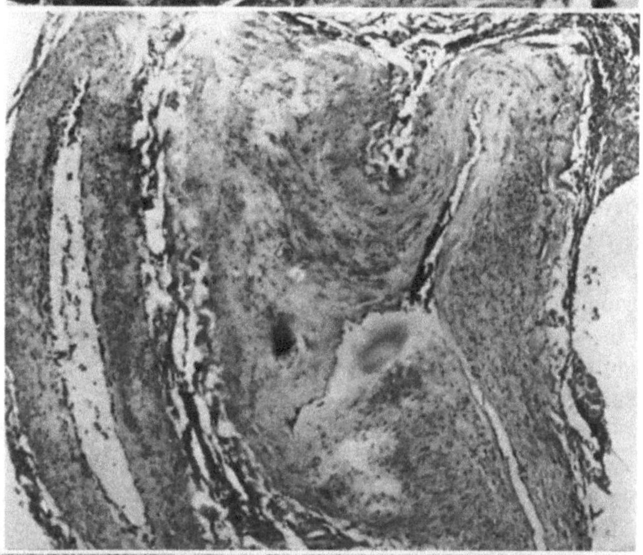
Fig. 1D

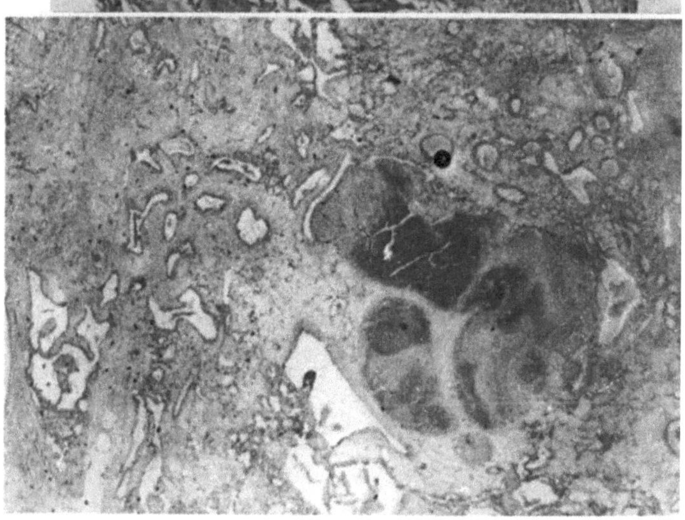
Fig. 1E

Clinical Aspects

Symptomatology of Spinal Angiomas

Hans Werner Pia

Spinal angiomas are no uniform type of disorder. They can be classified, according to their *location*, into

I. Vertebral angiomas
II. Extradural angiomas
III. Intradural angiomas, which can be subdivided into
  A. Subarachnoid
  B. Subpial
  C. Intramedullary angiomas

as well as according to their *histology*, into

I. Racemose arteriovenous angioma (*A. racemosum arteriovenosum*)
II. Cavernous angioma (*A. cavernosum*)
  and closely related or combined with
III. Angioblastoma

Besides the solitary angiomas, there are complex "mixed" angiomas to be distinguished, with simultaneous involvement of two or more structures of the vertebral column and spinal cord (Pia).

The features concerning the location and histology, which have scarcely been considered until the present time, determine the symptoms and course of the disease. These are also affected by the level of the lesion and, with the intradural angiomas, the relationship to the cord itself, viz., the posterior, anterior, and mixed group (Djindjian), the angioma type (single-coiled angioma, Glomus and juvenile type of Di Chiro), and also finally the age of the patient and other factors. For this reason most of the earlier larger series in the literature (Turner and Kernohan, 1941; Wyburn – Mason, 1943; Béraud and Meloche, 1965; Aminoff and Logue, 1974), as well as numerous publications with fewer cases, are of little or no value in evaluating the problem.

Occurrence

Spinal angiomas are rare; definite figures regarding their actual incidence are not available. The true figures are probably larger than is thought, as systematic post mortem examinations are not undertaken and a larger proportion were not recognized clinically. Some clues are given by the ratio of tumors to angiomas (Table 1). According to the available statistics, one can expect to encounter 4% - 5% of spinal angiomas in a group of spinal tumors. Deviations from these figures (Pia, and also Djindjian) are explained by a particu-

Table 1. Ratio of spinal tumors to angiomas

Literature	Spinal tumors	Spinal angiomas	%
(Rasmussen et al., 1940; Nittner and Tönnis, 1950; Newman, 1959; Klug, 1958; Umbach, 1962)	1224	69	5.6
Krayenbühl et al., 1969	961	43	4.5
Pia, 1975	570	60	10.5
		115	20.2

lar interest being shown in the problem. The relation of cerebral and spinal angiomas seems to be similar. In the material from Krayenbühl and Yasargil (1971), there were 186 cerebral angiomas among 4200 tumors (4.4%) and in our own material 201 angiomas among 3300 tumors (6%).

Personal Material and Types

In our material (Table 2), among 115 patients we found 149 angiomas. The latter figure indicates the inclusion of multiple angiomas, principally where there was a simultaneous occurrence in several tissue layers (skin, muscles, etc.). 83 angiomas (56%) were solitary and 66 (44%) were complex. Among the complex angiomas (Table 3), the combination of vertebro – extradural angiomas is the most frequent (N = 16) followed by the extradural – intradural angiomas (N = 7). With regard to the simultaneous occurrence of *segmental skin* (metameric) *angiomas*, several single observations have been published since the first description given by Cobb (1915). Cross (1947) reported on a personal case and five from the literature. Apart from a corresponding segmental incidence, they have also been described as occurring independently (Aminoff and Logue, 1974). Of four of our skin angiomas, two were combined with extradural angiomas, one isolated and three with complex intradural angiomas (Fig. 1A). Six global angiomas occupied an exceptional position, with simultaneous involvement of all layers including the subcutaneous and muscular tissue, the vertebra, and the extradural and intradural space; once, the skin was also

Table 2. Spinal Angiomas (Pia, 1953-1976)

	Number of patients	Number of angiomas	Solitary angiomas	Complex angiomas, Number	Complex angiomas, Percentage
Vertebral angiomas	7	23	7	16	70
Extradural angiomas	46	54	29	25	46
Intradural angiomas	51	60	43	17	28
Angioblastomas	11	12	4	8	67
Total	115	149	83	66	44
Lumbosacral extradural vascular anomalies	62	62	62	–	–
	177	211	143		

Table 3. Complex spinal angiomas (Pia, 1953-1976)

Location	No.	Cutaneous A.	Muscular A.	Vertebral A.	Extradural A.	Intradural A.	Angioblastomas	Complications	
Vertebral A.	16	–	1	X	16	2	–	Pathol. fracture	3
								Multiple vertebral angiomas	7
Extradural A.	25	2	5	16	X	7	1	Extradural hematoma	2
Intradural A.	17	3	5	1	7	X	7	Subdural hematoma	2
							aneurysms 1	Subarachnoid hemorrhage	29
								Intramedullary hematoma	4
Total	58	4	6	16	20	7	8		

affected. Comparable craniocerebral angiomas are not known. We give an example of a global angioma, which shows at the same time the closely related diagnostic and therapeutic problems:

Case 1: S.K. 218/66, aged 38, female.
At 4 years: acute (apoplectic) onset of a flaccid paralysis of the R. lower limb. Incomplete recovery. Atrophy and diminished growth.
Diagnosis: POLIOMYELITIS.
At 10 years: after an attack of measles, acute increase in the paralysis and disturbance of sensation.
Diagnosis: Infectious ENCEPHALOMYELITIS.
At 11 years: acute back pain and headaches. Complete atrophic paralysis, diminished growth, areflexia, anesthesia of R. leg, hyperreflexia in L. leg. Bilateral extensor responses. *CSF Bloody.*
Diagnosis: MYELITIS.
Improvement with mercurial inunction and orthopedic remedial measures. Development of a severe *kyphoscoliosis.*
At 16 years: within 2 months a *second* and *third subarachnoid hemorrhage, starting with back pain, followed by pain in the neck and headache and then coma.*
Bilateral carotid angiography – NAD. EEG – Negative.
Diagnosis: LEPTOMENINGITIS HEMORRHAGICA.
At 17 years: after *influenza,* 2 months later after a bruise on the head and after a further 2 weeks – *fourth, fifth and sixth subarachnoid hemorrhages.*
Diagnosis: Cerebral concussion (COMMOTIO CEREBRI).
Subsequently: increase in paraparesis, with atrophic right and spastic left lower limbs. Severe kyphoscoliosis. CSF: protein 40 mg%. Increased globulin.
Diagnosis: MULTIPLE SCLEROSIS.
At 18 years: on account of shortening of the leg, OSTEOTOMY performed. Increase in the paralysis (L). Pressure sores. Learnt tailoring.
At 19 years: disability in standing and walking.
At 20 years: presented for the first time in Neurosurgical Department. Almost complete transverse lesion at L 2. Right leg flaccid, left spastic. Sensation: complete loss. Bladder and bowel incompetence.
Lumbar manometry complete block. Lumbar CSF protein: 130 mg%.
X-ray: kyphoscoliosis. Vertebral angioma involving the laminae and pedicles of the second to fourth lumbar vertebrae.
Myelography: helmet-shaped block at L 1 and above this angiomatous and arachnoiditic changes.
First operation: November, 1958 *at age 20.*

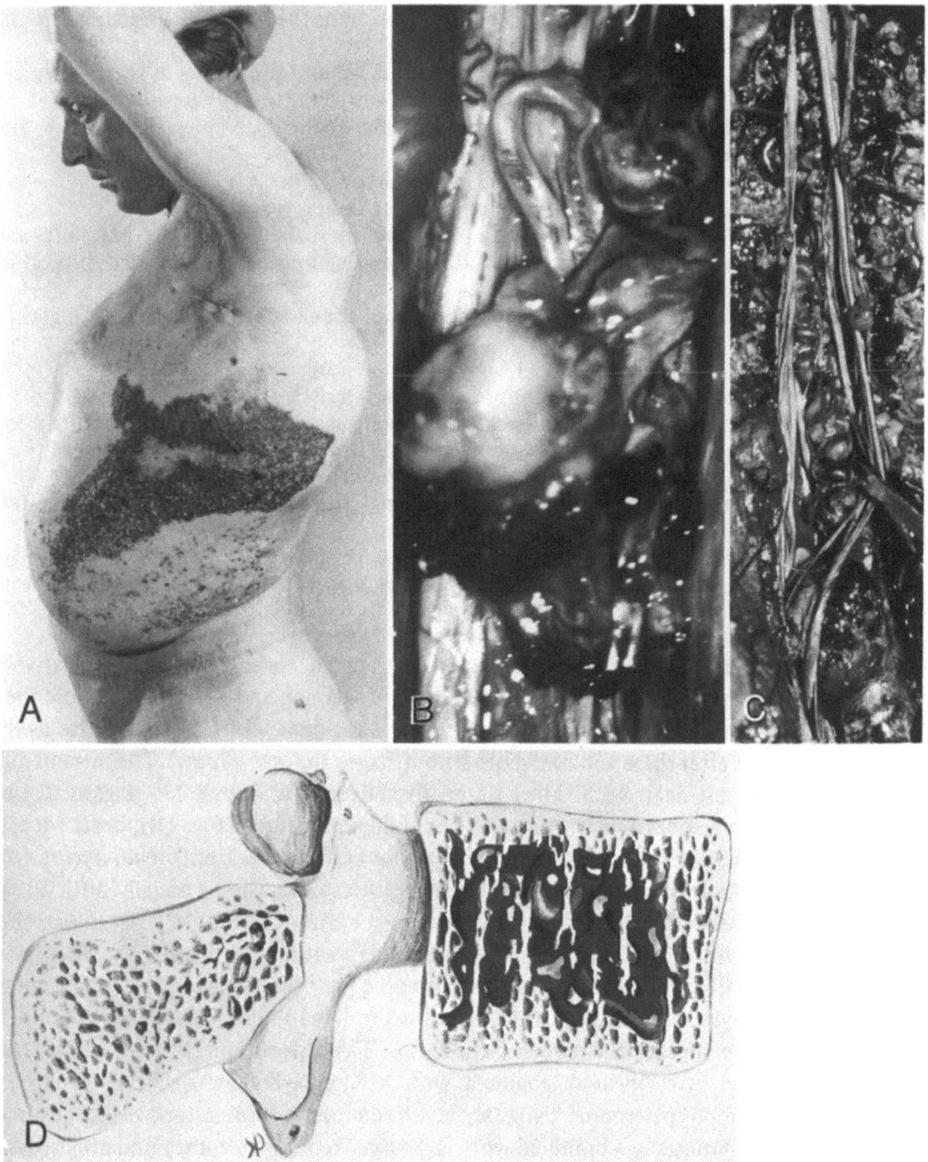

Fig. 1. (A) Segmental cutaneous angioma in a case of extradural-intradural angioma, (B) Arteriovenous angioma and aneurysm, (C) Arteriovenous angioma and angioblastoma of cauda equina, (D) Vertebral angioma

LAMINECTOMY L 1 – L 4. Extensive angioma of the soft tissues, muscles, bones, and extradural space. Copious arterial bleeding. Laminectomy was unavoidable. After blood loss of 6 liters, the operation was abandoned. Within a few months, improvement in the disability of gait and stance. Sensation returned to normal. Resumed work as tailoress. Retrained in evening classes for secretarial work. CSF block no longer present.
At 25 years: condition unchanged. Local low back pain.
Ossovenography: contrast medium seen intradurally – extensive angioma. In the same year: *seventh subarachnoid hemorrhage,* now with subsequent pains and a feeling of weakness in the L. upper limb. Then increased reflexes, which later could not be elicited.

At 27 years: with each menstrual period, intensification of the low back and leg pains and increase in the paraparesis.
At 28 years: 17th March, 1966, acute, violent lumbago and root pains in the D 8 region, also neck pain and headaches. Apoplectic episode. Complete transverse paralysis.
Eighth subarachnoid hemorrhage. Findings: a complete flaccid paraplegia below D 8, areflexia. Complete paralysis of bladder and bowel.
CSF cisternal: bloodstained. Lumbar: almost pure blood.
Ossovenography—thoracic: NAD. No angioma in soft tissues or extradurally.
Aortography: giant arteriovenous angioma in the region of the lumbar vertebrae, pre- and paravertebral, extending to just under the skin. Extending upward as far as D 8, typical intradural arteriovenous angioma.
Myelography: partial holdup at D 8, below that level appearances suggesting an angioma; complete block at D 12.
Second operation, 30th March, 1966 (13 days after hemorrhage).
LAMINECTOMY of D 7 - D 12. Subcutaneous tissues, muscles, and bones N.A.D.
Intradurally: subarachnoid: hemorrhagic, granulomatous arachnoiditis, with constriction of the cord in the whole area. Arachnoid excised. Dorsal arteriovenous angioma; very severe cord damage from a mainly R-sided *intramedullary hematoma and angioma.*
Total extent: 4 cm. Complete removal of the angioma and hematoma. Within a few months definite improvement.
Motor function: partial recovery. Limited mobility with splints.
Sensory functions: slight reduction in all modalities below L 1. Bladder and bowel controlled. No residual urine. Slight myositis ossificans around R. hip joint.
1976 at 38 years: condition unchanged, now married, does secretarial work.

Coexisting spinal angiomas and aneurysms are rare, in comparison to the relatively frequent association (7 – 10%) in cerebral lesions. Vogelsang and Dietz (1975) described a cervical aneurysm occurring with an intramedullary angioma, which was identified as the source of bleeding after three subarachnoid hemorrhages and was clipped. The intramedullary angioma was not dealt with. They found five aneurysms among 230 angiomas, i.e., 2.2%. An isolated personal observation, also in a child, unruptured (Fig. 1B), bears witness to their rarity. Djindjian (q.v.) reports on the important differences from *pseudoaneurysms.*

The differentiation of spinal angiomas from angioblastomas can be equally difficult, as can the simultaneous occurrence of *angiomas and* angioblastomas (Fig. 1C). Seven personal observations with histologic findings substantiate this relationship. Even if the discussion is by no means settled (Jellinger) and the angiographic pictures of angiomas and angioblastomas seem to be typical (Djindjian), there is at least no doubt about the close relationship and the progressive transition between both forms. The report from Förster and Kazner (1975) of a spinal arteriovenous angioma with a Klippel-Trenaunay-Weber syndrome (circumscribed osteohypertrophic varicose nevus syndrome, with arteriovenous fistulae or angiomas, not unusually combined with a Sturge-Weber syndrome) underlines these relationships.

Also of significance is the occurrence of spinal arteriovenous vascular malformations in the Rendu-Osler-Weber syndrome (multiple hereditary hemorrhagic teleangiectasia). On the basis of seven observations, Djindjian described their angiographic characteristics: pseudotumoral formations, pseudoaneurysms, and extreme venous development by which they are distinguished from typical arteriovenous angiomas. The occurrence with other congenital malformations is unusual. More definite relationships with dysontogenic or dysraphic states, as assumed by Nittner and Tönnis (1950) are not generally recognized. The occurrence of multiple lesions with vertebral angiomas (six personal cases) and with angioblastomas is not unusual (one personal case with intramedullary cervical and intrapontine angioblastoma; see also Yasargil), but it is not encountered with the spinal angiomas or in respect to the coexistence of spinal and cerebral angiomas.

Vertebral Angiomas

Vertebral angiomas (Fig. 1D) are *cavernomas*, or exceptionally *angiolipomas*. Their recognition in the x-ray films is simple due to their characteristic honeycomb, streaky porosity, between the residual trabeculae. According to autopsy material, 10% of the vertebral column may be affected. This finding is not supported either by radiologic or clinical evidence; their usual absence of symptoms accounts for the failure to diagnose them as frequently as these figures would suggest.

In our material, out of 23 cases 7 angiomas were *solitary* and 16 were *multiple*. Of the isolated forms, five cases were symptom-free. The angioma was demonstrated as an incidental finding.

Pathologic fractures in three vertebral angiomas complicated the vertebro-extradural angiomas. With the combined angiomas, it always involved a vertebro-extradural angioma and on two occasions there was in addition an intradural lesion. The associated extradural and intradural angiomas were responsible for the symptoms.

The preferential sites for the vertebral angiomas in our material are the lower thoracic and lumbar vertebrae (N = 16), with seven cases involving the remaining part of the dorsal region. *Multiple vertebral angiomas* with seven cases are not rare, five times with two vertebrae and once each with three and four involved. One patient had angiomas in the first and third lumbar vertebrae, the occipital bone, a rib, and the sacrum. As a rule, the angioma is found in the vertebral body with occasional extension into the arches; on three occasions, the arches were the site of the angioma.

Extradural Angiomas

These occur as vertebroextradural and purely extradural angiomas (Fig. 5A) and in general, like the vertebral angiomas they are cavernous angiomas, although one also finds angioblastomas. In our material (Table 4), about one-half were cavernous angiomas, 12 cases were classified as venous angiomas, two as capillary angiomas, five as arteriovenous cirsoid angiomas, and three as angiolipomas. In four cases no abnormality was found on exploration.

Extradural hematomas appear to be rare complications of angiomas. Among 49 spinal extradural hematomas, including one personal case, Liebeskind et al. (1975) did not find a single case. Among 19 angiomas, 13 suspected hematomas were not verified, apart from

Table 4. Histologic and operative appearance of extradural angiomas

	Histologic appearance		Operative/macroscopic appearance		
	Solitary	Mixed	Solitary	Mixed	Total
Cavernous	8	9	2	1	20
Venous	10	–	2	–	12
Arteriovenous	1	1	3	–	5
Capillary	2	–	–	–	2
Angiolipoma	2	–	1	–	3

one case (Cube, 1962). In our material, we found two hematomas among 54 extradural angiomas.

Extradural angiomas are reputed to be rare. Guthkelch (1963) who analyzed the literature up to 1948 found 14 cavernous angiomas and 14 angioblastomas associated with extradural hematomas and described eight personal cases, five solitary and three with vertebral angiomas. In our own material of 54 cases, there were 29 solitary and 25 mixed angiomas. The latter comprised 16 vertebroextradural, seven extradural-intradural, one cutaneous-extradural, and one angioma with an angioblastoma (histologically confirmed).

With regard to *location*, extradural angiomas can occur in all sections of the vertebral column; the cervical region is rarely involved and not at all with mixed angiomas, but they are equally common in the dorsal and lumbar vertebrae. With the solitary forms, the lower lumbar region and the lumbosacral junction are particularly affected.

The vertical extent is variable. It varies from the circumscribed forms (involving one vertebra) to the extensive angiomas (over six vertebrae). In the mixed forms, the angioma almost always extends beyond the limits of the vertebra involved in the angioma.

Lumbosacral Vascular Anomalies

Lumbosacral vascular anomalies are included as an interesting type of lesion which is not yet completely elucidated from the etiologic and pathogenetic point of view. Evidently, affinities exist with the verified extradural angiomas, and it is difficult or impossible to make any distinction from the clinical, macroscopic, or even histologic point of view.

These vascular anomalies have been well-known since the account of two cases given by Elsberg (1916) and have been more closely analyzed by us (Gümbel et al., 1969). They consist of isolated, convoluted, grape-like, or more lengthy dilatations of the ventral extradural venous plexus and more rarely of the dorsal plexus; the dilated vessels lie along the dura of the spinal roots and can even extend with them into the intervertebral foramen. Although there is no doubt that the vessels which predominate in the condition are veins, rather like varicose veins, one occasionally has the impression that they are arterialized.

In 22 cases which we have investigated *histologically,* the lesions seem to consist of a venous dilatation (ectasia) (Fig. 2B), with secondary changes in two-thirds, varying from a thinning of the intima with adherent thrombi to replacement of the musculature of the wall by fibrocollagenous tissue (intimal sclerosis). The sections of these angiomas which grossly seemed quite similar showed histologically venous dysplasia, cavernous angioma, angiolipoma, venous, and arteriovenous cirsoid angioma (Fig. 2C). The changes are not always easy to distinguish from the venous congestion which may accompany a prolapsed intervertebral disk. Among those with the latter diagnosis, operation usually followed and the diagnosis was confirmed. The assumption of a congestion of the venous plexus produced by posture can be excluded by the use of a special position on the table. Associations with a varicose condition in the lower limb or pelvis, or transmitted from larger veins, such as the inferior vena cava, were considered and discussed but excluded as far as possible. It is surprising that with solitary venous changes, as well as those combined with a prolapse, a spina bifida occulta is twice as frequent at 40% and root sheath anomalies are three times as frequent at 20% as with normal prolapsed disks. In the majority of cases, our own findings support the conception of a vascular anomaly and are against secondary vascular changes.

The frequency of extradural venous anomalies is 4.4% (1954–1964, 1091 intervertebral disk operations – 48 cases); according to a later series of 3000 operations, the propor-

Fig. 2 A-C

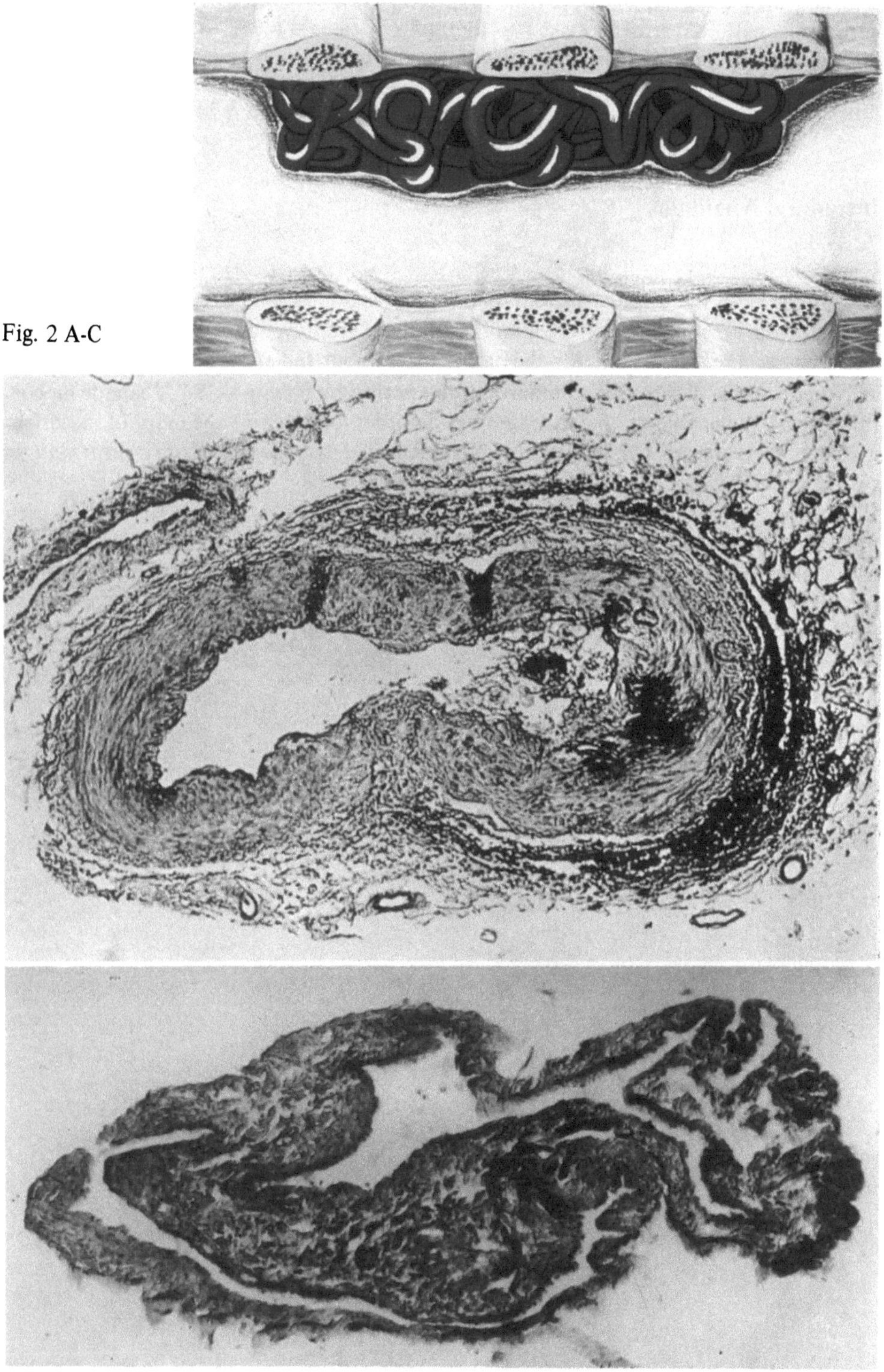

Fig. 2. Extradural angiomas. (A) Solitary extradural angioma, (B) Lumbosacral extradural phlebectasia, (C) Lumbosacral extradural arteriovenous angioma

tion is a little lower at 3% (Agnoli et al., 1976). The striking vessel changes associated with prolapsed intervertebral disks (up to 1967, 76 cases = 6.9%, to 1975 16%!), which may at least partially be attributed to the isolated form, also remains disregarded. Worth noting is one case record of a prolapsed disk associated with an arteriovenous angioma.

Intradural Angiomas

By analogy with the cerebral angiomas, the spinal angiomas can be regarded as congenital vascular malformations, which are almost exclusively arteriovenous racemose angiomas (A. *arteriovenosum racemosum*). All the earlier ideas about the etiology of spinal angiomas and their unique nature (see summarized description by Yasargil, 1962) cannot be confirmed by angiographic or operative findings. In order to underline the unity of the lesions wherever they are situated, they should all be regarded as *angiomas of the central nervous system* or *cerebrospinal angiomas*.

In spite of a possible histologic classification (four cases in our material), there are even today no *venous racemose angiomas*. During the 1950s, one personal observation (Fig.3) with partially thrombosed angioma vessels, in spite of the histologic findings, seemed from its gross appearance much more likely to be an arteriovenous angioma.

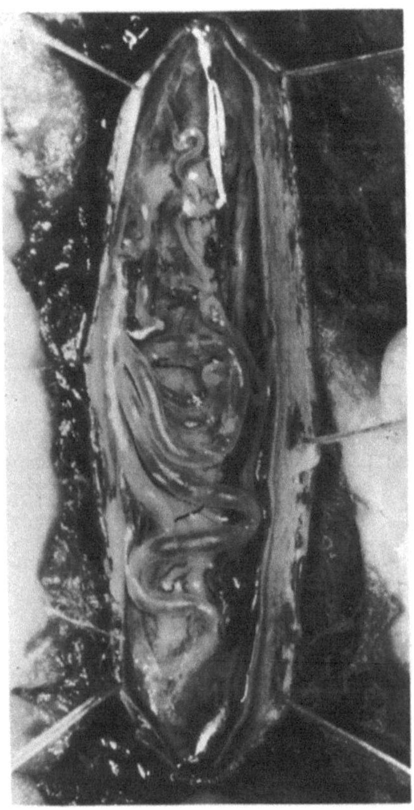

Fig. 3. Racemose angioma with partial thrombosis. Histologically: venous angioma. Naked eye appearances very suggestive of an arteriovenous angioma

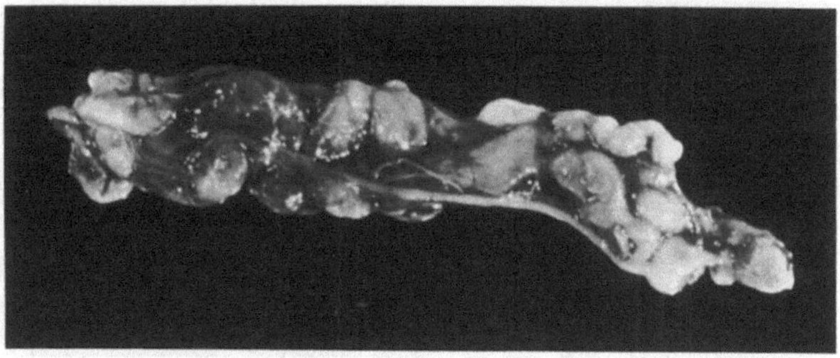

Fig. 4. Intradural cavernous angioma

Cavernous angiomas are extremely rare. We can only produce two observations, one circumscribed (Fig. 4) and a further subarachnoid cavernoma associated with a malignant intramedullary tumor (reticulum cell sarcoma?).

Subarachnoid Arteriovenous Cirsoid Angioma

The arteriovenous cirsoid (racemose) angioma is the best known type. It consists of greatly dilated (2 – 4 mm in diameter, occasionally even wider), twisted, convoluted vessels con-

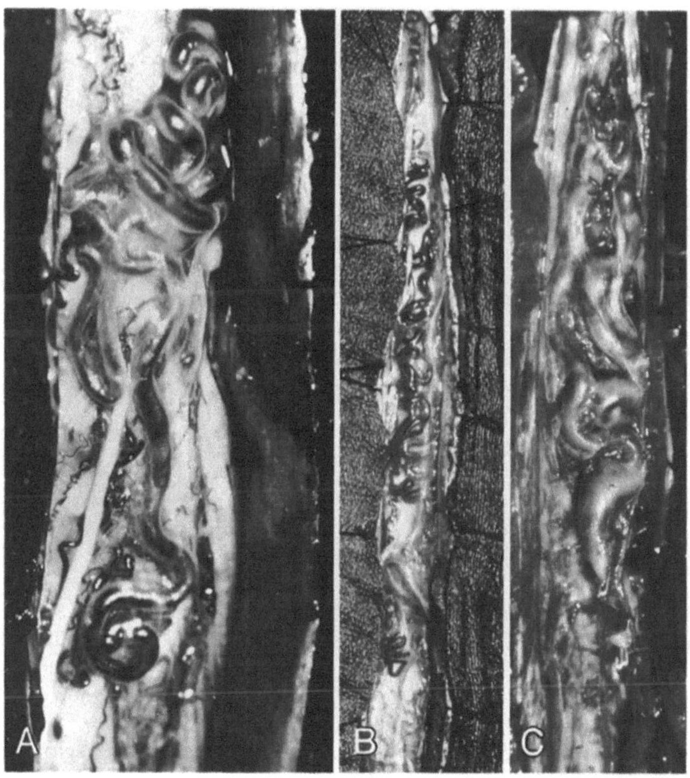

Fig. 5 A–C. Different types of subarachnoid arteriovenous angiomas

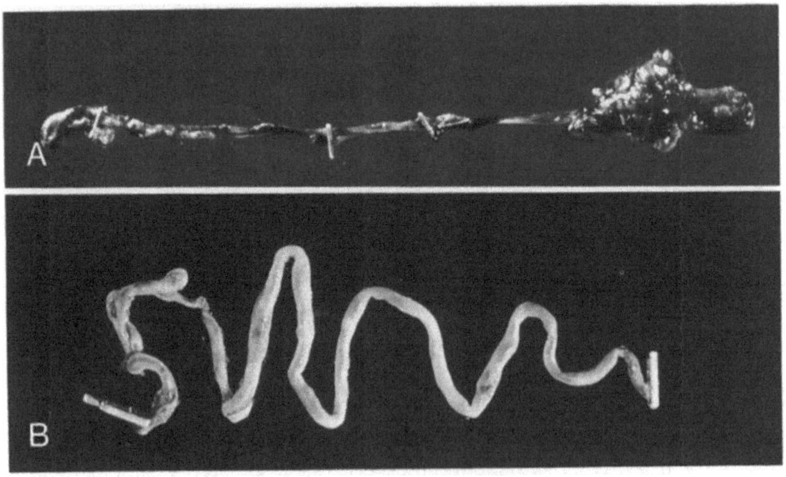

Fig 6 A and B. Extirpated arteriovenous angiomas

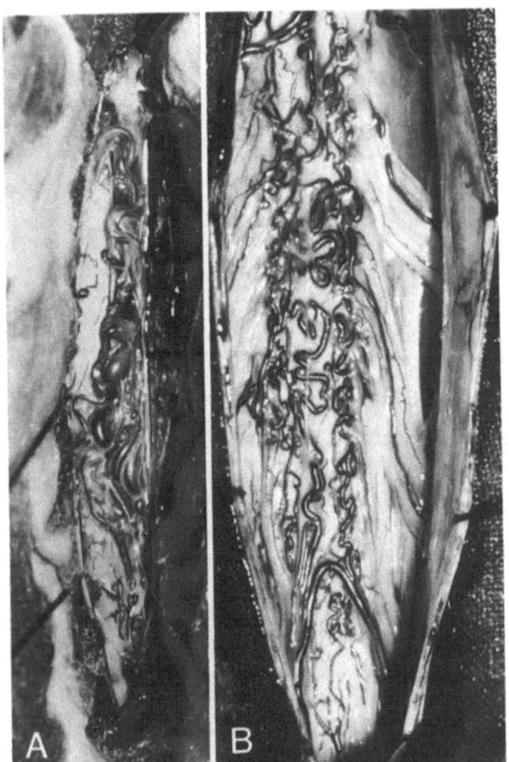

Fig. 7. Localized subarachnoid arteriovenous angioma. (A) Dorsolateral with marked kyphoscoliosis, (B) Cervical with subpial capillary angiomas, multiple feeders from dorsal radicular arteries

taining arterial blood. There is as a rule a centrally lying "glomus" formed out of one or several vascular convolutions (Fig. 5A, B, C). After their removal, they can be stretched out into a single vascular strand or into two vessels (Fig. 6A, B). From the central portion of the angioma, there are usually one or more similar dilated draining vessels running in a cranial direction, or less commonly caudally. More circumscribed arteriovenous angiomas are rarer (Fig. 7 A, B). The arteriovenous angiomas lie predominantly in the dorsal subarachnoid space, clearly separated from the pia and the spinal cord. Corresponding to this, they obtain their blood supply from dilated dorsal radicular arteries but with dorsolateral or lateral, and above all with the ventrally situated lesions, the supply is also from this source or it may be solely from the ventral radicular arteries.

Solitary arteriovenous fistulas, or a simple angioma attached to an afferent and efferent vessel, or a large angioma fed by one afferent (Taylor, 1964; Doppman et al., 1969 [single coiled angioma]; Djindjian et al., 1966), are unusual. Up to the present, we have not seen an angioma of this type. The participation of several large and small feeders, even when angiography has demonstrated a greatly dilated single afferent, is usual. As might be expected from this finding, the occlusion of the apparently solitary or most important afferent often has no effect on the size of the angioma or its filling (see Pia: "Operative Treatment").

Subpial Capillary Angiomas

As an equally important angioma type, we have described the circumscribed angiomas as capillary angiomas (Pia, 1965) and have analyzed them more closely. They are multiple and consist of small tortuous tangles of vessels which are normal in size or only slightly dilated or else of several elongated, pathologic vessels (Fig. 8 A, B). In contrast to the typical arteriovenous angiomas, they are situated predominantly subpial or they have so close a relationship to the pia that even under magnification it is not possible to differentiate them clearly. They seem quite regularly to share in the blood supply of the cord. Quite frequently, they run parallel and partly with the nerve roots or they may be wrapped all around them. In one case with a capillary angioma of the lower lumbar cord and conus, all the roots of the cauda equina were accompanied by small and large tortuous vessels. Such subpial capillary angiomas are either solitary or combined with the large angiomas. Their histologic picture is unknown, as one has never been removed at operation. Macroscopically, there is no doubt that it resembles an arteriovenous cirsoid angioma. They regularly contain arterial blood.

Intramedullary Angiomas

Intramedullary angiomas are also arteriovenous angiomas and are supplied by the ventral radicular arteries, principally the *arteria radicularis magna* (Adamkiewicz) or the *artery of the cervical enlargement.* Their structure is identical with the previously described arteriovenous angiomas. An important distinction is the isolated and localized, convoluted angioma nodule. It is precisely with these lesions that the differentiation between arteriovenous angioma and angioblastoma can be difficult or impossible. Mistakes are possible with mixed angiomas, with intramedullary, extramedullary, dorsal, and ventral subarachnoid extensions (mixed type (Djindjian)). In two personal cases, some 10 years ago, with extensive dorsal arteriovenous angiomas, the accessible portion of what was regarded angiographically as a pure dorsal angioma was excised; the intramedullary nodule was not seen, and was only later discovered.

Combined Intradural Angiomas

Out of 60 intradural angiomas, there were 17 complex angiomas. Their incidence, at 27%, is definitely smaller than with the vertebral and extradural angiomas. We found combined lesions as follows: with extradural angiomas – seven, muscular – five, cutaneous – three, and vertebral angiomas – one. The combination of spinal angiomas and tumors has already been mentioned and the problems commented on. In this context, it is merely necessary to put on record that of seven personal cases, six were histologically classified as arteriovenous angiomas and one as a cavernoma.

Location of Intradural Angiomas

The favored location for the intradural angiomas in the thoracolumbar and lumbosacral regions of the cord, i.e., the middle and lower dorsal and upper lumbar vertebral level, has long been known (Wyburn–Mason, 1943). This is confirmed in the latest reviews (see Yasargil). According to him, the segments D 6 – L 2 are involved in 80% with the segments C 4 – D 1 and L 4 – L 5 in diminishing frequency.

According to our own classification, related to the angioma types, the subarachnoid arteriovenous angiomas and subpial capillary angiomas occur preferentially in the lower lumbar and sacral cord, then in the lumbar cord, and only rarely in the cervical or cervicodorsal cord and the cauda equina. The cervical extent covers four to six vertebrae, although in isolated cases portions of the angioma appear to extend over the whole cord. Such a giant extension, which reached as far as the middle cranial fossa (N = 2) showed itself by a solitary, greatly dilated efferent channel. The angioma proper, the central portion of the angioma, is circumscribed in all cases. Because of this, the extension will be uncertain and problematic in its attachments. The capillary angiomas have basically the same location as the arteriovenous angiomas but they are always smaller and circumscribed (two to three vertebral bodies). Intramedullary angiomas have two preferential locations, thoracolumbar and cervical, which explains the already mentioned main blood supply through the *arteria radicularis magna* (Adamkiewicz) and *the artery of the cervical enlargement* (see contributions by Djindjian and Yasargil). The combined angioma/angioblastoma and the angioblastomas are numerically so small that their inclusion is disputed, and conclusions about their preferential location are not possible. *Solitary ventral angiomas* are unusual and we have not seen such a case.

Complications of Intradural Angiomas

Rupture of malformed angioma vessels with *spinal subarachnoid hemorrhage* (Fig. 9 A) is the most serious complication. Twenty-nine patients in our material had a total of 46 subarachnoid hemorrhages. One patient had eight (see case 1), another had four, two had three, and three had two hemorrhages. The remaining 18 patients each had one. Two patients had in addition a subdural hematoma and four an intramedullary hematoma (Fig. 9 B).

Spinal subarachnoid hemorrhages have been well-known for a long time, and they are met with in a variety of spinal diseases (Heidrich, 1970). Quite varying figures are given regarding their frequency in angiomas. Djindjian (p. 76) had 36 in 150 cases, Aminoff and

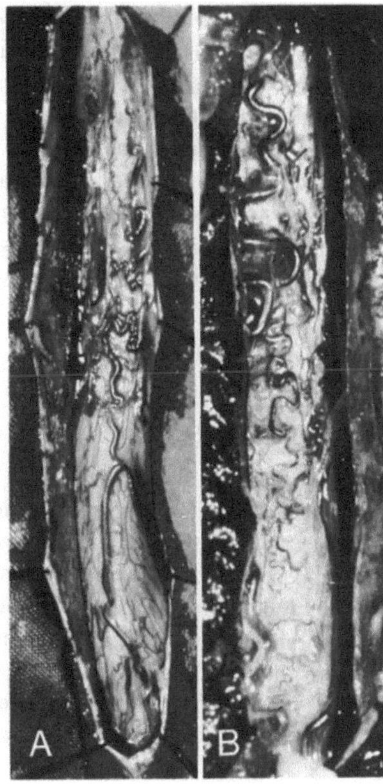

Fig. 8 A and B. Subpial capillary arteriovenous angiomas

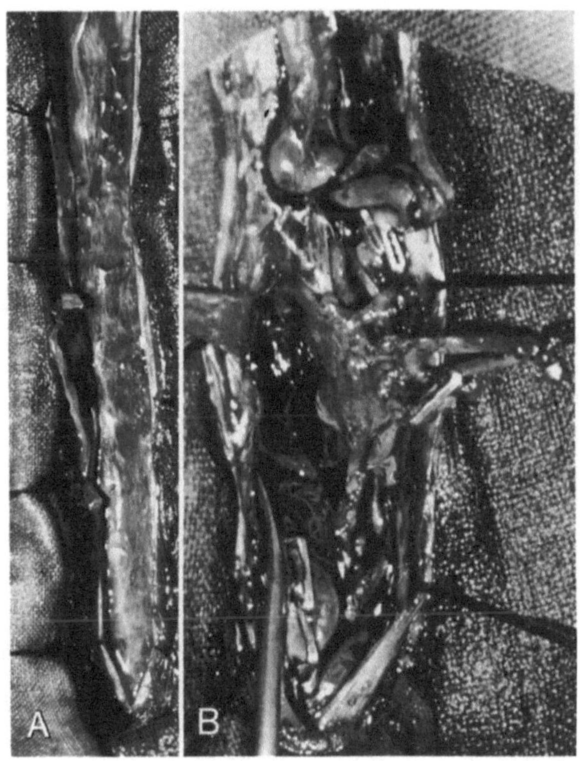

Fig. 9. Spinal hemorrhage. (A) Subarachnoid hemorrhage, (B) Intramedullary hemorrhage (case 1)

Logue (1975) six out of 60 cases, and Pia (1975) 25 in 60. They are particularly frequent in cervical angiomas: Bailey and Sperl (1969) 18 in 46 cases, Yasargil et al. (1975) eight in 11 cases. The reason for the diverse figures given for the frequency is the almost complete misunderstanding shown in the past, which even today is not unusual (see above).

Spinal subarachnoid hemorrhages are met with in all the types of angioma which we have described: in 25 subarachnoid arteriovenous angiomas 14, together with two intramedullary and two subdural hematomas; in 22 subpial capillary angiomas six cases of hemorrhage; in nine intramedullary angiomas four, together with two intramedullary hematomas, and in seven mixed angiomas with tumors three.

Late Complications

The late complications of subarachnoid hemorrhages are reactive changes in the leptomeninges which take the form of an *adhesive,* or *rarely, a cystic arachnoiditis.* These changes are seen even without any known subarachnoid hemorrhage. Their extent varies from a hemorrhagic type in fresh cases, slight adhesions and thickening in early cases, up to severe types with areas of calcification and extremely extensive scarring, which in the later stages strangles the cord like armor plating (Fig. 10 A, B). The secondary changes in the arachnoid exert an effect on the progressive myelomalacia, the prognosis, and not least, even on the possibilities of treatment and its outcome.

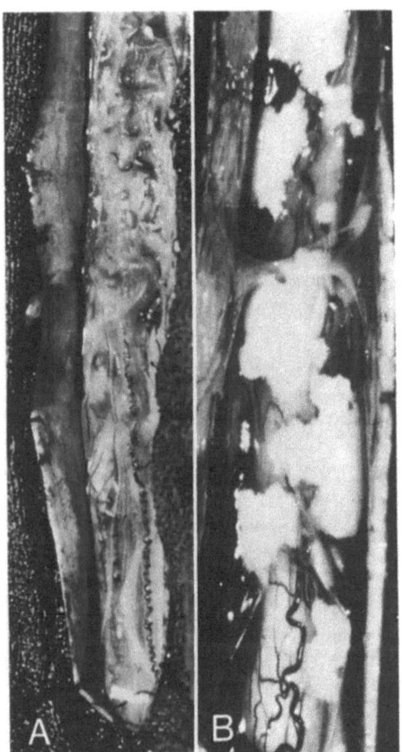

Fig. 10. Secondary arachnoiditis. (A) Very marked adhesive arachnoiditis 10 years after undetected spinal subarachnoid hemorrhage. Severe cord damage. Inability to walk. (Medical doctor), (B) Calcified arachnopathy

Table 5. Spinal angiomas (earlier diagnosis)

	Extradural angiomas Total 46		Intradural angiomas Total 51	
Correct diagnosis or suspect	2		10 (20%)	
Cerebral process with or without SAH	1		10	
Myelitis	4	= 24%	9	= 60%
Degenerative cord disease	1		7	
Multiple sclerosis	6 (13%)		15 (29%)	
Polyneuritis	1		4	
Spinal tumor	6 (13%)		11 (21%)	
Spinal trauma	2		1	
Spinal circulation disturbance	2		3	
Osteochondrosis,disc prolapse	19 (41%)		6	
Juvenile kyphoscoliosis	–		5	
Various	1		2	
Uncertain	4		2	

Symptomatology

In contrast to the tremendous advances in arteriographic diagnosis and treatment in the last decade, the general clinical diagnosis of spinal angiomas (extradural and intradural angiomas) is still unsatisfactory. The main diagnostic problem is "misdiagnosis" (Table 5).

A correct or suspect diagnosis was only exceptionally made with extradural angiomas and in 20% of intradural angiomas; in the former in five cases only after many years of misdiagnosis. The large number of intradural angiomas suspected to be cerebral lesions (20%) mainly presented symptomless subarachnoid hemorrhages. On the whole, the commonest misdiagnosis in extradural angiomas is a *disk lesion* (41%) and in intradural angiomas, inflammatory or degenerative cord diseases (60%). These latter were led by multiple sclerosis at 29%, as compared with 24% and 13% respectively in extradural angiomas. The course, clinical picture or prominent signs, e.g., a severe scoliosis, can explain such errors in diagnosis. The diagnosis of tumor is suggestive in 13% and 21% respectively, in such corresponding clinical histories. This is not really serious in comparison with the other diagnosis mentioned, as it is likely to lead to special investigations and treatment.

An analysis of the various forms of intradural angioma did not show any significant variation, with the qualification that in the tumor cases, which will not be considered any further here, the diagnosis of tumor was increasingly made or suspected.

Sex and Age Distribution

All published series, including our own, confirm a *preponderance of males* to females in a ratio of 60 – 70% to 30 – 40%. No further conclusions can be drawn from this. The distribution (Table 6) with regard to the age and onset of the illness and the age of treatment shows important variations between extradural and intradural angiomas and also within the two locations. The extradural angiomas, with an average of 42 years are 10 years older but present for treatment after a shorter period of illness. Among these, the onset of the illness and its treatment are definitely later for the vertebro-extradural angiomas than for the solitary forms.

Intradural angioma patients are affected earlier, and among them those with mixed angiomas are the earliest, followed by arteriovenous angiomas, and lastly those with capillary

Table 6. Age at onset of symptoms and receiving treatment

	Age at onset	Age when treatment given
Extradural angiomas	42.5	44.5
Solitary extradural angiomas	42	43.5
Vertebroextradural angiomas	44	50
Intradural angiomas	33.5	38.2
Arteriovenous angiomas	31.3	37.5
Capillary angiomas	42	46
Complex angiomas	21.5	24.5

Table 7. Age in decades at onset of symptoms and receiving treatment (figures in percentages)

Years	Extradural angiomas		Intradural angiomas	
(up to)	Onset	Treatment	Onset	Treatment
0–10	–	–	13	7
11–20	11	9	20	19
21–30	16	7	15	13
31–40	23	18	15	13
41–50	16	20	7	13
51–60	20	23	22	19
> 60	13	22	7	15

angiomas. Strikingly, with the same average distribution, the duration of the illness with typical subarachnoid arteriovenous angiomas is significantly the longest. Further information is provided by the grouping of the patients according to decades (Table 7).

Extradural angiomas do not fall ill before the 2nd decade, 50% up to the 40th year, almost 40% between 40 and 60, and 13% after that. Fewer than 20% were treated before the age of 30, a third up to 40, and two-thirds only after that, of whom more than 20% were in the 7th decade or later.

Nearly two-thirds of intradural angiomas are affected before the 40th, one-half before the 30th, and one-third before the 20th year. Also the age of receiving treatment is about equally divided before and after the age of 50, yet one-quarter have already been treated before the age of 20. These figures agree with those given by Djindjian and Yasargil for the intradural angiomas. In the earlier series from the literature (Béraud and Meloche, 1965) and the cases of Aminoff and Logue (1975), the age of diagnosis is substantially later. Of the 60 cases (25-year follow-up) of the latter, the diagnosis was in no instance made before 20, 11 times by the 40th year, 33 times by the 60th year, and later than that 16 times. These figures no doubt reflect the improvement in diagnosis, but still more, however, they show the great delay between the onset of the disease and the start of treatment.

It thus becomes apparent, as with the cerebral angiomas, that the intradural spinal angiomas – in spite of variations between the particular types – represent an illness that favors the first half of life. *Hemorrhage,* the most serious complication, occurs essentially in the first 3 decades. The average age of patients who have a hemorrhage is 22 years, while that of the uncomplicated angiomas is 50 years.

Duration of Illness

The individual duration of the illness, when considered in relation to the age of onset, the location, and type of the angioma promises to yield greater information.

Extradural Angiomas

Solitary extradural angiomas may have not only the shortest but also the longest histories. Two cases with extradural hematomas were admitted immediately, whereas in the 2nd to the 4th decades particularly long histories, up to 24 years, can occur. In the subsequent age groups a course of a few months is most usual.

In patients with vertebro-extradural angiomas, the onset is later and the illness of medium duration from 2 – 4 years. On the other hand excessively long histories are less common than formerly. With regard to the site of the lesion any clear-cut correlation with the duration of the illness is less evident. It is about the same for both angioma types in each location, with the exception of their preferred locations, which have already been discussed.

Lumbosacral vascular anomalies have a still more chronic course than the angiomas in this region. The peak lies between 5 and 10 years, but very frequently there are significantly longer histories, up to 30 years. The age of onset is likewise variable. The peak is shifted almost one decade, to nearly 50 years.

Intradural Angiomas

With intradural angiomas and particularly with the subarachnoid arteriovenous angiomas and the mixed types, the onset of the illness is definitely earlier than with the subpial, capillary angiomas. The length of the illness varies so widely that no clear differentiation is possible. In all groups up to the age of 40, short, medium, and above all very long histories predominate; with the capillary angiomas, there is a strikingly higher age of onset and a relatively short previous history. Any more definite correlation between location and length of history cannot be detected.

In Yasargil's 11 cases with *cervical angiomas* (one extramedullary, one intramedullary, and nine mixed), the onset of the illness was between 7 and 45 years, and they were diagnosed and operated on between the ages of 14 and 48. The longest histories were 15 years (from 7 to 22 and from 20 to 35 years). The various series show that apart from certain differences, neither the age of onset nor the location of the angioma is of great significance for the diagnosis in any individual case.

Course of the Illness

The pattern of the illness is more important and characteristic than the duration in making a diagnosis. Three clinical types can be distinguished with the extradural and intradural angiomas, viz., the apoplectiform, the remitting, and the progressive.

Extradural Angiomas

Twelve patients (27%) with extradural angiomas (Table 8) had an apoplectiform course, of whom two showed a subsequent remission and progression, 19 (42%) had a remitting course, once with a later spinal apoplexy, and 14 (31%) showed a progressive pattern. Only

Table 8. Onset and course of extradural angiomas

	No.	Complication	Immediately	Admission -1 y.	-2 y.	-5 y.	-10 y.	> 10 y.
Acute or apoplectiform	12 (27%)	Vert. fract. 2 Extradur. 2 H'ge	6	2	2	–	1	1
Remitting	19 (42%)	Vert. fract. 1	–	2	2	10	3	2
Progressive	14 (31%)	–	–	9	3	–	1	1
Total	45	5	6	13	7	10	5	4

six patients with an apoplectiform course were admitted immediately, including two with pathologic vertebral fractures and one with an extradural hematoma. The second hematoma had acute spinal symptoms with a partial recovery 10 years before admission. Thirteen patients came for treatment within the first year, the majority surprisingly with a chronic progressive picture, those with a remitting course only very much later. The main reason is the specially favored misdiagnosis of multiple sclerosis. Vertebro-extradural angiomas, as with the solitary angiomas, favored a remitting and only exceptionally an apoplectiform course. Solitary angiomas show as their main method of presentation either apoplectiform or progressive patterns.

Intradural Angiomas

Twenty-two (37%) of the intradural angiomas (Table 9) had an apoplectiform onset, including three with remissions and six with a progressive course, 13 (22%) had a remitting course, three of whom had a later spinal apoplexy, and 25 (41%) had a progressive course, including four with later apoplexy. By collecting together all the patients with acute spinal symptoms, 29 patients (48%) are obtained, i.e., nearly one-half had definite or suspected symptoms of a spinal angioma. Four intramedullary and 16 spinal subarachnoid hemorrhages come into the apoplectiform group, but only the four former and two subarachnoid hemorrhages were admitted immediately. Two subarachnoid hemorrhages occurred in the

Table 9. Onset and course of intradural angiomas

	No.	SAH IMH	Immediately	Admission -1 y.	-2 y.	-5 y.	-10 y.	> 10 y.
Acute or apoplectiform	22 (37%)	16 IMH 4	5	5	2	3	5	2
Remitting	13 (22%)	2	–	1	1	8	3	–
Progressive	25 (41%)	7	–	8	6	5	3	3
Total	60	29	5	14	9	16	11	5

remitting and seven in the progressive groups. As in the extradural angiomas, the course of the illness is unusually long in all three groups. This is true particularly for the first group. The three angioma types do not differ from one another with respect to the pattern of the disease.

The site of the angioma seems to have no effect. Our own results for cervical angiomas are confirmed (Yasargil, et al., 1969). The latter found in 37 cases a progressive pattern in 21 and a "more rapid course" in 16. Ten patients had episodes of relapse.

The patterns of behavior described in relation to extradural angiomas have been discussed and analyzed by us (Pia and Vogelsang, 1965) but have not otherwise been evaluated in the literature. As regards the intradural angiomas, the essential features of these have been well-known since the classic contribution of Wyburn–Mason (1943). In contrast, Aminoff and Logue (1974) in their 60 cases observed a predominantly chronic progress in 48 cases, with fluctuations in several. Twelve showed an acute presentation, five times with an immediate severe spinal cord lesion and seven times without any later progress.

Spinal Bleeding

Among the various types of spinal bleeding, subarachnoid hemorrhage has the greatest significance. Among 29 cases, 23 were "pure" bleeds while four were accompanied by an intramedullary and two by a subdural hematoma (Table 10). As a rule, subarachnoid hemorrhage is misdiagnosed or not recognized at all. Among 25 cases, including two with accompanying subdural hematomas, on ten occasions a cerebral cause, i.e., an aneurysm, was assumed and cerebral angiography undertaken. Among these were all the seven cases with recurring hemorrhages. Nine subarachnoid hemorrhages were not recognized. A spinal lesion was suspected five times (two tumors, myelitis, anterior spinal syndrome, trauma). In three patients, a correct diagnosis was arrived at in each case only after the last of three subarachnoid hemorrhages. In four cases with subarachnoid hemorrhage and hematoma, the acute paraplegia dominated the clinical picture, so that the symptoms of the subarachnoid hemorrhage were obscured. Subarachnoid hemorrhage occurs in half of the cases as the presenting symptom, very rarely in the later course of the disease (three times), and practically never as a terminal episode.

In cases where it was the first symptom, only three of these were verified at once. Bleeding in the course of the disease within 2 years (one) and after 10 years (two) was recognized immediately on one occasion, within 1 year and 10 years, respectively.

Hemorrhages as a terminal symptom have a greater importance on account of the associated manifestations. They occurred after illnesses lasting from 2 years (four) up to 5

Table 10. Spinal haemorrhage and course (No. = 29)

SAH	No.	Occurrence			Admission				
		- 2 y.	> 5 y.	> 10 y.	Immediately	- 1 y.	- 2 y.	- 5 y.	> 10 y.
1st symptom	15	-	-	-	3	5	2	4	1
During the course	3	1	-	2	1	1	-	-	1
Last symptom	11	4	3	4	9	2	-	-	-
Total	29	5	3	6	13	8	2	4	2
Intramed. h'ge	4	2	1	1	4	-	-	-	-
Subdural h'ge	2	1	-	1	1	1	-	-	-
Isolated SAH	23	2	2	4	8	7	2	4	2

years (three), and more than 10 years (four). Nine patients were admitted at once, two after several months. Among these were four patients with intramedullary hematomas with the clinical picture of paraplegia and two with associated subdural hematomas, in whom a space-occupying lesion (i.e., a tumor) was considered to be the cause of the symptoms. Recurring subarachnoid hemorrhages (seven cases) are frequent; they followed in a few months or days in two cases, but five times at longer intervals, up to 7 and 18 years.

In spite of the difficulty of diagnosing pure spinal subarachnoid hemorrhage, in general the course of the illness is significantly shorter than in uncomplicated angiomas. The frequency of bleeding is high and involves all types of angiomas. Intramedullary hematomas were seen in three intramedullary angiomas (of which two were mixed) and in one angioma-tumor case. Spinal hemorrhages occur in more than 50% of subarachnoid arteriovenous angiomas, in a third of subpial capillary angiomas, and in half of the complex (mixed) angiomas and of the angioma-tumor group.

Precipitating Factors

Apart from the pattern of the disease and the hemorrhages, extrinsic and intrinsic conditions as precipitating and exacerbating factors are of importance in the understanding of the angiomas. Such factors which have been well-known for a long time from individual descriptions have been subjected to a detailed analysis by ourselves and others (Pia and Vogelsang, 1965; Aminoff and Logue, 1974). In addition, the comparison (Table 11) shows that extradural and intradural angiomas behave similarly.

Among the extrinsic factors, trivial or irrelevant trauma is incriminated in some cases. In spite of the temporal relationship with later development of symptoms, which was quite definite in five cases of Aminoff and Logue (1974), the association is open to question. There is scarcely any doubt regarding the influence of physical stress including lifting and straining, as the increased symptoms recede again after resting. We are not satisfied that we have seen any effect produced by physical position, as mentioned in some comparative surveys. The authors in both papers cite sitting, standing, and bending forward and a diminution when lying; in contrast, our three cases showed increased troubles solely when recumbent. Of seven patients with exacerbations in a particular body position and exertions, six patients had a specific stimulus which was always effective. The effect of heat or cold

Table 11. Provocation and exacerbation of the symptoms of spinal angiomas

	Extradural a.	Intradural a.	
	Pia, 1975 No. = 46	Pia, 1975 No. = 60	Aminoff and Logue, 1974 No. = 60
Irrelevant trauma	2	3	5 (5?)
Physical exertion	5	9	19 exercises
Straining and lifting	6	5	-
Posture	1	2	14
Heat	2	2 (improved 3)	-
Cold	2	1	-
Infections	-	2	3
Menstruation	3	4	-
Pregnancy	1	1	1

is puzzling, the more so because of five intradural angiomas, three showed an improvement and two a worsening. Five patients had aggravation of symptoms in relation to mild infection. Menstruation and pregnancy have a greater influence, more especially menstruation. Even if the number of precipitating and exacerbating factors is not great, there is no doubt about their effect. Above all, this holds true for the large group of patients who, as a result of the same "stimulus", develop a permanent intensification or regression. This was the case with all our patients with deterioration precipitated by menstruation, and the majority of those where there was aggravation associated with physical stress. An impressive individual example is the aggravating influence of pregnancy; in one instance, seven times out of eight pregnancies, and in three pregnancies among the patients of Aminoff and Logue (1974). In our patients, every such effect was abolished after the removal of the angioma.

Signs and Symptoms

The symptoms differ between the extradural and intradural angiomas, and even within the individual groups. Table 12 summarizes the essential facts in the main groups.

Table 12. Symptoms (percentage incidence)

		Extradural a.	Intradural a.
Pain	None	9	18
	Local	70	46
	Radicular	59	28
	Funicular	9	33
	Meningeal	-	46
Motor deficit	None	24	9
	Spasticity	37	28
	Flaccidity	35	18
	Combined	6	35
	Atrophy	15	39
	Inability to walk	13	46
Sensory deficit	None	30	20
	All modalities	46	39
	Dorsal columns	2	22
	Spino-thalamic tract.	-	15
	Radicular	22	-
Bladder and bowel disturbances	None	63	29
	Deficit	11	29
	Paralysis	26	42

Extradural Angiomas

For all practical purposes, *pain* is never absent in extradural angiomas. Local and root pains, almost always combined, are very suggestive. On the other hand, long tract pains are not of any significance. Root pains are less common in the solitary than in the mixed forms. A relapsing character is particularly frequent with a lumbosacral location.

Motor deficits are absent in one of four patients (25%). The paralyses can be either spastic or flaccid. Flaccid paralyses are predominantly associated with lesions of the cauda equina and roots. The same applies to atrophy. Combined spastic-flaccid palsies are of no practical value. Only a few patients are unable to stand or walk at the time of admission. Nearly all the patients with normal or impaired gait, and the majority of those with flaccid cauda equina or radicular paresis, are associated with the solitary extradural angiomas.

Sensory deficits may be absent or are radicular, and with cord damage all modalities are involved. Radicular symptoms are also prevalent in the solitary angiomas.

Bladder and bowel disturbances are certainly not a prominent feature. The main causes are anterior compression of the cord, as well as uni- and multiradicular disturbances.

Lumbosacral vascular anomalies do not differ substantially from angiomas in this location. Frequently, there is no significant back pain, but isolated sciatica in one-quarter of the patients and bilateral sciatica in nearly 30% stresses the bilateral root involvement; particularly frequently, there is aggravation with stress, and a relatively large number (30%) of obvious motor deficits.

Intradural Angiomas (Excluding Tumor Cases)

Pain is absent in only about one in five of our patients but is particularly frequent in those with a chronic progressive course. Root and long tract pains were about equally frequent, but no difference existed within the individual groups.

Meningeal irritation (pains) as a result of subarachnoid hemorrhage is almost always present, although in our own mild cases the symptom is only elicited on direct enquiry. Spinal subarachnoid hemorrhage is easy to diagnose if the initial pain is localized to the back at the level of the angioma, and only secondarily involves the neck or the head. Such an onset applies in our material to half of the patients and in Djindjian's to 27 out of 36 (75%). Nearly all cervical cases start without neck pain, so that they are difficult to distinguish from cerebral subarachnoid hemorrhages. Among 16 spinal tumors with subarachnoid hemorrhage (Prieto and Cantu, 1967), all started with backache, and headaches developed later, often only days or weeks after the original low back pain. First bleeds are rarely accompanied by neurologic deficits, secondary bleeds regularly so. Coma is unusual.

Motor deficits were practically always present in our material. In nearly one-half, these were so severe that the patients were unable to stand or walk at the time of admission. Accordingly, nuclear pyramidal, combined pareses, with or mostly without atrophy are commoner than solitary spastic or acute flaccid paralyses. We have not noted any difference between typical subarachnoid and subpial angiomas.

Sensory deficits are absent in 20% of patients. The commonest feature was an involvement of all modalities or a dissociated loss, with isolated posterior column loss more frequent than isolated involvement of the anterolateral tracts. Thus, posterior column lesions predominated in dorsal subarachnoid arteriovenous angiomas.

Bladder and bowel disturbances are absent in nearly one-third. The remainder had deficits determined by the size and location of the cord lesion and not varying according to the type of angioma.

Mixed angiomas, extradural-intradural, and global angiomas do not present any particular course or symptoms which would make any clinical differentiation possible.

Of the *intramedullary angiomas,* six showed a relapsing, apoplectiform and three a chronic progressive course. From the outset, there were severe, initially fleeting, or extensive remitting deficits in the progressive group, with the pattern of an advancing tumor predominating. We have never seen an intramedullary syndrome with involvement of the motor system and the anterolateral tracts.

Bruit

An audible fistulous bruit over the angioma is described in certain cases, but in general, however, it is of no practical significance (Yasargil, 1971). There was no case in our material, although omission of the investigation in the majority of patients must be taken into account. In the series of Aminoff and Logue (1974) out of 12 patients examined, a bruit was present in two. The demonstration of a bruit is pathognomonic.

Natural History

The natural history pattern of the symptoms is variable, but is does show certain consistencies which should at least give occasion for suspecting the diagnosis. A chronic progressive course is very suggestive of a developing tumor and cannot be distinguished clinically from it. In the apoplectiform pattern with solitary or repeated serious exacerbations and less clearly in the early stage with remitting course, it is possible to distinguish an early, middle, and late stage.

The early stage is recognized as a group with fleeting or almost completely remitting, slight, or severe deficits. Here also one includes the subarachnoid hemorrhages without neurologic (i.e. spinal) symptoms and a second small group with immediately occurring obvious deficits.

By the *middle stage,* unequivocal spinal deficits are already observable, viz., incomplete or slight motor symptoms, often already apparent, spastic paraparesis, and partial sensory deficits, which can persist unchanged over the years.

Finally, in the *late stage* after many years or decades, severe and still more severe deficits as already described determine the clinical picture. Then or later, a spinal apoplexy, more frequently, however, without an intramedullary hematoma, leads on to an acute transverse lesion of the cord.

Aminoff and Logue (1974) in their material, 6 months after the start of the illness, found deficits which were slight in 34 and severe in 11 patients. After 3 years, only six remained in the former group, while 28 had become severely disabled, altogether 59%. Thus the most severe deterioration took place within 1 year. In the remaining groups, the progression was not so marked. Of 12 patients with an apoplectiform onset, five showed a progressive deterioration while seven remained static after the elucidation of the diagnosis; three were without any deficit after 5, 8, and 17 years, two slightly impaired after 13 and 16 years, two paralyzed after 4 and 6 years. Twenty were dead at the time of the publication, seven had died from undetermined and three from extraneous causes, nine from complications of the paraplegia, and one after a subarachnoid hemorrhage.

Cervical angiomas appear to behave in a similar manner. Of ten cases reported by Yasargil (1975) five were ill for between 4 and 22 years without progress; the remaining five had progressively deteriorated.

In spite of the differing pattern of behavior, there is absolutely no doubt about a progressive deterioration. Only 9% of the cases of Aminoff and Logue (1974) remained symptom-free or without progression, and in our own material there were none.

Cerebrospinal Fluid Findings

As in all spinal lesions, a full examination of the cerebrospinal fluid should be undertaken in spinal angiomas. In our material (Table 13), the fluid was normal in one-half of the extradural and in one-quarter of the intradural angiomas. Raised cell counts up to more than 100 as an isolated finding can be misinterpreted; this is only exceptionally the case. The same holds true for the microscopic demonstration of erythrocytes in three of our cases where there was no macroscopic sign of blood.

Pathologic increases of protein are extremely characteristic, and in one-half of the cases of intradural and about one-third of the extradural angiomas, they were related to a narrowing or restriction of the fluid pathways. All the mixed intradural angiomas and also the tumor-angioma cases, which are not under consideration here, always showed a manometric block and greatly increased protein levels. As a rule, this was between 60 and 100 mg%. With lumbosacral angiomas, the cerebrospinal fluid is normal, and a manometric investigation is not undertaken.

Table 13. CSF-findings in spinal angiomas (in percentage)

	Extradural a.	Intradural a.
Normal	50	23
Increase in cells	6	28
Erythrocytes	-	13
Protein increased	41	70
Manometry (normal, i.e., no block)	72	45
pathologic, (i.e., block)	28	55

Summary

The clinical diagnosis of a spinal angioma can only rarely be made with certainty. On the other hand, it should already be suspected in the early stages on the basis of definite or suspicious findings and evidence, and even more easily in the middle stage when the nature of the disease can be established by radiologic investigations and when, by removal of the lesion, irreversible damage can be prevented or diminished. This applies equally for extradural and intradural angiomas (Table 14).

Extradural Angiomas

A vertebral angioma which has spinal symptoms and signs strongly suggests a vertebro-extradural angioma. Urgent signs are an apoplectiform and remitting course with local root involvement, with or without spinal or radicular deficits, and repeated intensification or exacerbation as a result of extrinsic or intrinsic stimuli (physical stress, menstruation,

Table 14. Clinical diagnosis of spinal angiomas

	Extradural angiomas	Intradural angiomas
Accompanying signs	Cutaneous angioma (+) Vertebral angioma (++)	Cutaneous angioma (+)
Complications	Pathologic vertebral fracture (+) Extradural hematoma (+)	Spinal subarachnoid hemorrhage 50% in the first 4 decades Intramedullary hematoma (+)
Age at onset	Middle age Middle and later age: vertebroextradural a.	Early and middle age ++ Middle and later age: subpial cap. a.
Course	Apoplectiform 30% Remittent 40% Progressive 30%	Apoplectiform 50% Remittent 20% Progressive 30%
Provocation and exacerbation	Exertion 32% Pregnancy	Exertion 32% Pregnancy
Pain	Local and radicular 60%	Radicular 30% Funicular 30% Meningeal 50% First back pain!
Motor deficits	Not typical	Spastic atrophic 40%
Sensory deficits	Not typical	Dissociated 35%
Diff. diagnosis Earlier diagnosis	Chron. cord disease 25% Disk lesions 40% Spinal tumor 25%	Cerebral lesion 20% Chronic cord lesion 60% (MS 30%) Spinal tumor 20%
Spinal bruit	-	+
CSF	Pathol. 50% Protein increased 40% Manometric block 30%	Pathol. 75% Protein increased 70% Manometric block 55%

pregnancy). The condition can occur at any age with predominance in the first 4 decades for solitary extradural, and in the later decades for vertebroextradural angiomas. Angiomas of the cauda equina and the lumbosacral junction are almost invariably confused with intervertebral disk lesions; when there was a remitting course, chronic inflammatory or degenerative spinal cord diseases were often suspected for many years. A progressive pseudotumoral pattern usually suggested a tumor.

Intradural Angiomas

Fairly definite symptoms of an intradural angioma are the rarely detectable angioma bruit and, more important, spinal subarachnoid hemorrhage at an early age (10 - 40 years), with onset of pain localized in the back! Scarcely any doubt exists when there are associated spinal symptoms and deficits; these are often absent with the first bleed but never with recurrences. An apoplectiform pattern is strongly suspect, but less so a remitting course which is mostly misdiagnosed. A progressive course leads to a suspicion of a tumor. Intensification or deterioration as a result of physical stress and during menstruation or pregnancy increases the suspicion, above all if there is a regular and repeated appearance associated with the particular stimulus, with the subsequent disappearance of the manifestations. Root and tract pains, amyotrophic paraparesis, and dissociated sensory disturbances with predominating posterior column loss are certainly characteristic but, at the same time, because of the remitting pattern, they are the cause of years of misdiagnosis. Among these, chronic cord diseases are of the greatest importance, more particularly multiple sclerosis. In three-quarters of the cases, the CSF is abnormal, with increased protein and a manometric block being the most frequent. Each suspicion, even of a supposedly definite spinal cord disorder, demands the use of special investigations, whenever possible spinal angiography, otherwise myelography. The consideration of clinical data and progress, and the CSF findings, can so decisively improve the early diagnosis that cures are no longer the exception but can become the rule.

Clinical Symptomatology and Natural History of Arteriovenous Malformations of the Spinal Cord

A Study of the Clinical Aspects and Prognosis, Based on 150 Cases

Michel Djindjian

The arteriovenous malformations of the spinal cord, mistakenly regarded as a rare condition, are more frequent than is thought. The more routine use of spinal angiography has allowed the revelation of minimal malformations which were not seen on myelography, or the revision of such erroneous diagnoses as myelitis or myelomalacia. Thus, 150 malformations have been collected in 15 years from 3000 spinal angiographies.

These malformations, like their intracranial counterparts, are more frequent in males (68%). The situation is the same with respect to the age of presentation, where they are more frequent in children and young adults. Statistically, 30% of the cases have been diagnosed before 20 years, 30% between 20 and 40 years, 30% between 40 and 60 years, and 10% from 60 to 75 years. The extremes range from 18 months to 74 years.

The delay in diagnosis is variable and at present is tending to diminish, thanks to a more rapid diagnosis. It is made early, in under 1 year, in 26% of cases, but also late, taking over 10 years in 14% of cases. The diagnosis is, therefore, often delayed in relation to the first clinical signs – in 60% of the cases, the malformation is only discovered 1 - 10 years after its development. The effect of this on the prognosis is, therefore, obvious.

The age at onset of the clinical manifestations is the most important criterion, as this alone can serve as a guide line for establishing the natural history of these malformations. It is remarkable to note that 50% of the malformations reveal themselves before 30 years of age (Table 1).

Table 1. Age at onset of the clinical manifestations of arteriovenous malformations

Age at Onset by decade	Number of cases	Percentage
0 - 10	31	20%
10 - 20	29	20%
20 - 30	12	8%
30 - 40	20	13%
40 - 50	24	16%
50 - 60	20	13%
> 60	14	10%
Total	150	100%

The clinical symptoms are quite variable on account of a number of factors which include the anatomy of these malformations which can penetrate the cord or remain extramedullary, their longitudinal extent, and their mechanisms of decompensation. But, among the numerous clinical presentations which may proclaim the presence of the arteriovenous malformations, two are characteristic: spinal subarachnoid hemorrhage and focal syndromes of the spinal cord and roots.

Spinal Subarachnoid Hemorrhage

Spinal subarachnoid hemorrhage suggests first of all a vascular malformation, more especially if there are localizing spinal signs. Nevertheless, its frequency is less than in the cerebral lesions, where bleeding is seen in three quarters of the cases.

We have seen it 36 times (24%), 32 times as the presenting symptom, 20 times appearing as a pure bleed, with misleading cerebral signs on five occasions. On 16 occasions, factors involving stress were involved, including two pregnancies. One must emphasize the fact that with one exception, all our subarachnoid hemorrhages occurred in those malformations which were partly or completely *intramedullary*.

With regard to age, it is essential to specify that 55% of the subarachnoid hemorrhages were in subjects younger than 15 years, that in 85% of cases it was the presenting symptom, and finally that in half of the cases it appeared to be a straightforward hemorrhage. It therefore seems logical to think that in the general setting of subarachnoid hemorrhage in children, which is actually not a common occurrence, arteriovenous malformations are underestimated as a cause, as long as one fails to use angiography as a means of investigating the spinal cord.

The recurrent types are frequent, being accompanied as a rule by root and cord signs; on the other hand, the occurrence of a second isolated subarachnoid hemorrhage, although a possibility, is very rare.

Nevertheless, these recurring hemorrhages are not serious enough to present a risk to life; one patient only died in the seventh episode as a result of raised intracranial pressure, three others had valves inserted for hydrocephalus, the spinal cause of which was not discovered in two of them until later.

If the diagnosis of spinal subarachnoid hemorrhage is easier when there are some cord or root signs, even if these are not fully developed, it is necessary to think of it all the more in the pure forms, because they sometimes lack the onset with back pains or preexisting root signs. A posteriori, in 27 cases out of 36, the presenting symptoms were elicited on questioning, objective signs were found on the clinical examination, or radiologic anomalies were found on the routine radiographs of the spine.

The Syndromes with Spinal Cord or Root Deficits

In contrast to the cerebral arteriovenous malformations which, apart from hemorrhages and epileptic attacks, only involve slight focal deficits, those in the spinal cord, after a more or less lengthy clinical course, can lead finally to a total paraplegia.

Different clinical pictures may be produced, among which the most suggestive is that of a *localized cord and root syndrome* which develops spasmodically (69%). This evolution by fits and starts is typical, its frequency variable, and often encouraged by some precipitating factor (effort, pregnancy, trauma). Commonly, the clinical picture is associated with a subarachnoid hemorrhage at the time of the first episode. The spinal level involved always remains the same, which is an important fact in excluding episodes of disseminated sclerosis. Although at the start any remission may be complete, most often it is only partial, and as a rule each episode leaves behind some aggravation of the neurologic deficit. It is apparent that at any time in such a process of evolution, a fresh episode in a patient who until then has been slightly or moderately handicapped may lead to a permanent paraplegia or tetraplegia.

The cord and root syndromes with a *progressive* course (30%) are the types, above all, which are the least suggestive of an arteriovenous malformation, all the more so because they are seen, as a rule, in older subjects. The clinical state sometimes advances progressively in the manner of a spinal compression from a tumor but sometimes by successive episodes.

The *apoplectic forms* producing a catastrophic onset of cord damage which develops in a few hours, showing no remission, are very rare (1%), if one makes a careful study of the clinical histories.

Apart from these clinical factors, the diagnosis of spinal arteriovenous malformations may be helped still more if one finds an associated dysplasia, from an examination of the straight films and the study of the cerebrospinal fluid. The study of the dysplasias and of the plain films is given in detail in the Chapter "Angiography in angiomas of the spinal cord."

The examination of the cerebrospinal fluid may reveal a bloody fluid, an albuminocytologic dissociation, a raised protein associated with a more or less marked pleiocytosis, and even a normal fluid. One may conclude from this that although a bloody fluid is a weighty argument in favor of a spinal angioma (1/4), and a dissociation (1/2) as presumptive evidence, a normal fluid should never allow one to reject this diagnosis.

Classification

The classification of the spinal arteriovenous malformations derives indirectly from the angiogram, since all the malformations fed by the anterior spinal artery system have, with some exceptions, an intramedullary component, and on the other hand, every malformation fed by the posterior spinal system is extra- and retromedullary. This leads one to classify these malformations in terms of their blood supply and the three main spinal vascular territories described by Lazorthes (cf. Table in "Angiography in angiomas of the spinal cord", page 123).

In summary:

Posterior supply – retrospinal (RAVM)	60 cases (40%)
Anterior or mixed feeders	90 cases (60%)
Intramedullary (IAVM)	84 = 93%
Extramedullary	6 = 7%

This classification into two main types (IAVM and RAVM) which we have introduced, and which is based on arteriographic and anatomic criteria, is amply supported by the natural history of the lesions, their mechanisms of decompensation, and the problems of operation. It is, therefore, possible (Tables 2 and 3) to suspect the type of malformation

Table 2. Anatomic subdivision of the arteriovenous malformations in relation to their arterial supply

	Anterior	Mixed	Posterior	Total	%
Cervical (C 1 - D 1)	5	15	1	21	14%
Middorsal (D 2 - D 6)	10	11	12	33	22%
Dorsolumbo-sacral (D 7 - Cauda)	17	32	47	96	64%
Total	32	58	60	150	100%
%	21%	39%	40%	100%	

Table 3. Factors in the differential diagnosis between intra- and retromedullary arteriovenous malformations

AVMs 150 cases	Intra- or Mixed Medullary AVMs 90 cases	Retromedullary AVMs 60 cases
Sex: Male	57%	87%
Sex: Female	43%	13%
Age at onset of symptoms	86% before 40 years	85% after 40 years
Associated malformations	29%	6%
Subarachnoid hemorrhage	41%	1.6%
Progressive	20%	60%
Pattern: by fits and starts ("strokes")	80%	40%
Abnormalities in straight x-rays	40%	2.5%

before the stage of arteriography, provided that the possibility of the diagnosis has been considered beforehand. The youth of the patient, the presence of a subarachnoid hemorrhage, and of a dysplasic element are the particular arguments for suspecting an intramedullary component in the malformation; on the other hand, an advanced age and a progressive course are characteristic of a retromedullary malformation.

It is remarkable to note that, with the exception of one cervical lesion, all of our subarachnoid hemorrhages occurred in those malformations with an anterior spinal component (AVM + SAH = IAVM). These characteristic criteria – age at onset, subarachnoid hemorrhage – are clearly shown in the three diagrams, according to the three different spinal levels (Figs. 1 - 3).

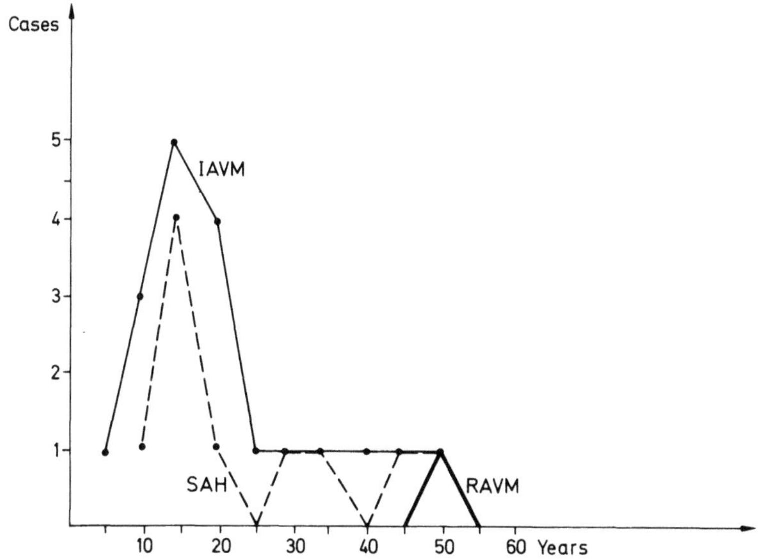

Fig. 1. Subarachnoid hemorrhages in the cervical region vs. age at onset

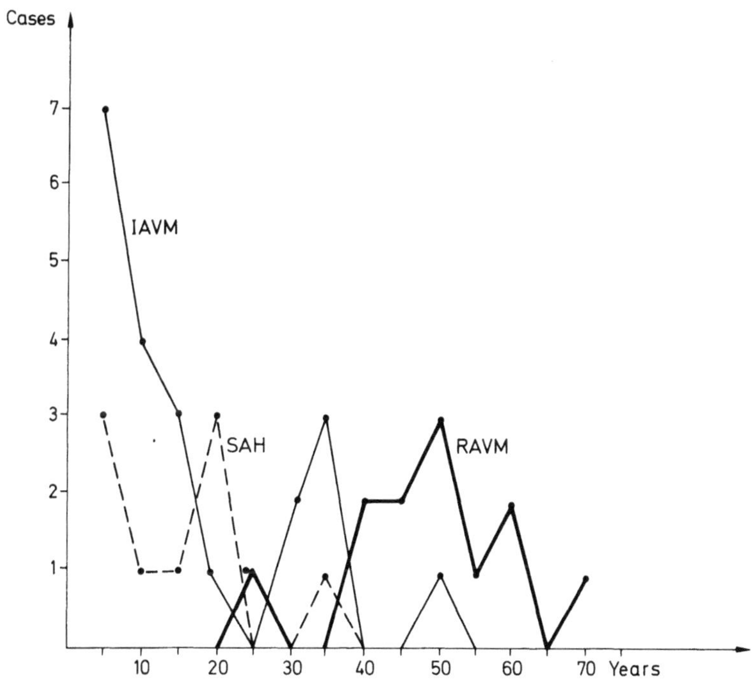

Fig. 2. Subarachnoid hemorrhages in the dorsal region vs. age at onset

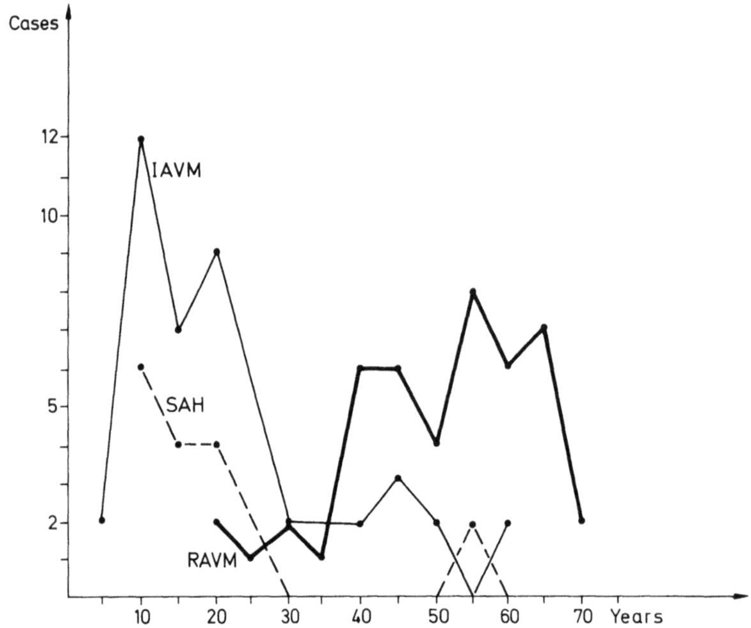

Fig. 3. Subarachnoid hemmorrhages in the dorsolumbar region vs. age at onset

Natural History and Prognosis of the Arteriovenous Malformations

If we review the whole of our statistics, it seems difficult to us to translate into figures the natural history of the arteriovenous malformations of the spinal cord (as has been done by Aminoff and Logue, 1974) because, as the years go by, the number of nontreated cases falls to a level that is no longer statistically significant. Two factors undoubtedly influence the course: the existence or nonexistence of penetration into the cord and the segmental level of the malformation. Nevertheless, we have attempted to plot out a "natural history" of these malformations by including with them the cases treated by palliative methods (posterior excision, ligation) in order to secure a larger number of cases. In particular with the cervical lesions, where these measures seem the most effective, it is certain that this grouping of cases falsifies to some extent the true pattern of development of these lesions.

Posterior Malformations

In the case of the *posterior malformations* (RAVM), their spontaneous evolution follows most frequently a progressive course (60%) and leads, in an average of 6 years, to a bedridden state. These eminently curable lesions, therefore, have quite a serious prognosis if left untreated.

Intramedullary Arteriovenous Malformations

Figs. 4, 5 and 6 represent the clinical state, as seen over 20 years of natural development, in the intracervical, dorsal, and dorsolumbar malformations. The clinical condition of the patient is divided into six stages numbered from 0 to 5:

Stage 0: Normal condition
Stage 1: Minor troubles
Stage 2: Impairment of function interfering with social and professional activities
Stage 3: Considerable handicap. Walking with two sticks. Independent life still possible
Stage 4: Bedridden
Stage 5: Transverse lesion of the cord

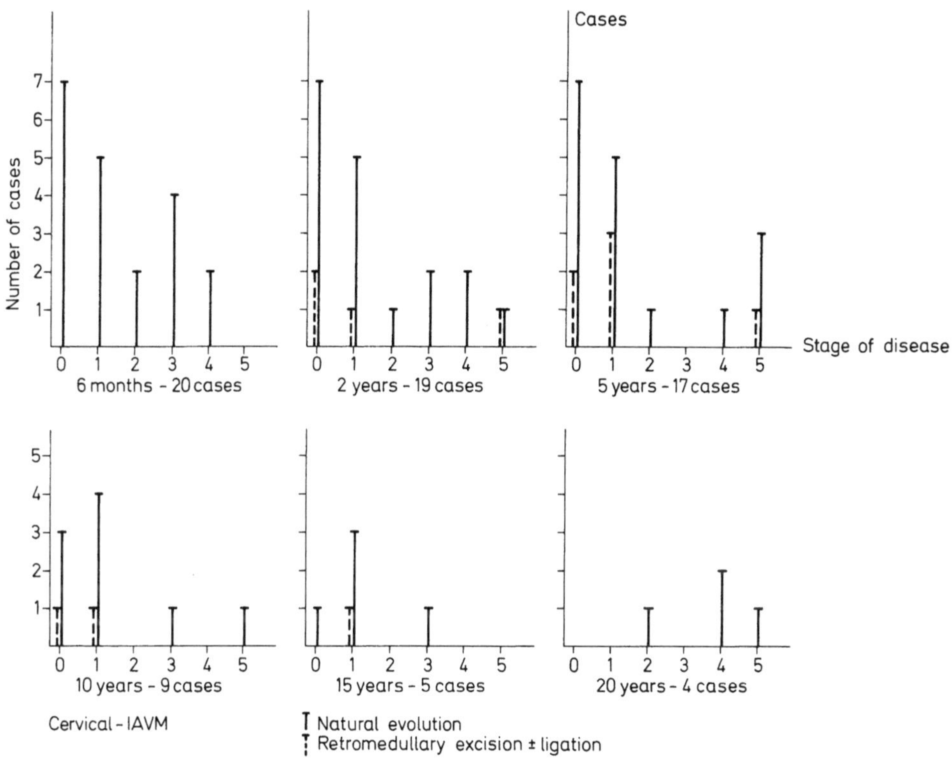

Fig. 4. Clinical state seen over a 6 month - 20 year period of the natural development of cervical malformations

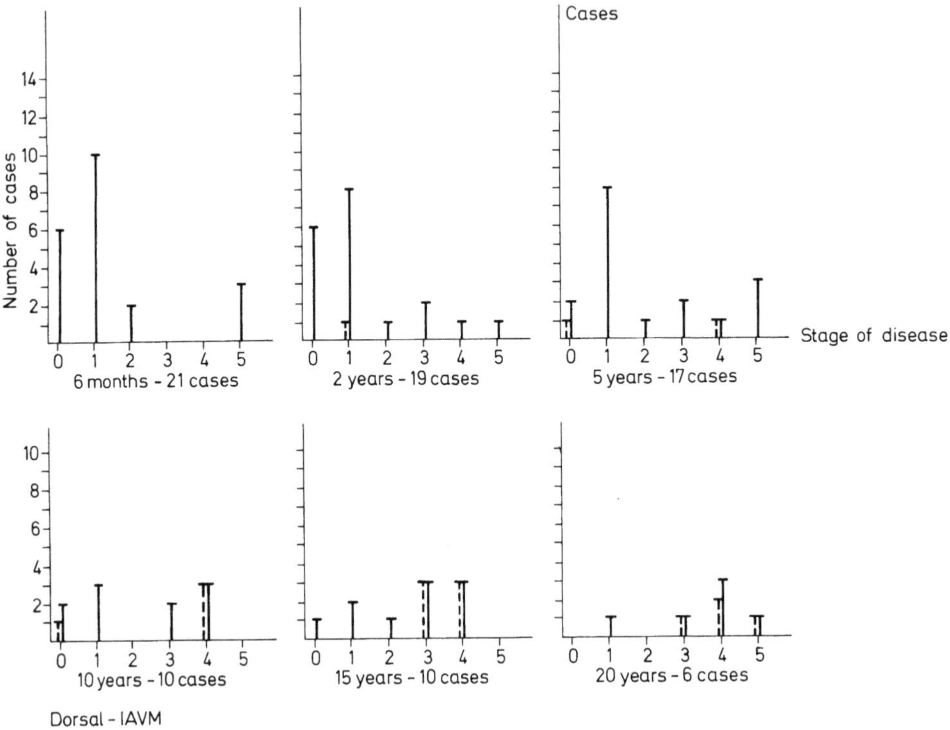

Fig. 5. (legend see page 83) ▲

Fig. 6. (legend see page 83) ▼

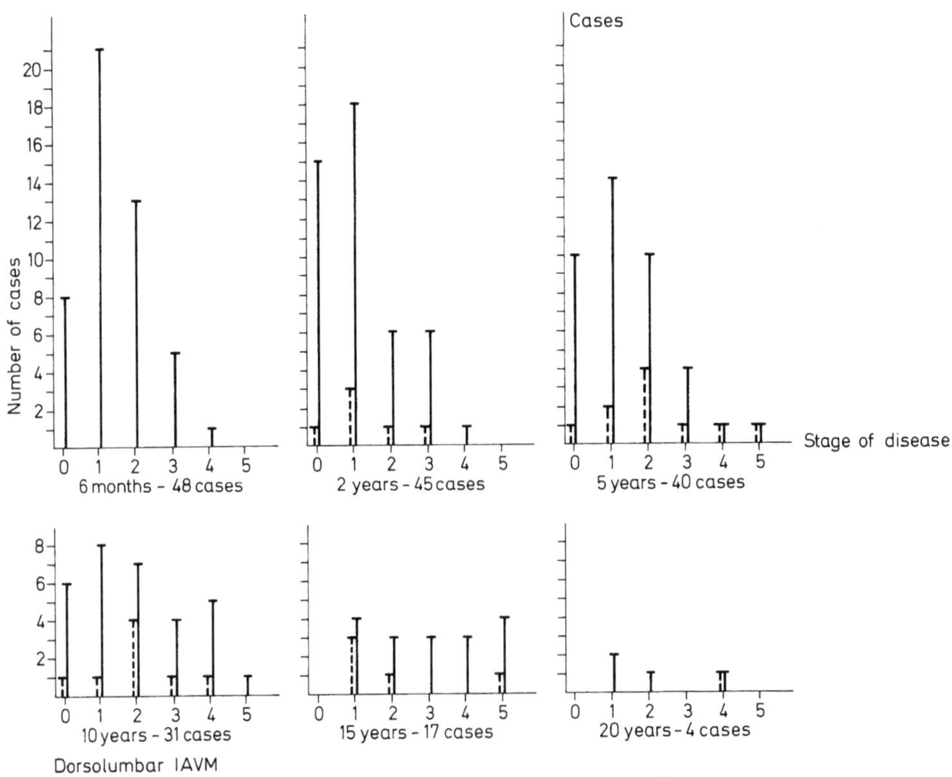

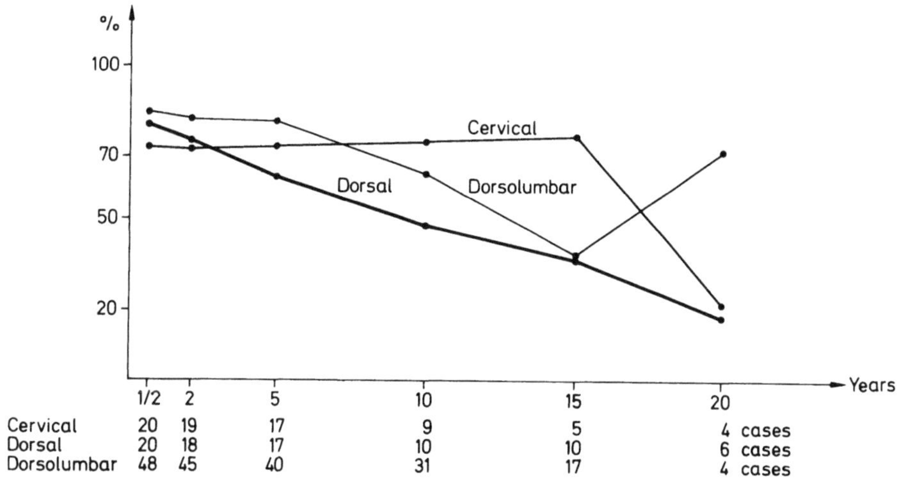

Fig. 7. The comparative natural history of IAVM in the three vascular territories (Group A)

Fig. 7 shows the comparative natural history of the IAVM in the three vascular territories. The first three stages (0, 1, 2) – i.e., the patients who are normal or slightly handicapped (Group A) – are grouped and contrasted with the last stages (3, 4, 5) where the patient is bedridden or housebound. These different diagrams lead us to make several observations:

A mere five out of 90 IAVMs were only slightly or moderately handicapped, after 20 years of progression of the disease. Apart from this, one of our patients died in the 20th year of his history, from a catastrophic bulbocervical hematomyelia.

The relative tolerance of the cervical forms is probably explained by the rich vascular supply of the cervical cord, which permits a better adaptation and response to ischemic episodes.

The gradient of the graph in the dorsal region bears eloquent testimony to the sensitivity to ischemia of the dorsal segments of the cord and indicates a particularly serious pattern of progress at this level.

As for the dorsolumbar lesions, they have a gradient of deterioration intermediate between those of the cervical and dorsal arteriovenous malformations.

Whatever the vascular anatomy of the malformation, the patient progresses in the long term toward a bedridden state, which is unpredictable in any individual case. This is certainly the best argument in favor of radical excision of the lesion, whenever the anatomic configuration of the malformation appears to be suited to such a course of action.

We regret to report *four spontaneous deaths* which must be put down to the dysplasia, three of whom were children (17, 7, and 3 years). There was one case of cervicodorsal softening, one case of raised intracranial pressure resulting from a recurrent hemorrhage, one death caused by visceral hemorrhages in the case of a tetraplegia in the setting of a Rendu-Osler-Weber syndrome, and one case of a bulbocervical hematomyelia in an adult, after a history of 20 years.

◄ Fig. 5. Clinical state seen over a 6 month - 20 year period of the natural development of dorsal malformations

Fig. 6. Clinical state seen over a 6 month - 20 year period of the natural development of dorsolumbar malformations. ⊤ = Natural evolution; ⊤ = Retromedullary excision ± ligation

Radiologic Findings in Spinal Angiomas - Plain X-Rays, Myelography, and Spinal Phlebography

Agnolo Lino Agnoli, Albrecht Laun, Hans Werner Pia, and Heinzgeorg Vogelsang

Introduction

Selective spinal angiography is now the procedure of choice for the diagnosis of intradural spinal angiomas. It has largely displaced the other radiologic investigations of the spinal canal. However, the diagnostic significance of straight films and tomography, myelography, and spinal phlebography has not been diminished. With vertebral, extradural, and some intradural angiomas these investigations give characteristic or suggestive findings, or they provide the indication for and supplement the findings of selective angiography. A further and more important reason for discussing them is the fact that such painstaking and specialized angiography is only possible in a few departments, and the classic investigative procedures are still undertaken in most cases. For this reason, they are indispensable in achieving an improvement in early diagnosis and, hence, early treatment.

Straight Films

The x-ray investigation of the vertebral column by plain films and tomography yields specific findings in angiomas of the vertebrae and may disclose localized or more extensive pressure effects and anatomic changes. For the actual diagnosis of the angiomas it is of no value.

Angiomas of the Vertebrae

Vertebral angiomas are easy to recognize on account of the streaky and honeycomb cavitation of the spongiosa between the residual trabeculae (Fig. 1A). As a rule, the vertebral body is involved, more rarely parts of the vertebral arch, either in addition, or on their own. Multiple involvement of vertebrae and other bones is not unusual. In our material, out of 23 cases there were seven with multiple vertebral involvement. *Pathologic fractures* seen three times in our material (Fig. 1B) are easy to recognize and have pathogenetic significance when associated with an apoplectiform clinical course. If there are spinal symptoms, with radiologic evidence of a vertebral angioma, one can reasonably suspect a vertebroextradural angioma. Further investigations are then indicated (Pia and Vogelsang, 1965; Pia, 1975).

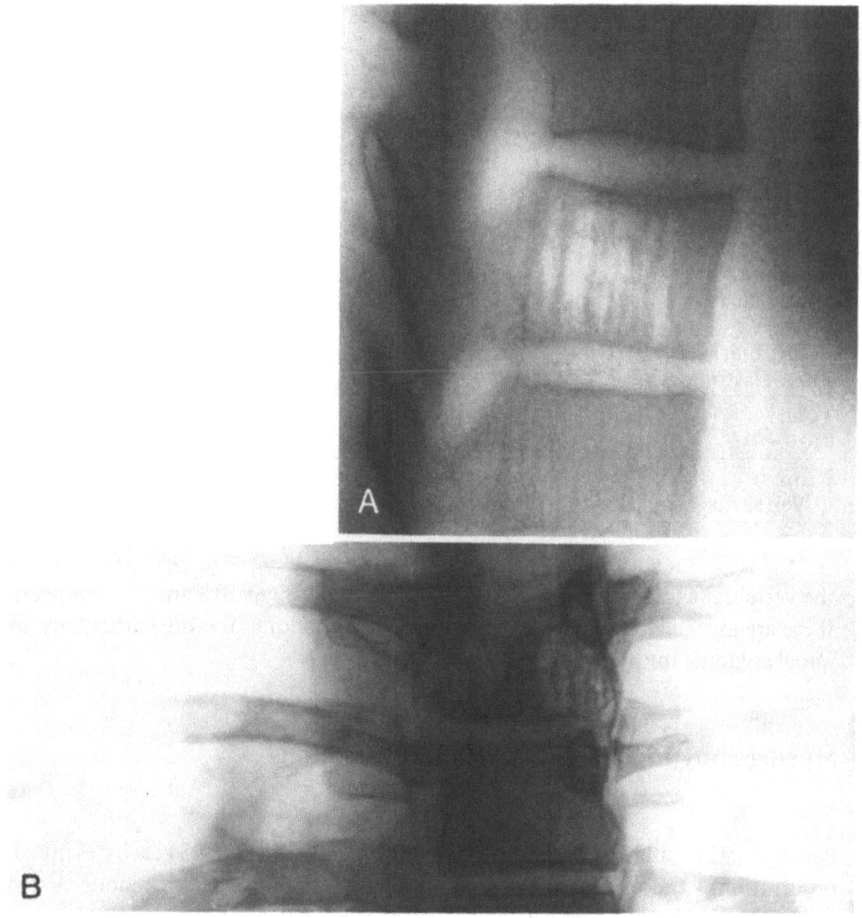

Fig. 1. (A) Vertebral angioma, (B) Vertebral angioma with pathologic fracture

Pressure Signs

These include expansion of the spinal canal, radiologic atrophy of the articular processes, widening of the interpedicular distance with large space-occupying angiomas, pressure defects in the dorsal margins of the vertebral bodies, and parts of the vertebral arches; widening of the intervertebral foramina in the cervical region is uncommon. Besides one personal case with widening of the cervical spinal canal further individual cases were described by Djindjian, 1962; Doppman et al., 1969; Langmaid, 1963; Lombardi and Miglivacca, 1959.

Scoliosis and kyphoscoliosis are quite frequently found (Dalloz et al., 1963; Djindjian et al., 1970; Pia and Vogelsang, 1965; Umbach, 1962) (Fig. 4C). The causes of this deformity are multisegmental or radicular lesions of the anterior horn, or anterior nerve roots, with atrophy of the corresponding musculature.

Calcification in the angiomas is unusual. In our material (Table 1), local abnormalities, seen in 21%, are produced usually by vertebral and vertebroextradural angiomas. Without these, the proportion only amounts to 4%. Relatively more frequent, without considering

Table 1. Plain x-ray findings in spinal angiomas

	Number	Normal	Local abnormalities	Scoliosis or kyphoscoliosis
Vertebral a.	7	-	7	-
Vertebro-extradural a.	16	-	16	-
Extradural angiomas	29	26	-	3
Intradural angiomas	59	44	2	13
Global angiomas	6	1	1	4
Angioblastomas	12	8	1	3
Total	129	79	27	23
(%)		61%	21%	18%
Without vertebr. a.	106	74%	4%	22%

the vertebral angiomas, are scoliosis and kyphoscoliosis at 18% and 22%, respectively. When these are associated with spinal symptoms, an extradural or more particularly an intradural spinal angioma must always be considered.

Myelography in Spinal Vascular Malformations

Perthes (1921, publ. 1927) and Guillain and Alajouanine (1925) each described, as a "first observation," the myelographic findings in an intradural, arteriovenous cirsoid angioma. Later communications from Globus and Strauss (1929), Puusepp (1938), and Bassett et al. (1949) confirmed the typical findings, which portrayed the dilated vessels as negative shadows in the myelogram. With the commencement of the operative treatment of spinal angiomas, particularly after the second World War, myelography continued to be the most important diagnostic procedure. Comparable results are found in all the articles about the diagnosis and treatment of angiomas. Apart from the "vascular" filling defects in the myelogram, the pulsation of the vessels seen during the screening turned out to be a further pathognomonic sign. Wyburn-Mason (1943) in three myelograms found a complete block in one and a free flow of the contrast medium in the other two. In six cases reported by Epstein et al. (1949), of which four were confirmed by autopsy, there were typical myelographic findings in three, although on the other hand Brion et al. (1952) reported four cases with atypical findings. Odom et al. (1957), Teng and Shapiro (1958) and Teng and Papatheodorou (1964) found in an equally small number of cases the typical "vascular" filling defects in the myelogram. A collection of larger series (Newman, 1959; Djindjian et al., 1962; Baker et al., 1967; Doppman et al., 1969; Pia and Vogelsang, 1965; Yasargil, 1968) by Yasargil (1971) of 108 myelograms in intradural angiomas showed typical findings in 63%. Five percent had a complete and 4% a partial block. The findings were suspicious in 14% and indefinite in 4%. Finally, in 10% there was the appearance of an arachnoiditis, Djindjian et al. (1970) in a later series saw tortuous vessels and pools of contrast in 48%. According to the experience of Aminoff (1976), these vascular defects converge to a point which possibly corresponds to the arteriovenous shunt.

The myelographic findings become all the clearer as one increases the amount of contrast medium used. The optimum amount is 10 - 12 ml of oily contrast medium. More limited experiences with air myelography (Svien and Baker, 1961; Hindmarsh, 1974; Liliequist, 1976; Poole and Larsen, 1971) confirm its expected inferiority as compared with positive contrast media.

Extending the investigations of Wyburn-Mason (1943), Pia and Vogelsang (1965) tried to distinguish the myelographic findings in different types of extradural and intradural angiomas. The findings which had for so long been regarded as typical were only shown by the large subarachnoid arteriovenous cirsoid angiomas, while the other types showed divergent appearances. With the introduction of spinal angiography, myelography was written about much less in the literature. Thus, in spite of the increase in operatively verified angiomas, the systematic investigation of the myelographic findings in the various types of spinal angiomas was unfortunately no longer discussed.

The myelographic findings in our own material were examined in accordance with the classification of Pia (1975) and grouped into vertebroextradural angiomas, extradural angiomas, extradural lumbosacral vascular anomalies, intradural angiomas, and their subsidiary forms, global extraintradural angiomas, and angiomas and angioblastomas. Tracings of all the findings were made and collated for each type in order to be able to identify their characteristics.

Extradural Angiomas

We divide the true extradural angiomas into solitary extradural angiomas and the mixed vertebroextradural angiomas. Involvement of the extradural space is also found in the mixed intraextradural angiomas and the global angiomas. Lumbosacral extradural vascular anomalies are also discussed on account of their doubtful angiomatous nature and the difficulty of distinguishing them from true angiomas in this region.

Solitary Extradural Angiomas

Solitary extradural angiomas are predominantly cavernomas and venous angiomas; they are rarely arteriovenous cirsoid angiomas. Among 29 cases, there were four cervical, ten thoracic, eight lumbar, and seven lumbosacral. Myelography was done in 22 patients, with an oily contrast medium in 16 and a water-soluble medium in six.

Complete Block

In angiomas with a complete block, the margin of the contrast medium at the upper and lower pole was shown as irregular and streaky or finger-like (Fig. 2A). It was not possible to detect afferent and efferent vessels, with filling defects in the contrast. In no cases were the borders of the column of contrast smooth, convex, or concave.

Partial Block

Angiomas with a partial block showed a similar picture. The filling defects in the contrast were multiple and multiform, always irregular and blurred, and they extended usually over several vertebral bodies. Broad and finger-shaped margins were also found in these cases (Fig. 2B, C). Particularly evident in the lateral views were pointed processes through which the contrast medium leaked away. Occasionally, filling defects were seen, which made one

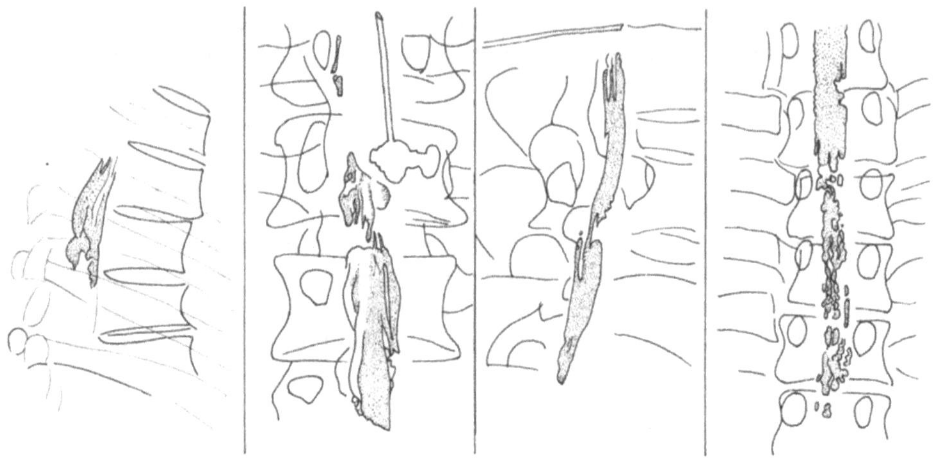

A B C D

Fig. 2. Myelographic findings in extradural arteriovenous angiomas. (A) With complete block. Enlarged vessels? (B, C) Incomplete block. Atypical defects of vascular type, (D) Vertebroepidural angioma without block. Atypical defects of vascular type

think of a dilated angioma vessel. Operative confirmation was not successful because artificial conditions are created by the laminectomy and decompression. However, the suspected true findings are not excluded by this.

No Block
On many occasions, the flow of the contrast medium was only slightly hindered. Repeated partial blocks or defects of larger or smaller drops, with lateral and anterior compression were the usual finding. No changes were found which would suggest dilated or convoluted vessels.

Lumbar and Lumbosacral Angiomas

Angiomas in the lumbar or lumbosacral region were usually investigated with water-soluble medium, as they are often suspected clinically of being medial or lateral lumbar disk lesions. The findings were not typical and gave the impression of an extradural malignant tumor, a prolapsed intervertebral disk, or a root sheath defect. Occasionally, the filling defects could not be categorized and were reminiscent of the previously described changes.

Vertebroextradural Angiomas

Of 23 patients with vertebral angiomas, 16 had combined vertebroextradural angiomas. In all cases the lesions were cavernomas. In the latter, it is spinal neurologic deficits which furnish the indications for a contrast investigation. Out of 16 patients, ten had myelography, one with air, three with water-soluble, and six with oily contrast medium. As with the solitary extradural angiomas, the changes were recognized by irregular, multiple defects in the column of contrast medium, which were reproducible and not confined to the vicinity of the vertebra affected by the angioma. Occasionally one had an impression of vessels, dilated or in clusters. Our operative experience, that with combined vertebroextradural angiomas the extradural portion regularly extends beyond the vertebrae involved, in both directions, was confirmed by myelography (Fig. 2D). In the rare cases where there was a complete block, the changes in the adjoining segments of the contrast medium were correspondingly altered, so that it appeared unlikely to be a tumor. Lumbosacral angiomas can show changes like a prolapsed intervertebral disk.

Lumbosacral Extradural Vascular Anomalies

The etiologic, pathogenetic, and clinical significance of lumbosacral extradural vascular anomalies have been considered and evaluated in the chapter on "Symptomatology of Spinal Angiomas." Although a prolapsed intervertebral disk is almost always suspected on clinical and etiological grounds, it is virtually impossible to distinguish between them in the myelogram. This has already been pointed out in an earlier paper (Gümbel et al., 1969). Apart from the typical findings for a prolapsed intervertebral disk, solitary root sheath defects without signs of compression were predominant. A further investigation and reappraisal of the myelograms and myelotomograms of 17 patients confirmed these findings and showed at the same time a particularly high percentage of associated anomalies of the caudal dural sac and the root sheaths. Five patients had a megacauda (Pia) and two further had in addition widening of the nerve sheaths. These findings also indicate that the extradural lumbosacral vascular anomalies – histologically they are usually varicose dilatations of the veins – represent one of the types of lumbosacral anomalies of the dura and extradural tissues (fat and vessels).

Intradural Angiomas

Intradural angiomas are, almost without exception, arteriovenous cirsoid angiomas. The typical types are the subarachnoid dorsal arteriovenous angioma with preferential site in the lower thoracic, lumbar and sacral cord, intramedullary angiomas, predominantly cervical and lumbar and extraintramedullary. The extramedullary portion can be dorsal, lateral, or ventral or can completely surround the cord. Solitary ventral arteriovenous angiomas are rare. In contrast to these large arteriovenous angiomas, it is also necessary to distinguish the small subpial or partially subpial capillary angiomas (Pia). They can likewise be combined with the intramedullary portion of an angioma. It is important for the interpretation of myelographic findings to be aware that the subpial capillary angiomas constantly and the large subarachnoid arteriovenous angiomas in the late stage, particularly after spinal subarachnoid hemorrhages, are sometimes associated with a severe adhesive arachnoiditis; the cystic variety is seen more rarely. In the latter, they are absent in the early stages. One should also take note of the complicating subdural and intramedullary hematomas which also play a part in determining the myelographic findings. Special types are the mixed intradural and extradural angiomas, global angiomas with simultaneous involvement of the vertebral column and soft parts, and finally angioblastomas and angiomas combined with these.

Solitary Intradural Angiomas

Of 59 intradural angiomas, myelography was done in 39 patients, for the most part elsewhere. For the last 10 years, in all suspected cases, selective angiography is done first of

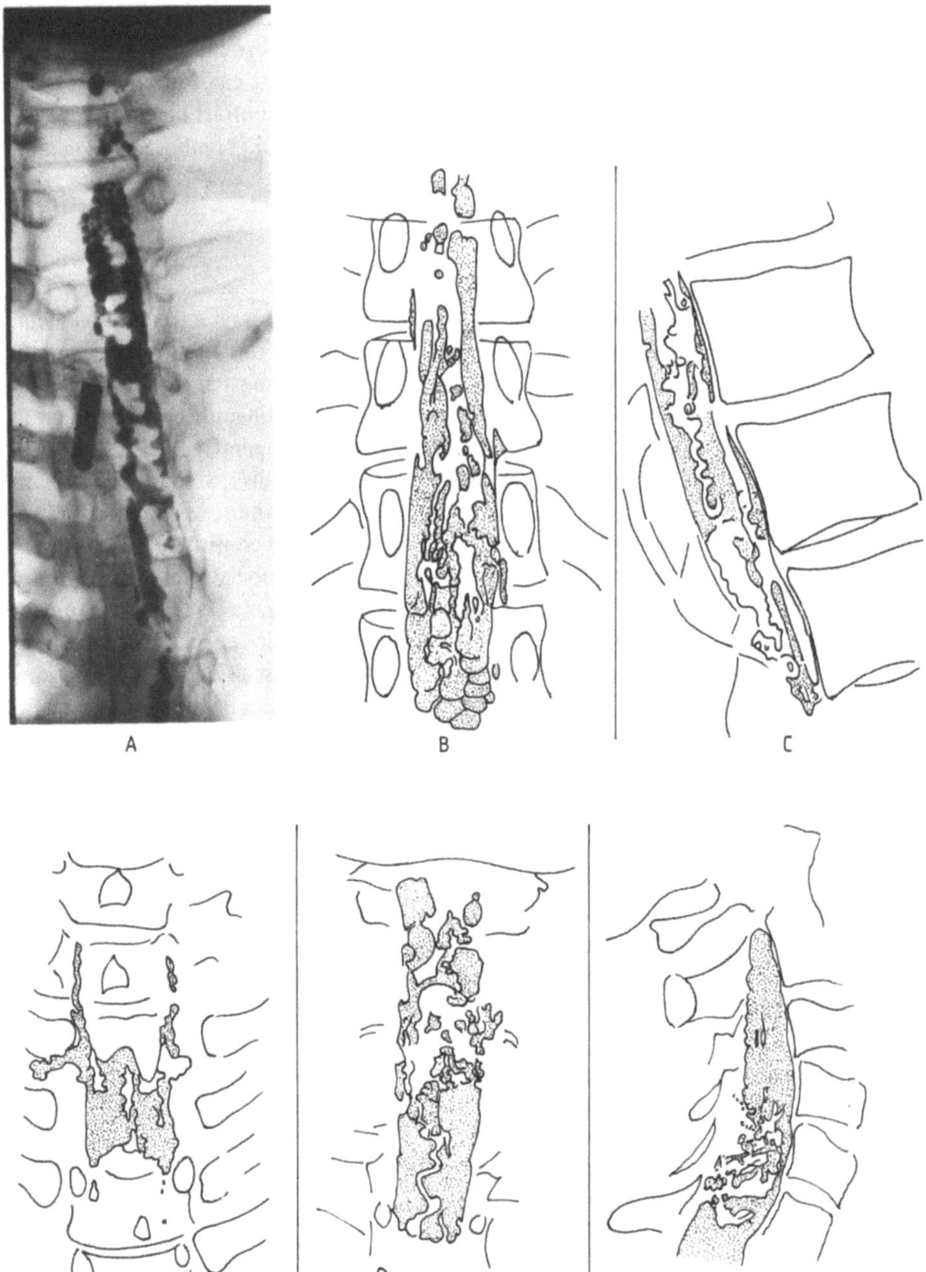

Fig. 3. Myelographic findings in intradural angiomas. (A) Typical large and extensive subarachnoid arteriovenous angioma, (B, C) dorsolateral and intramedullary arteriovenous angioma, (D) intramedullary hematoma with suspicion of angiomatous vessels, (E, F) left-sided dorsolateral extramedullary and intramedullary arteriovenous angioma of the cervical cord. Note the enlarged efferents

all, and only if the findings are negative, is myelography done. In transferred patients with the myelography already done, angiography was done straight away.

The classical picture of large subarachnoid arteriovenous angiomas is so typical that it does not require any further description. The angioma with all its components, viz., the large and small clusters of vessels in the center and the greatly dilated tortuous vessels and the draining vessels, shows itself as a negative image so that the whole extent of it can be comprehended (Fig. 3A). In early cases without arachnoiditis, the subarachnoid space is free and the relationship of the angioma to the subarachnoid space and the spinal cord are clearly recognizable. For this reason, lateral angiomas and dorsal and extraintradural angiomas can frequently be identified (Fig. 3B, and C). Even with the largest arteriovenous angiomas, the spinal subarachnoid space may remain free.

Our own material consisted predominantly of late cases with extensive arachnopathy. Among 28 cases where the operative and myelographic findings could be compared, adhesive arachnoiditis predominated over the cystic form (Table 2). The surprising thing is the very large number of typical and atypical angioma findings.

Table 2. Operative and myelographic findings in intradural angiomas

	Arachnopathy seen at operation	Typical angioma vessels	Atypical angioma vessels	Isolated arachnopathy
Adhesive arachnopathy	23	14	5	4
Cystic arachnopathy	5	3	2	-
Total	28	17	7	4

Complete Block

Angiomas with a complete block make up one-third of our material. The most frequent cause is arachnoiditis, which causes the subarachnoid space to be closed off at the site of the central angioma nodule after possibly many years of progress. The pattern of the myelographic block is irregular, yet altogether smooth and never digitate, as in the extradural angiomas. In the rarer cystic arachnopathy, its pattern is rounder and more uniform. The adjacent angiomatous changes allow one to differentiate them from arachnopathies of other origin. They are typical or atypical according to the size of the angioma (Fig. 4A).

One *intramedullary hematoma* with small extramedullary and intramedullary angiomas was distinguished by the typical appearances of an intramedullary block with a suspicion of vascular filling defects above it (Fig. 3D).

With the *intramedullary arteriovenous angiomas,* the angiographic distinction between solitary intramedullary or extramedullary location can be difficult. This myelogram of a cervical angioma shows clearly that it consists of a dorsal, left lateral extramedullary and also intramedullary angioma, extending ventrally (Fig. 3E, F). Angiographically, it was more apparent, on account of the main vascular supply which was coming from the right, that it was an intramedullary angioma predominantly on the right side. The operative removal confirmed the myelogram. The differential diagnosis between intramedullary arteriovenous angiomas and angioblastomas is not possible.

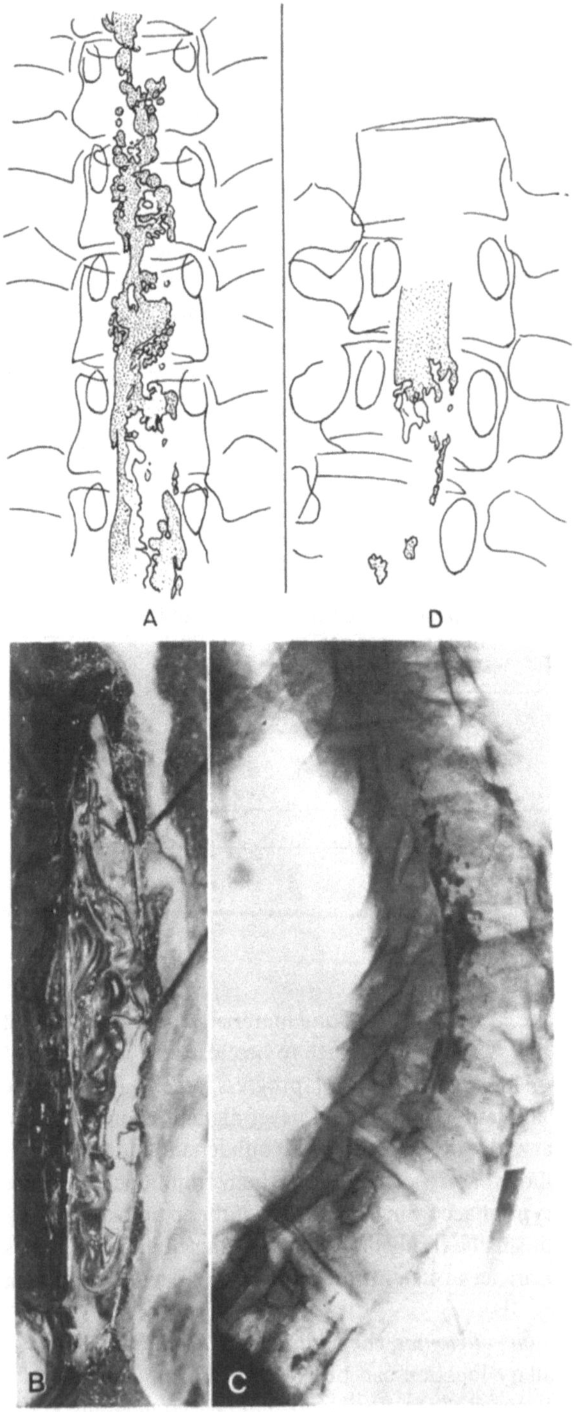

Fig. 4. Myelographic findings in intradural and combined angiomas. (A) Huge arteriovenous angioma with severe arachnoiditis. Note the atypical vascular defects, (B, C) operative and myelographic findings in a dorsolateral circumscribed arteriovenous angioma with marked arachnoiditis (mostly removed). Defect in the center. Global and atypical vascular defects in the peripheral parts. Marked kyphoscoliosis, (D) combined intra- and extradural angioma with complete block and atypical suspicious defects

Partial Block

An incomplete myelographic block is the rule with the late cases of dorsal subarachnoid arteriovenous angiomas and the subpial capillary arteriovenous angiomas. The principle cause is the pseudotumoral form of secondary arachnopathy not seen with the complete block. As the arachnitic changes do not remain restricted to the region of the angioma nodule, but can extend over the whole angioma and even beyond that, they produce secondary changes in the typical angioma myelogram. The filling defects become less tortuous and corkscrew-like and less "vascular" in appearance. However, with the large subarachnoid angiomas they remain, at least partially, so clear that a diagnosis can be made with some certainty (Fig. 4A). Usually, the contrast medium flows in drops through the irregularly constricted subarachnoid space. Because of the arachnoiditis, the angioma vessels are stuck together into larger or smaller units, although they may remain isolated; they and the arachnoid membrane then give rise to lacuniform and typical angioma defects of varying shape and size. In circumscribed angiomas with arachnopathy, the interpretation can be difficult for the inexperienced. As an example of this, a thoracic lateral angioma with ventral and dorsal extension showed a mixed pseudotumor appearance near the adherent center of the angioma, while above, there were multiple filling defects from dilated angioma vessels. Note especially the severe kyphoscoliosis (Fig. 4B, C).

Subpial capillary angiomas provide the greatest diagnostic difficulties. Out of 25 cases, we have never been able to make a definite diagnosis. Spinal angiography was negative in eight cases and suspicious in two. Myelography still remains the most important special diagnostic procedure. The problem in demonstrating them myelographically is the very small size of the angioma and the pathognomonic arachnoiditis which is usually quite extensive. In our first paper (Pia and Vogelsang, 1965), we described the appearance of arachnoiditis in the myelogram as typical for capillary angiomas. An up-to-date review of a larger series essentially confirms the earlier findings of multiple partial holdups. Larger defects in about one-half of the cases are uncharacteristic and do not allow any type diagnosis to be made. In the remainder one finds extensive, streaky filling defects. They are not typically corkscrew-shaped, but still have outpouchings suspicious of angioma and a suggestive serpentine course. The association of the clinical picture of an apoplectiform or remitting course, and a spinal subarachnoid hemorrhage confirms the supposed diagnosis. If the clinical and myelographic localization of the lesion are in agreement, operation is indicated.

Mixed Intradural-Extradural and Global Angiomas

Mixed intradural-extradural angiomas (7) and global angiomas (6) with simultaneous involvement of vertebrae and soft tissues are also arteriovenous cirsoid angiomas. Myelography was done in six patients. Five had an atypical block or partial holdup with irregular borders. It was neither pseudotumoral nor did it correspond to the findings described in the extradural angiomas. Only in one case with a free passage was the lateral compression suggestive of an extradural lesion. First of all the block made one think of an obstruction from an intradural angioma. Typical and atypical angioma filling defects are found regularly. Apart from these findings, the large number of complete blocks should be noted. (Fig. 4D).

Angioblastoma and Angioma

Without going into the problem of combined angioma and angioblastoma (see "Symptomatology"), the myelographic findings in eight out of eleven cases will be discussed. Five

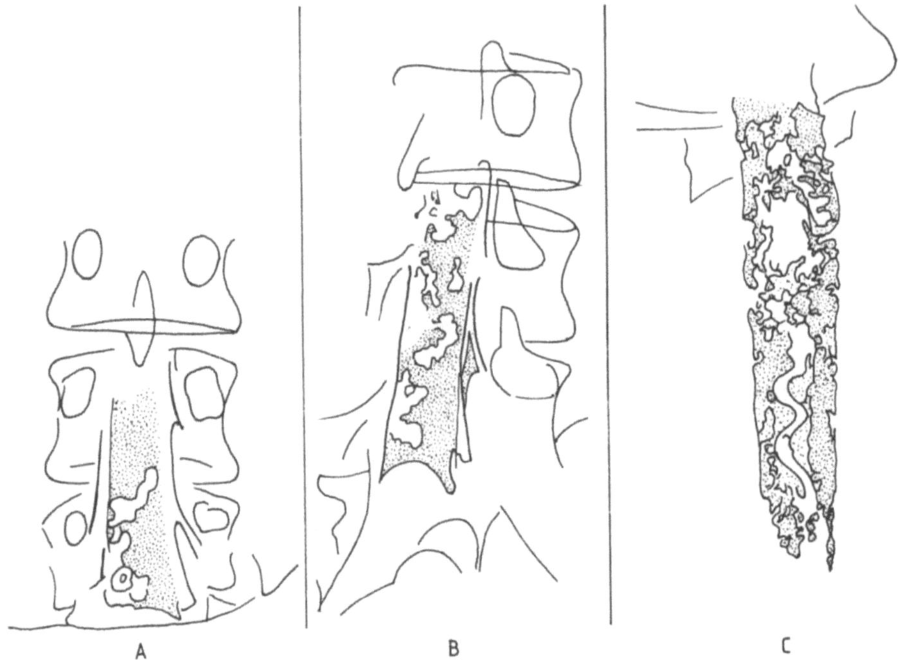

Fig. 5. Myelographic findings in angioblastomas and combined angiomas and angioblastomas. (A, B) Arteriovenous angioma and angioblastoma of cauda equina. Typical tumor block and vascular defects, (C) intramedullary angioblastoma of the cervical cord with extramedullary angiomatous portions

Table 3. Myelographic findings in spinal angiomas

	Number	Complete block	Incomplete block	No block	Typical angioma vessels	Atypical angioma vessels	No vessels demonstrated
Isolated extradural angiomas	22	7	9	6	-	1	21
Vertebro-extradural angiomas	10	2	2	6	-	-	10
Intradural angiomas	39	13	19	7	21	11	7
Combined intrad.-extrad. angiomas	6	4	1	A	2	3	A
Angioblastomas	8	5	3	-	4	4	-
Total	85	31	34	20	27	19	38

patients had a complete and three an incomplete block. The border was usually smooth and curved or helmet-shaped, but could also be irregular with digitate branching. One-half showed typical dilated angioma vessels which corresponded to those of the large subarachnoid arteriovenous angiomas (Fig. 5A, B). With the intramedullary angioblastomas and angiomas, the picture corresponded to that of the solitary intramedullary angiomas. In typical cases, apart from the expansion of the cord, it showed dilated angioma vessels in the region of the tumor and, at the same time, the very dilated efferents (Fig. 5C).

The result of our investigations (Table 3) has established that, without reference to the site and nature, a typical myelographic finding with dilated vascular loops was only present in 27 out of 85 patients (32%). If only the intradural angiomas are considered, the proportion amounts to nearly 50% and with the large subdural angiomas alone, to almost 80%. In 19 cases (20%), there were atypical angioma findings, in 39 (48%), variable evidence of compression. The proportion is particularly high in those with complete and partial blocks. It shows once more the large number of arachnopathies. More important than the mere figures are the varied findings.

Extradural angiomas, as cavernomas, produce particularly frequently a complete or nearly complete obstruction of the spinal subarachnoid space. The margins of a complete or partial block are irregular, streaky, or digitate and cannot always be distinguished from a tumor. More important are irregular lateral, ventral, and dorsal filling defects over a large area, which with vertebroextradural angiomas extend beyond the actual vertebra involved. Occasionally, the edge and the finger-like defects make one think of angioma vessels. Lumbosacral angiomas and also the lumbosacral vascular anomalies produce uncharacteristic appearances, which often resemble those seen in prolapsed intervertebral disks.

Intradural subarachnoid angiomas show the typical finding of the angioma and its efferents, displayed as a negative shadow. The anatomic relationships with the spinal cord are often easily recognizable, so that it is possible to distinguish dorsal, ventral, lateral, and extraintramedullary types. The typical finding remains identifiable, even in the more uncommon cases with a partial block. The myelographic diagnosis of the smaller arteriovenous angiomas and of all late cases is much less clear on account of the associated arachnoiditis. The vessels are adherent to, and merge with, larger filling defects. The picture of the twisted vascular loops becomes less distinct and finally is completely lost. However, atypical vascular defects may be recognizable.

Subpial capillary angiomas which represent about 30% of our intradural angiomas show uncharacteristic arachnoiditic findings, and only occasionally atypical vascular filling defects in addition.

Intramedullary angiomas, hematomas, and angioblastomas have the same sort of myelographic findings as the intramedullary tumors. The angiomatous nature of the lesion becomes clearer, as the more extensive extramedullary portion of the angioma is demonstrated in the myelogram. In these cases, type diagnosis and localization are possible. It is not usually possible to distinguish between angiomas and angioblastomas. However, it must be taken into consideration that even in the other intramedullary tumors – ependymomas and astrocytomas, etc. – dilated vessels in the contrast column are not uncommonly visible (Wyburn-Mason, 1943; Krayenbühl and Yasargil, 1963).

Intra-extradural and global angiomas are distinguished by typical subarachnoid angioma findings, owing to the large number with a complete block.

As selective spinal angiography is only undertaken in a few specialized departments, myelography is the most frequently used contrast investigation. It is still of the greatest significance especially for the early recognition of these lesions. Our experiences show that typical and atypical findings are significantly common and even allow a certain differentiation of the various types. The *decisive thing is* that *there are no negative myelographic findings.* Findings such as tumor and arachnoiditis predominate and indicate the need for further investigation or for operation.

Spinal Phlebography

Spinal phlebography undertaken by transosseous injection or catheter technique is of little significance for the recognition of spinal angiomas (Fishgold et al., 1952; Svien and Baker, 1961; Greitz et al., 1962; Djindjian et al., 1962; Pia and Vogelsang, 1965; Vogelsang, 1963, 1970, 1975). A system of valves in the intradural veins at the point where they perforate the dura interferes with the retrograde injection and demonstration of the intradural venous system (Vogelsang). Thus, even with the use of very considerable pressure, it is not possible to make intradural angiomas visible. Indeed, we have never managed to demonstrate a solitary vertebral angioma. Spinal phlebography shows positive results only with solitary or mixed angiomas of the extradural space, i.e., in solitary extradural, vertebroextradural, and intradural and extradural angiomas. In global angiomas with simultaneous involvement of the soft tissues, the dilated veins in the muscles and connective tissues may be demonstrated.

Characteristic findings are greatly dilated and increased veins, also more rarely convoluted clusters in the extradural space and the paravertebral region (Fig. 6A). In global angiomas, they encroach on the muscles and other soft tissues and here they can form an extensive venous network (Fig. 6B, C). Likewise, besides a possible or doubtful dilatation, one often finds stenoses and interruptions of the extradural veins resulting from the compressive effects of the angioma, which is usually a cavernoma.

Our own experiences with 42 spinal phlebograms in verified angiomas (Table 4) show that 25 (60%) were without pathologic findings. Among the pathologic findings there were nine (21%) extradural angiomatous venous dilatations, usually paravertebral and eight (19%) with uncharacteristic interruption of the extradural venous plexus. The positive findings were particularly frequent in extradural (3/9) and in mixed intraextradural angi-

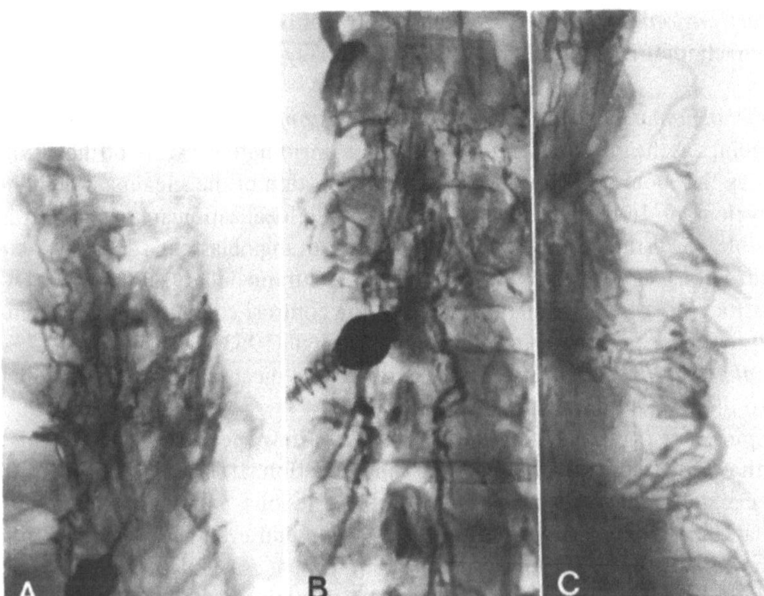

Fig. 6. Spinal phlebographic findings in extradural angiomas. (A) Typical angiomatous venous enlargement, (B, C) global angioma with angiomatous veins extradurally and in the muscle layers

Table 4. Phlebographic findings in spinal angiomas

	Number	Normal	Pathologic findings	
			Pathologic veins	Block
Vertebroextradural angiomas	7	5	1	1
Isolated extradural angiomas	9	4	3	1
Intraextradural angiomas	4	1	3	-
Intradural angiomas	19	13	2	4[a]
Angioblastomas	3	2	-	1
Total	42	25	9	8
%		60%	21%	19%

[a] One patient with postop. phlebography.

omas (3/4); they were uncommon in intradural angiomas (2/19). In spite of the subordinate role of spinal phlebography, when a spinal angioma is suspected clinically, one should not necessarily discard this method of investigation, which is technically simple, is well-tolerated, and free of discomfort. In those departments which are unable to perform selective spinal angiography, its use is recommended before the myelogram is done and in the others, after negative angiography.

Summary

Selective spinal angiography (Djindjian, Di Chiro) is the procedure of choice in the investigation of spinal angiomas and has largely displaced the other contrast studies. Our own experiences confirm this statement, as far as intradural and extradural angiomas are concerned. We have not yet succeeded in demonstrating the small subpial capillary angiomas and the extradural venous angiomas, so that in these cases, after negative selective angiography the indication is to proceed with spinal phlebography and myelography. If there are no technical facilities for performing selective angiography, then myelography is, all the more, the most important method of investigation.

Addendum

Meanwhile water soluble and totally absorbable contrast media (Metrizamide) are available for checking the whole spinal canal. Our findings prove that even small spinal angiomas can be detected with great accuracy. We believe that the use of these contrast media for the initial examination and before angiography will help to achieve an early and correct diagnosis.

Angiography in Angiomas of the Spinal Cord

René Djindjian

Historical Aspects

Since they were originally described around the end of the 19th century, vascular malformations of the spinal cord have been made the object of many classifications, the variety of which is easily understood if one considers that they have been based on the evidence of anatomic observations, both macroscopic and microscopic, and also operative descriptions.

Arteriography has the advantage of showing these malformations in situ and provides a dynamic analysis of the lesions which enables one to consider them from three different aspects.

1. *Classification:* these malformations have one or more arteriovenous shunts and, as in the case of the brain, they are as a rule arteriovenous aneurysms.
2. *Anatomic and clinical factors:* The study of the structure and the different components of these lesions (viz., afferent pedicles, angiomatous tangle of vessels, and drainage pathways) highlights the preferential locations, which are probably related to the embryology, and the clinical characteristics which are common to the malformations in similar locations.
3. *Treatment:* Finally, the preliminary knowledge of the anatomic details of these angiomas offers the possibility of a logical and effective treatment, which is now completely upsetting the prognosis of malformations, which until quite recently were deemed inoperable in the majority of cases.

The angiomas of the spinal cord, mistakenly considered to be a rare condition, are more common than would be thought from the accounts in the literature. The more routine use of selective spinal angiography has allowed one to reveal minimal malformations which escaped demonstration by myelography or total (midstream) aortography and also to revise diagnoses such as disseminated sclerosis or myelitis. One hundred and fifty cases of angioma have been collected in more than 10 years.

Anomalies Suggesting the Diagnosis

Apart from the neurologic findings, the existence of a spinal angioma may sometimes be suspected either because of dysplasic anomalies or else from a study of the plain radiographs or the myelogram.

Discovery of an Associated Dysplasia

The dysplasic origin of the angiomas themselves explains the frequency of associated dysplasias, which we have met with 41 times. The association of a segmental cutaneous or bony angioma (Figs. 4A,B,7C) is the most suggestive. On twelve occasions we have seen a cutaneous angioma, five times a vertebral angioma, and three times the triple association in skin, vertebra, and cord (Cobb's syndrome). Four times the cutaneous angioma has not been segmental and has been of no localizing value.

Among other malformations, the most frequent has been the angiomatosis of Rendu-Osler-Weber (multiple hereditary hemorrhagic telangiectasia) found on eight occasions (Figs. 1A, B, 2A, B); elsewhere we have noted a complex malformation of the lymphatic system (Fig. 4C) in a case of von Recklinghausen's disease, five cases (5) of Klippel-Trenaunay-Weber syndrome (Figs. 5A, B, C, 6A, B, C, D), and also hepatic and splenic angiomatosis.

Straight Radiographs and Tomographs

Analysis of the plain films is able to bring two types of argument to the diagnosis of a spinal angioma.

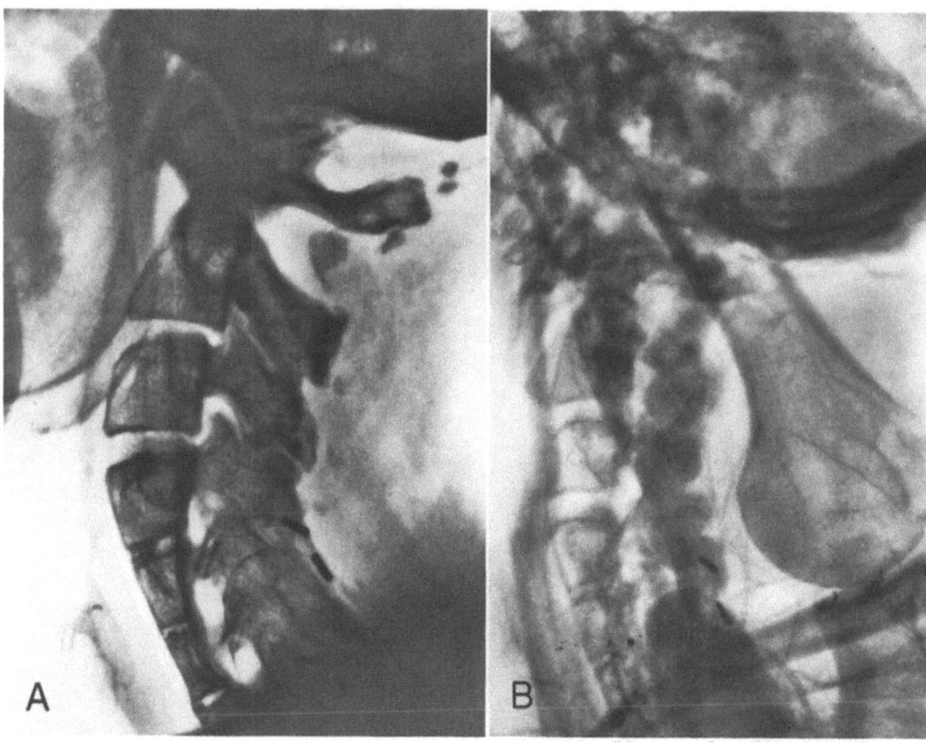

Fig. 1. Diffuse angiomatosis (syndrome of Rendu-Osler-Weber). (A) Marked erosion of the 4th, 5th, 6th and 7th cervical vertebrae (spinal synostosis), (B) Aortography. Huge vascular sac, which explains the bony erosion

1. Some merely reveal the existence of an expanding intraspinal lesion.
2. Others are more specific and indicate the possible presence of a malformation.

The signs of an expanding lesion bear a relation to the size of the malformation and of its draining veins.

1. Enlargement of the spinal canal is the most common (15 times) the size of the malformations in the cervical region explaining the preponderance at this level (ten times) (Figs. 1A, B, 3A, B, C, D).
2. Erosion of a pedicle (eleven times) (Fig. 2A, B) is basically due to the size of the draining veins. Erosion of the posterior aspect of a vertebral body is more uncommon (four cases).

In fifteen patients, a scoliosis or a kyphoscoliosis was significantly related to the lesion.

The etiologic localizing signs are epitomized by the segmental vertebral angioma met with on only five occasions, even though the appearance was not characteristic. One may mention the possibility of calcification in the center of the malformation (one case) and

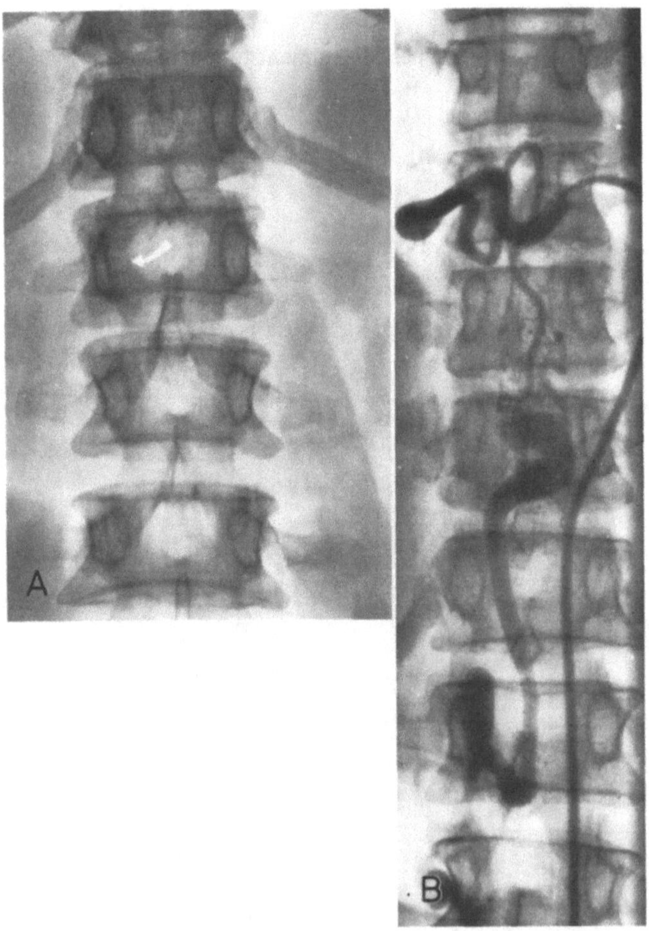

Fig. 2. Diffuse angiomatosis (Rendu-Osler-Weber). (A) Erosion of the pedicle of L 1 on the right (arrow), (B) Spinal angioma with a huge vascular sac supplied by the dilated artery of Adamkiewicz (coming from the 10th R. intercostal artery) and draining into a dilated radiculomedullary vein, which is eroding the vertebral pedicle

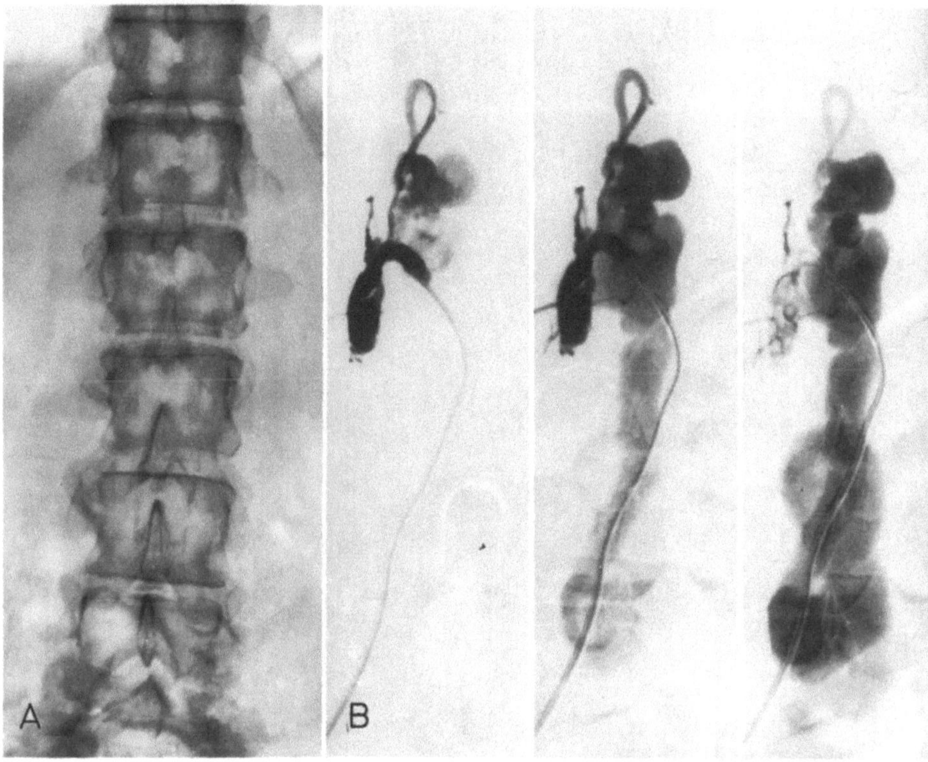

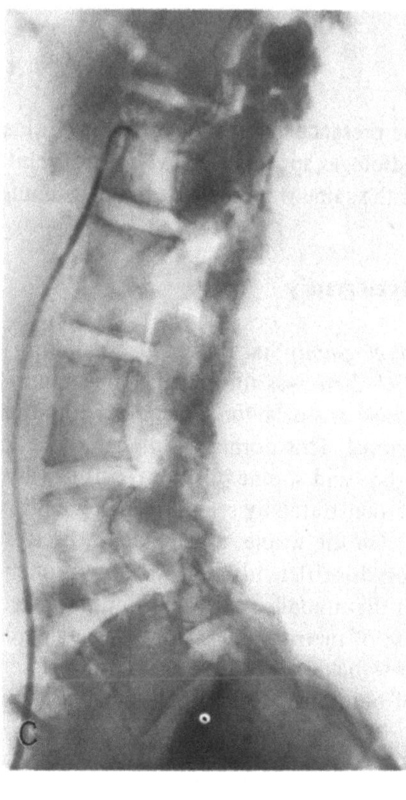

Fig. 3. Spinal angioma with marked bony erosion simulating a giant tumor of the cauda equina. (A) Routine plain films (AP) showing marked widening of the interpedicular distances, (B) Anteroposterior arteriogram filling a huge angioma fed by the 2nd right lumbar artery, (C) Erosion of the vertebral bodies at five levels, (D) Lateral arteriogram. The venous dilatations explain the bony erosions

Fig. 3 D. see reverse side

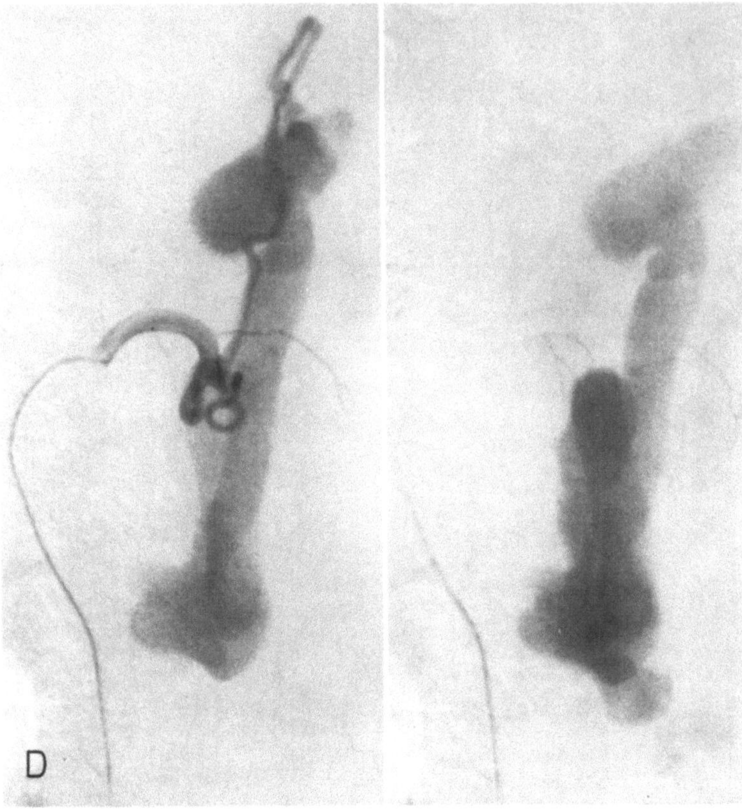

Fig. 3D

the presence in five cases of a spina bifida in its neighborhood. With regard to these various radiologic appearances, we would point out that in *one-third* of *the cases* the radiographs of the spine were of value in determining the anatomic localization.

Myelography

Myelography has proved to be abnormal in 93% of the cases in which it has been done; in 62% there was the specific appearance of an angioma; and in 31% there was evidence of a block or a delay on screening, without any typical appearance. In 7% the appearances were normal. This normal result cannot be confirmed until after repeated screening in both the prone and supine positions. It is usually seen in those smaller angiomas which can only be demonstrated by selective angiography.

On the whole, myelography often leads to the diagnosis of angioma, but when the history is sufficiently suggestive, it is much preferable to consider angiography straight away, as the myodil is a serious hindrance to obtaining subtraction films of the angiograms. The use of metrizamide* is now changing certain of our ideas. Apart from the fact that it is absorbable and thus does not interfere with subsequent angiography, it has the advantage of outlining perfectly the spinal cord, and by screening in supine and prone positions, one

*Metrizamide (Amipaque = 2- (3-acetamido-5N-methyl acetamido-2, 4, 6- tri-iodobenzamido)-2 deoxy-D-Glucose. Synthesized by Nyegaard & Co., Oslo.

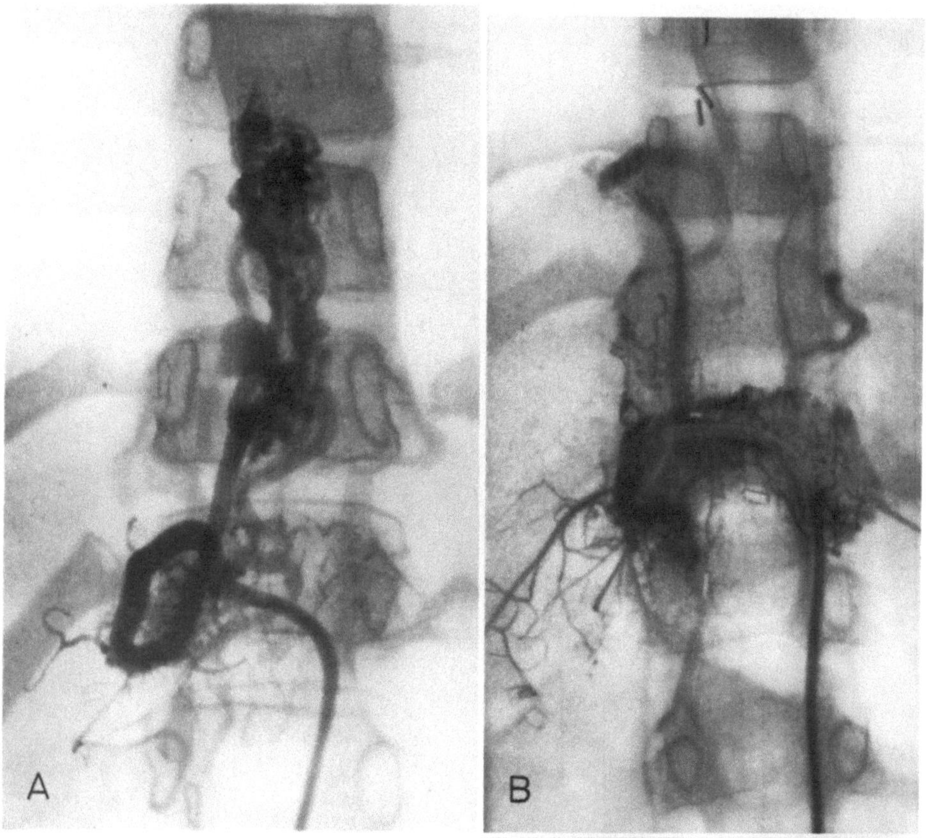

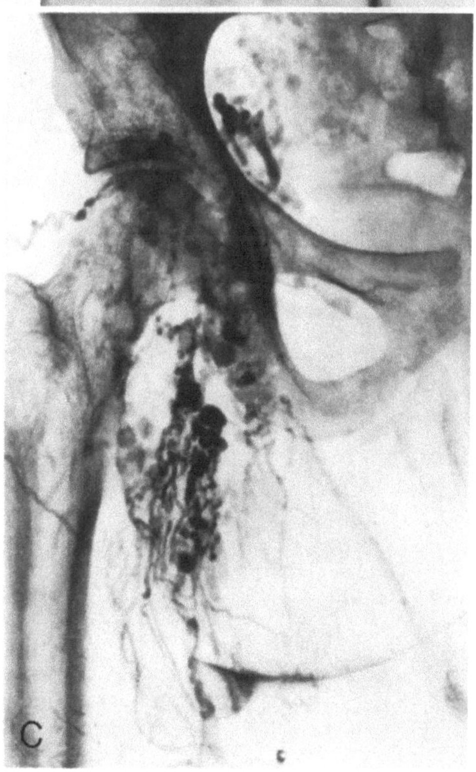

Fig. 4. Spinal angioma with lymphatic dysplasia and an angioma of the vertebral body, in a case of von Recklinghausen's disease. (A) Posterior spinal pedicle of the angioma arising from the 12th right intercostal artery, (B) After excision of the angioma, one is able to see much more clearly the diffuse opacification of the angiomatous vertebra, (C) Lymphography. Very large, varicose iliac and crural lymphatics on the right, with lymphoedema of the right lower limb. Also rectal, vesical, and vaginal lymphorrhagia

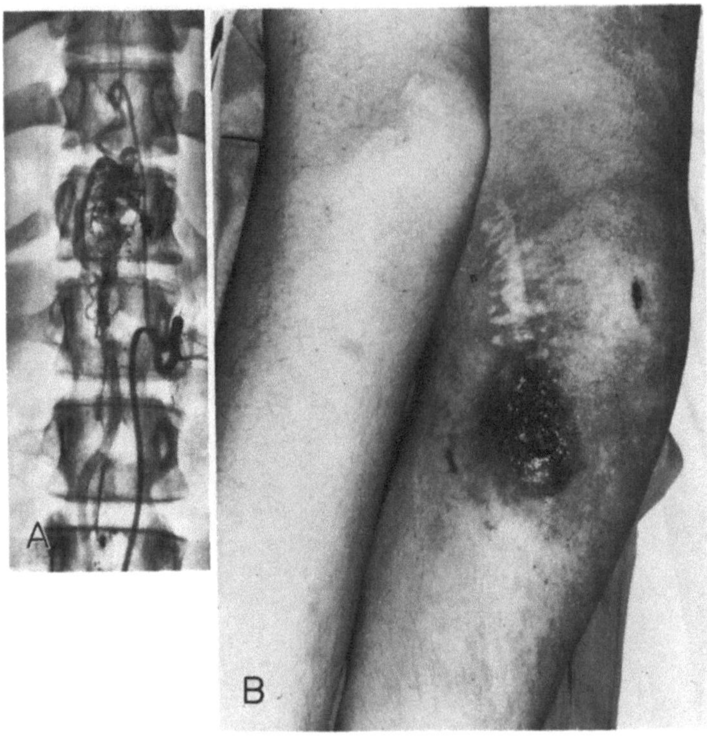

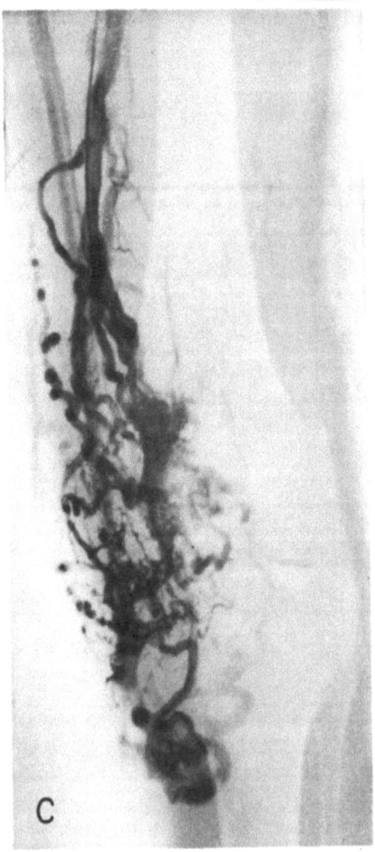

Fig. 5. Spinal angioma and a Klippel-Trenaunay syndrome. (A) Intramedullary angioma fed by the artery of Adamkiewicz, arising from the first left lumbar artery, (B) Marked edema of the left lower limb with ulceration resistant to all treatment, (C) Huge angioma of the leg, filled from the left femoral artery

can sometimes see malformations of quite small size. In this way, when it is positive, it encourages one to perform angiography more readily on a patient who may have been reluctant to undergo this examination.

Actually there are no pathognomonic myelographic appearances for a spinal angioma. If the myelogram is positive, it may equally well suggest an angioma as a vascular tumor (hemangioblastoma, Fig. 8A, B, or ependymoma); furthermore, myelography does not claim to have any localizing value and still less for locating the feeding vessels of the malformation. The worm-like patterns at the level of the cauda equina can simulate a vascular malformation, angiography has been negative, and at operation a typical "redundant nerve root" has been found (Fig. 8C).

Air Myelography

Air myelography (Fig. 8D, E) is contraindicated whenever the diagnosis is suspected because the withdrawal of a large amount of CSF is dangerous. Carried out eight times in our series, it has caused a sudden and serious deterioration in the condition of two patients. Its only positive contribution is to demonstrate the swollen appearance of the cord in certain very large intramedullary angiomas.

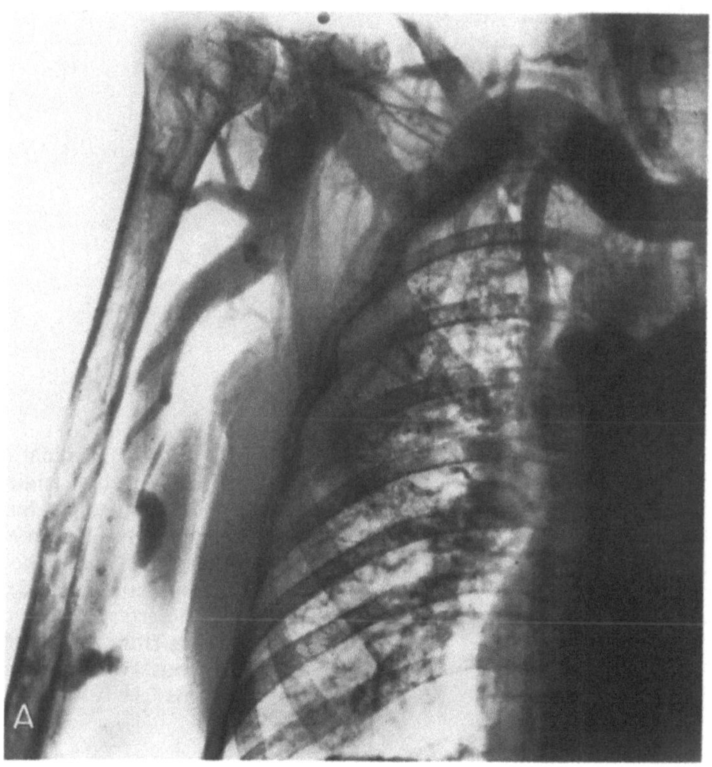

Fig. 6 A.
Legend see next page

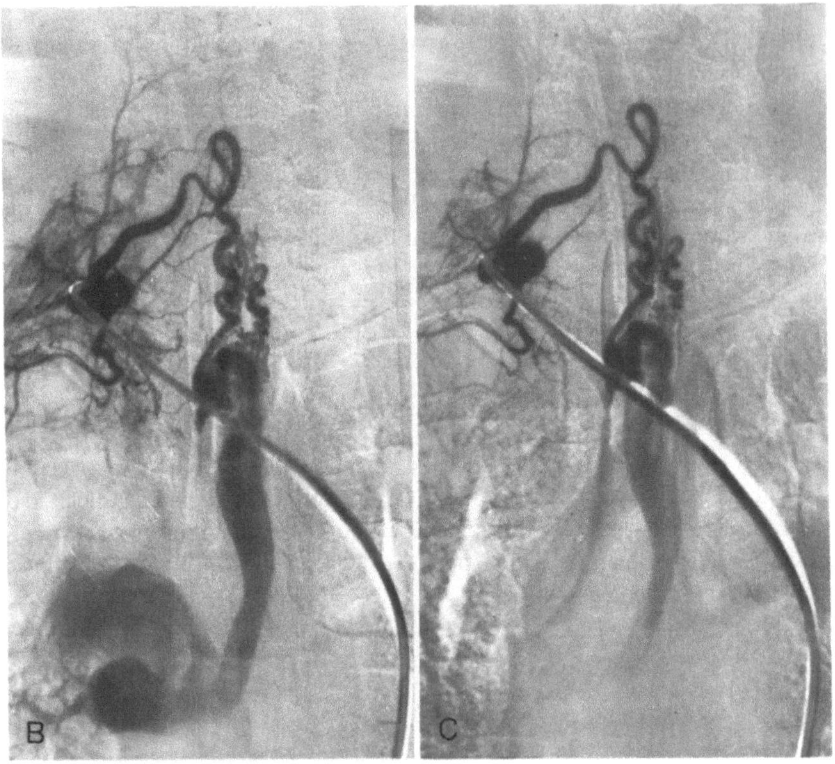

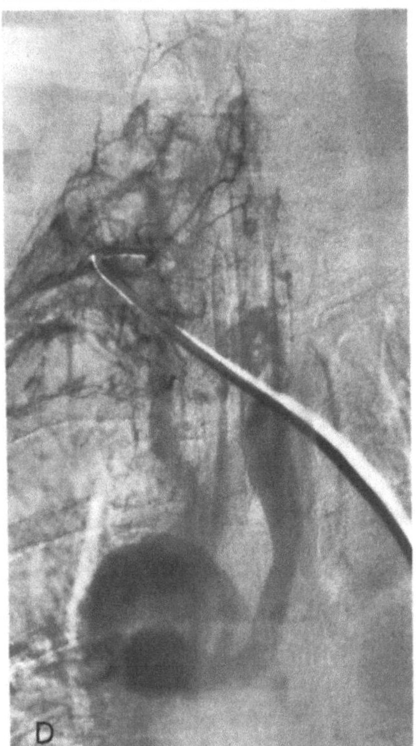

Fig. 6 B-D. Spinal angioma associated with a vertebral angioma and an angioma of the right upper limb. (A) Dilatation of the subclavian artery and of the brachial artery explaining the excavated lesion of the humerus, (B,D,C) Spinal angioma fed by the artery of the cervical enlargement arising from the deep cervical artery (R). Copious venous drainage toward the azygos

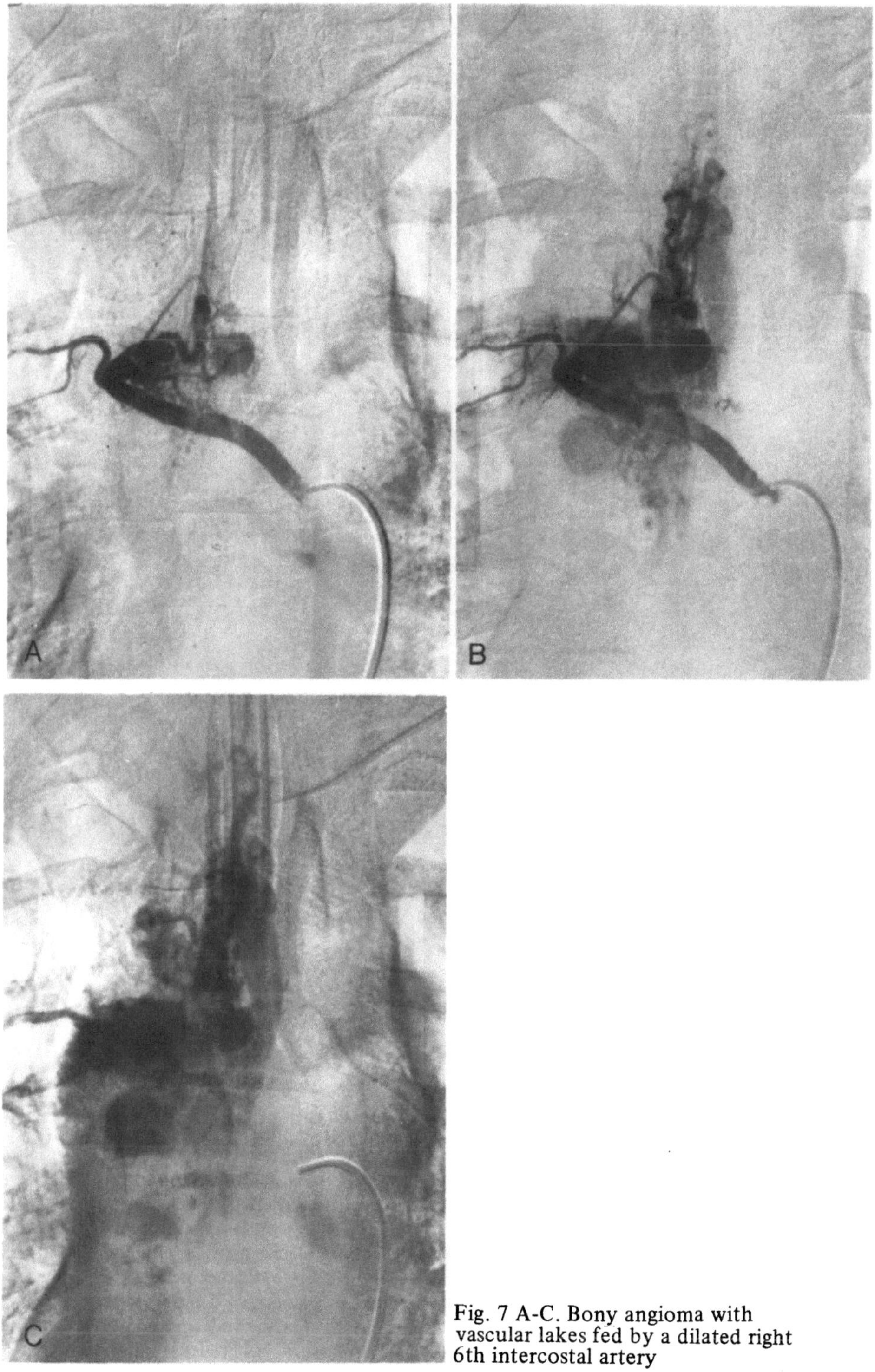

Fig. 7 A-C. Bony angioma with vascular lakes fed by a dilated right 6th intercostal artery

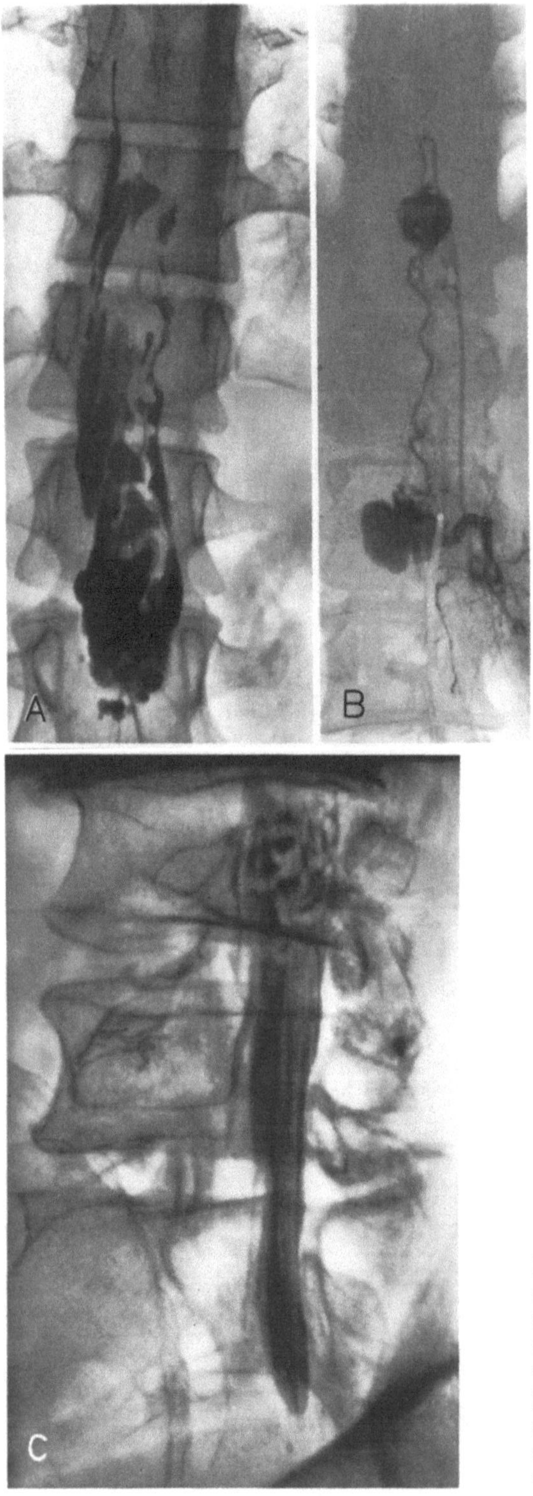

Fig. 8 A - C. Myeolography (positive contrast). (A, B) Vascular patterns due to two tumors without any blockage of the contrast. Hemangioblastomas with huge draining veins, (C) Worm-like patterns (dimer-X) at the level of L 3. Normal angiography. At the operation a "redundant nerve root" was found

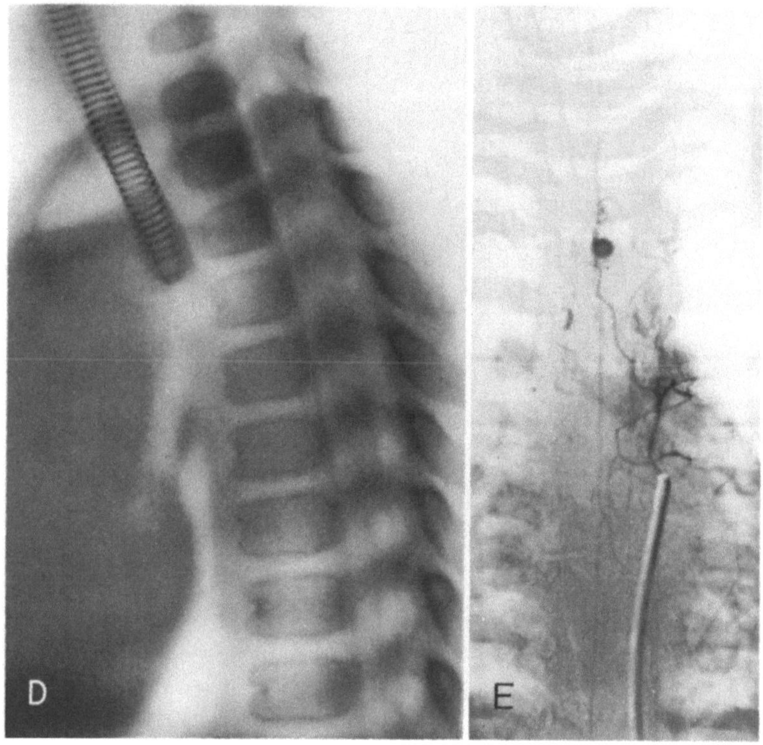

Fig. 8 D and E. Normal air myelography associated with a small pseudoaneurysmal angioma in the upper dorsal region

The Angiographic Investigation

Angiography is the essential step in the investigation and study of the malformation. Regardless of context, it constitutes the indispensable examination. Just as one would not consider exploring and treating a cerebral angioma without angiographic studies, one cannot conceive the diagnosis and discussion of treatment of a spinal angioma without arteriography. The diagnostic precision of this method is very great, the only cause of failure being represented by the extremely rare malformations which are excluded from the circulation as a result of total or partial thrombosis of the feeding vessels. The dynamic impression of the malformation on the successive films of the series allows one to verify the true nature of the lesions (arteriovenous aneurysms), while at the same time it locates the constituent parts (afferent arterial pedicles, angiomatous mass, venous efferents) with a remarkable anatomic precision which is indispensable in making decisions about treatment.

Spinal angiography allows one to make an assessment of the angioma. The results of this study are set out diagrammatically showing tracings of the arteriographic films, and it will include the afferent pedicles with their level of entry and their anterior or posterior destination, the malformation, the extent of the venous pedicles and efferents, and the

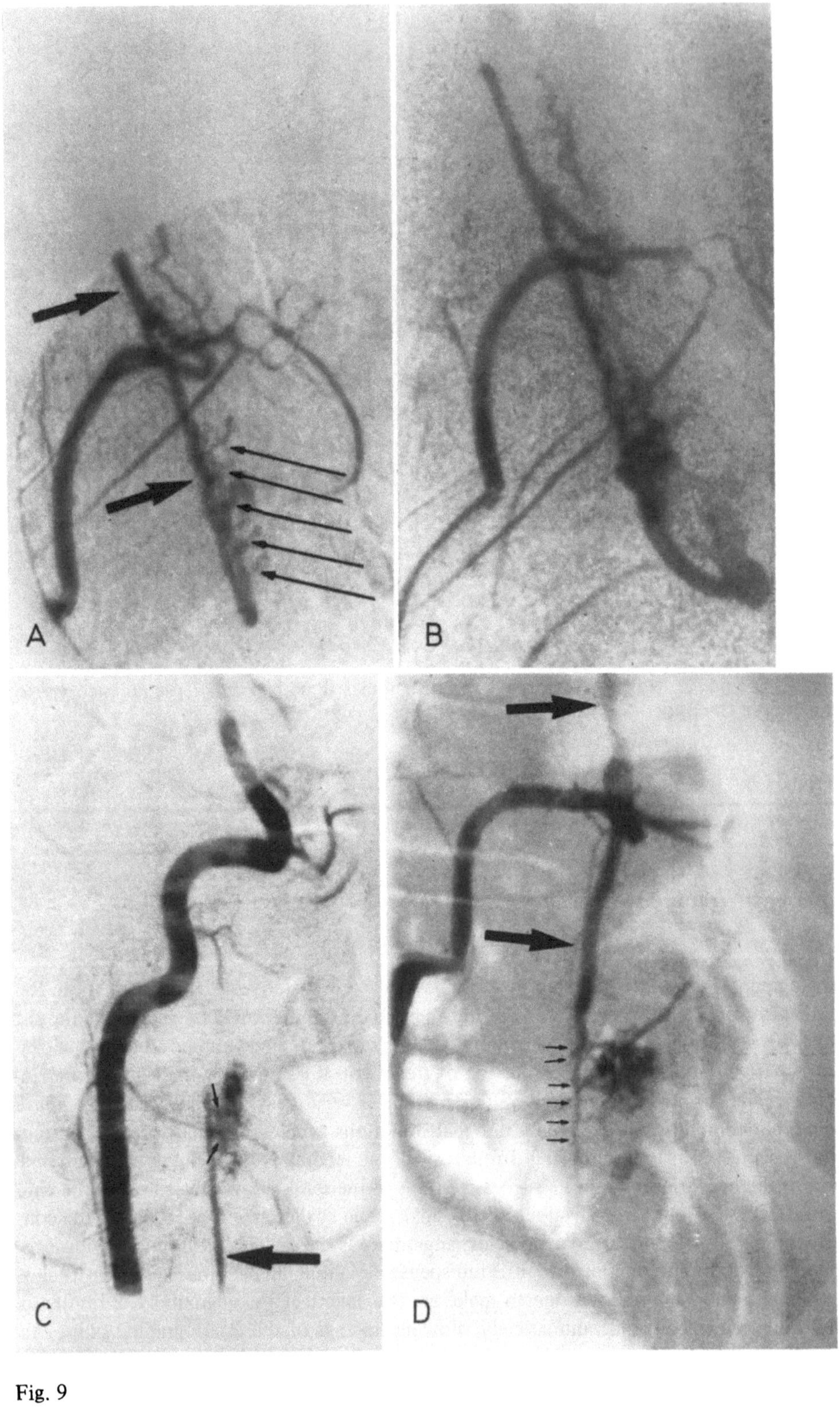

Fig. 9

origin, penetration, and appearance of the spinal (radiculomedullary) arteries in the neighborhood of the angioma. The results of treatment (operation or embolization) are controlled later, by a further angiogram.

Analytic Study

Feeding Vessels

Number
In 30% of cases, there is one feeding artery; in 70% of cases, there are several. In certain cases, we have found up to ten feeding arteries. In the midthoracic region, we have seen feeders ascending from the first lumbar artery or descending from the vertebral artery.

Diameter
1. In general the cervical, intercostal, or lumbar artery supplying the feeding vessel (anterior or posterior radiculomedullary) is dilated, constituting a real "mega-artery" (Fig. 2B). The ascending and descending branches of the feeding vessels are often very tortuous and are superimposed on a dilated anterior or posterior spinal vein (Fig. 12A, B, C); this fact accounts for the vascular patterns with a double outline which one sometimes sees on myelography.
2. Sometimes the pedicle is normal in size and the spinal artery is not dilated either; it feeds an angioma of moderate size. The demonstration of bifid intercostal arteries with a common trunk encourages the search for a malformation (Figs. 12B, 14C, D), because an angioma may very well be attached to such an abnormal vessel.
3. Exceptionally, the pedicle is stenosed, and in these cases, it is necessary to make serial exposures over a long period in order to demonstrate the draining veins, which may appear quite late.

Origin
1. Intramedullary angiomas are fed by *the anterior spinal arteries*. The increase in size of these arteries enables one to opacify the dilated sulcocommissural arteries (Fig. 9A, B, C, D). Well-localized lateral films on a rapid serial angiogram allow one to see these arterioles, usually three to six in number, which are entering the anterior aspect of the cord and opacifying the intramedullary angioma on the later films.

In the cervical region, the anterior feeding arteries are: the anterior spinal artery, originating from the terminal portion of the vertebral, the radicular arteries C 3, C 4, C 5, and C 6 (Fig. 10A) which come from one or both vertebral arteries, and the artery of the cervical enlargement (Fig. 6B, C, D), which may arise either from the vertebral or the deep cervical arteries. Furthermore, it is not unusual in the lower two-thirds of the cervical cord

---

◀ Fig. 9. Sulcocommissural arteries. Their dilatation in the angiomas allows them to be demonstrated by arteriography (serial pictures, 3 at the start of the injection). (A, B) Dorsal intramedullary angioma fed by an upper dorsal radiculomedullary artery. The sulcal arteries can be seen (arrows). On the later films the angiomatous mass can be seen and a draining vein leaving the inferior pole of the angioma, (C) Cervical intramedullary angioma fed by the ascending branch of the artery of the cervical enlargement (large arrow). (D) Dorsolumbar intramedullary angioma fed by the artery of Adamkiewicz (large arrows). Sulcal arteries (little arrows) opacifying the angioma

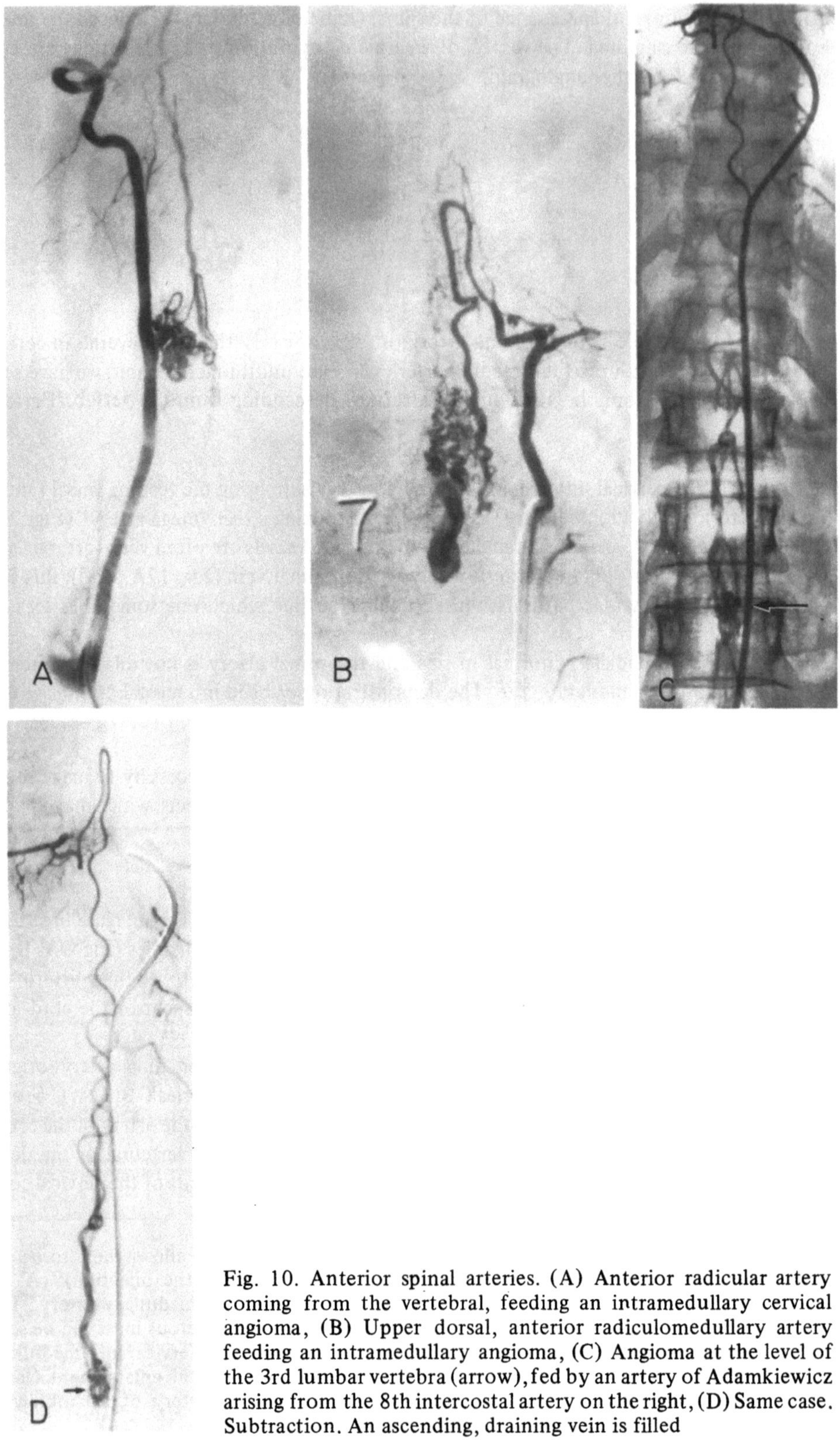

Fig. 10. Anterior spinal arteries. (A) Anterior radicular artery coming from the vertebral, feeding an intramedullary cervical angioma, (B) Upper dorsal, anterior radiculomedullary artery feeding an intramedullary angioma, (C) Angioma at the level of the 3rd lumbar vertebra (arrow), fed by an artery of Adamkiewicz arising from the 8th intercostal artery on the right, (D) Same case. Subtraction. An ascending, draining vein is filled

to find the anterior afferents originating from the highest intercostal arteries, afferents which are reaching the lower pole of the malformation. As a general rule, the cervical angiomas have multiple pedicles, and it is quite common to observe the development of fresh pedicles after ligation or embolization of the angioma, if a complete excision of the angiomatous mass is not performed.

In the dorsal region, the feeding artery is the anterior superior radiculomedullary artery which may arise on the right or the left, from the third, fourth or fifth intercostal arteries (Figs. 7A, B, C, 10B); very often these arteries arise from a common trunk, ascending from the fourth or fifth intercostal artery and from this trunk the fourth, third, and second intercostal arteries arise. The radiculomedullary artery is often dilated, and its ascending branch may opacify an angioma in the region of C 6 - C 7; its descending branch may opacify an intramedullary angioma sometimes situated as low as D 6 or D 7; this shows the necessity of demonstrating this artery in order to avoid missing an angioma. Filling of the artery of the cervical enlargement and the artery of Adamkiewicz may not opacify an upper dorsal angioma.

In the dorsolumbar region, the feeding artery is the artery of Adamkiewicz (Fig. 10C, D). Sometimes a veritable mega-artery, it may opacify an intramedullary angioma extending from D 5 to the conus medullaris. The presence of a supplementary artery of Adamkiewicz around D 7 or D 8, when the artery of Adamkiewicz is low, is often difficult to demonstrate, on account of the vascular "steal" caused by the angioma. In the lower dorsolumbar region, the angioma may be fed by the artery of Adamkiewicz coming from an intercostal or lumbar artery and also by a lumbosacral radicular artery coming from the common iliac.

2. The posteriorly situated angiomas are fed by *the posterior spinal arteries.* The pedicle may be very dilated and tortuous or, on the contrary with the small angiomas, it may be nearly normal in size.

In the cervical region, the feeding vessels are multiple, most frequently coming from both sides simultaneously, from the vertebral and the deep cervical arteries. In the upper third of the cervical cord, the posterior spinal artery coming from the vertebral artery often takes part and in the lower two-thirds, the ascending branches of the posterior spinal coming from the highest intercostal arteries take part.

In the dorsal region, it is not unusual to find several posterior spinal pedicles (Fig. 11A), but in certain cases, we have observed one solitary posterior spinal feeder opacifying an angioma with large draining veins. This is to stress the importance of demonstrating without exception all the intercostal arteries from D 2 - D 7; the omission of the injection of one of these branches which may be difficult to catheterize because their orifices are small and very close to each other, risks missing the angioma.

In the dorsolumbar region, the feeding vessel may be a solitary posterior spinal artery (Fig. 11B) in the little malformations, or several posterior spinal arteries in the large ones. Anastomoses between the posterior spinal arteries are not uncommon in this region, when one considers the frequency of the posterior vertebral anastomoses.

3. *The mixed angiomas* are those which are both intramedullary and retromedullary in the same segment, thus forming a huge angiomatous mass. On the lateral films, this angiomatous mass is often shown in two separate parts, one anterior fed by the anterior radiculomedullary artery and the other posterior, fed by a posterior spinal artery. Mixed angiomas are fed either by an artery of the lumbar or cervical enlargement comprising an anterior and a posterior spinal artery coming from a common trunk, or by one or several posterior spinal arteries and an artery of Adamkiewicz arising at another level, sometimes quite remote.

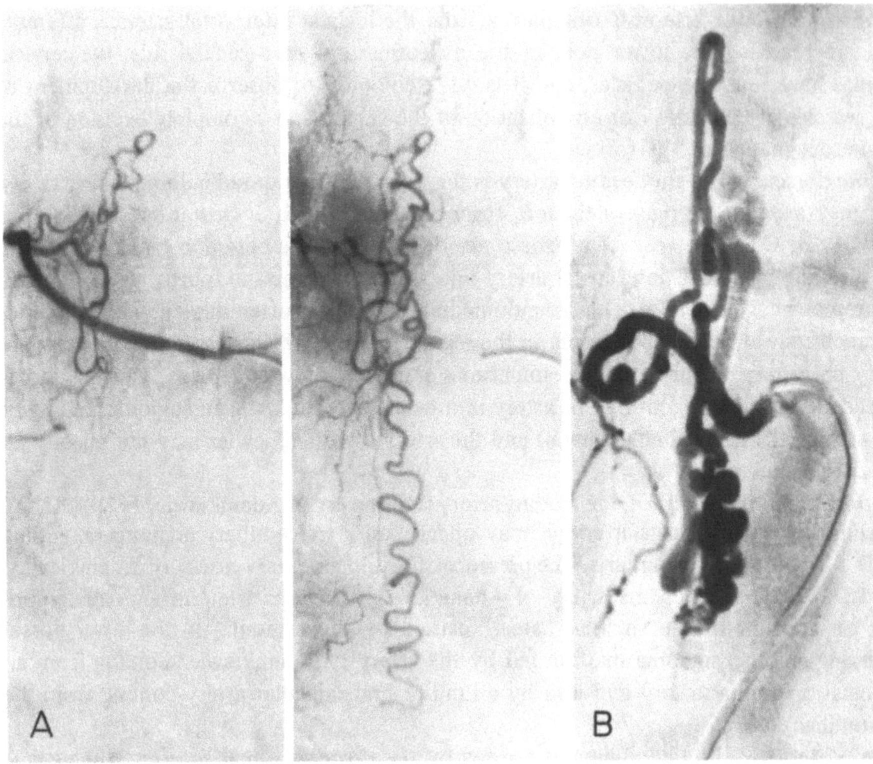

Fig. 11. Posterior spinal arteries. (A) Upper dorsal, retromedullary angioma, fed by a posterior spinal artery coming from the 6th intercostal artery (R), (B) Dorsolumbar retromedullary angioma, fed by a posterior spinal artery coming from the 1st right lumbar artery

The Angiomatous Mass

This appears in the form of dilated vessels intermingled one with the other, having a mulberry-like appearance.

1. It is of variable size, sometimes small and difficult to see, especially if it is obscured by myodil residues. Sometimes there is a simple arteriovenous fistula without any detectable angiomatous mass (Fig. 12A, B, C). Most often the angioma is of a moderate size, although sometimes it is very large, covering several segments. In these cases the feeding vessels are multiple.

2. In cases of *Rendu-Osler-Weber's disease* (eight cases), the angiomatous mass is often huge with greatly dilated feeding arteries and draining veins which are also very dilated, covering the whole length of the spinal cord. In all the cases we have seen very large venous lakes, sometimes huge and eroding the bony pedicles, sometimes even scalloping the posterior aspect of the bodies of two to three vertebrae (Figs. 1, 2, 13D). This spinal pattern where the arterial dysplasia is associated with a venous dysplasia seems characteristic of the spinal angiomas seen in this condition.

3. In a few cases we have seen spontaneous thrombosis of intramedullary angiomas, either a partial thrombosis with obstruction of the draining veins or a total one. In these cases it is not possible to demonstrate the angioma by angiography, but its existence has been con-

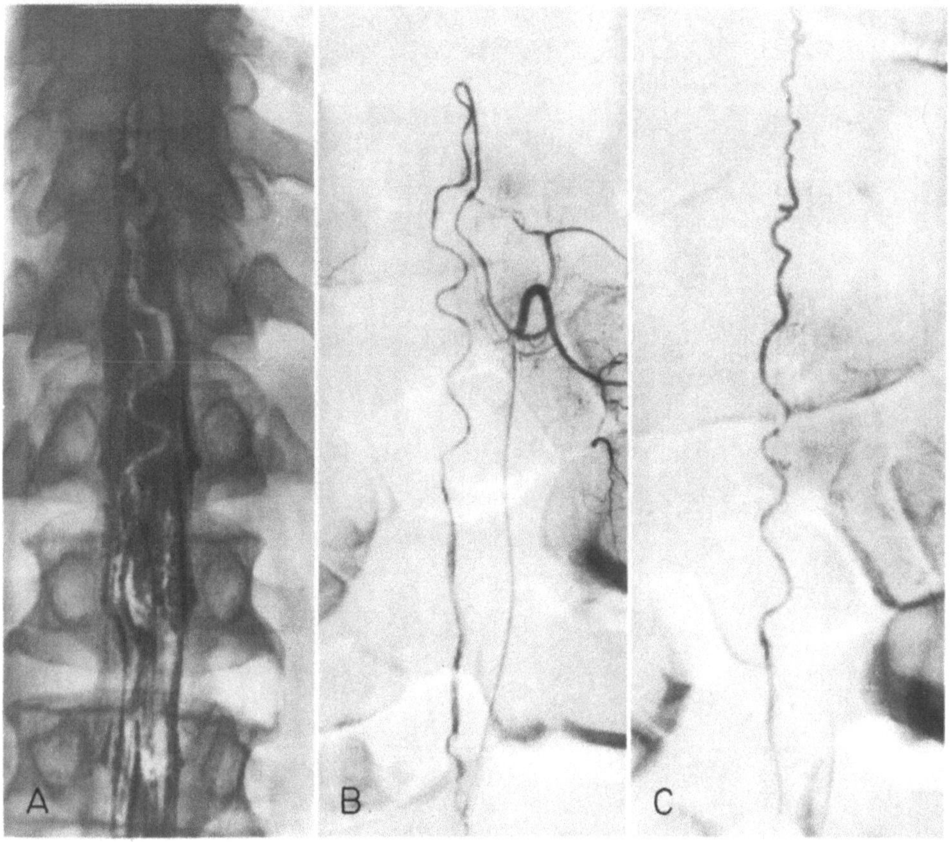

Fig. 12. Simple arteriovenous fistula. (A) Myelography. Double vascular pattern corresponding to the arteries and the veins, (B) Very large artery of Adamkiewicz coming from a bifid intercostal D 11, D 12 (L). Tortuous descending branch, which changes in size and opens directly into a vein, (C) Draining vein

firmed by exploratory laminectomy prompted by the appearance of huge vascular patterns on the positive contrast myelogram.

*Arteriovenous Malformations and Spinal Arterial Aneurysms**

The protean appearance of these arteriovenous malformations explains the wide disparity in the angiographic appearance, which may just as much present a classic appearance as to be simplified to the extreme as a simple arteriovenous fistula, or by reason of its size to mimic a tumor or else a "pseudoectasia" simulating an arterial aneurysm (Fig. 13C, D). Recent publications (Di Chiro and Wener, 1973; Vogelsang and Dietz, 1975; Merry and Appleton, 1976) have given accounts of arterial malformations which were isolated or associated with arteriovenous malformations, and do not agree with the observations in our series of 150 cases.

*This section is by the courtesy of Dr. Michel Djindjian.

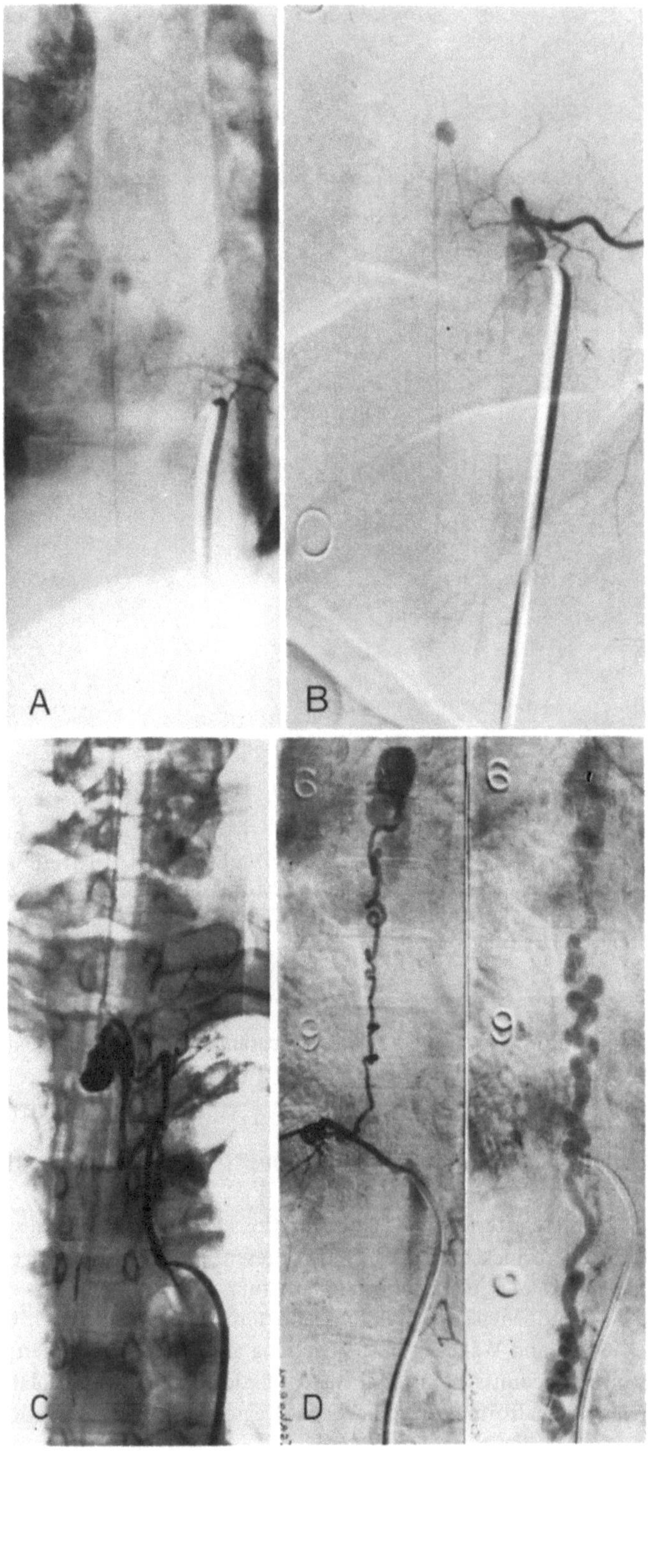

Fig. 13 A - D

In actual fact, in more than 3000 spinal arteriograms, we have only come across one case of a pure arterial aneurysm (Fig. 13A, B). On the other hand, in our series of 90 arteriovenous malformations, we have found pseudoectasic appearances 18 times (20%); in eight their exact nature has been histologically confirmed after a radical operation (Fig. 13C), and in the other ten cases which have been treated palliatively it has been suspected from the angiograms. In three cases, the appearance at arteriography and at operation was that of an arterial globe or sac connected to an adjacent arteriovenous malformation (Fig. 14A, B); in the five other cases, the sac represented the center of the arteriovenous malformation with arterial pedicles and venous efferents. We were able to observe in two cases structural modifications in these intramedullary angiomas. The discovery of an angioma with a branching angiomatous mass on the anterior spinal axis has made us postpone operation or embolization. Two years later, one of these patients presented with a complete flaccid paraplegia and at angiography the angioma had an aneurysmal appearance (Fig. 14C, D).

If arterial aneurysms occur in the spinal canal they can only be regarded as exceptional and we cannot detect any association – arterial aneurysm / arteriovenous malformation – in any of the eight cases where we have had histologic verification (i.e., of a dysplasic vessel and not an arterial aneurysm).

We do not share the opinion of Di Chiro and Wener (1973) on the almost constant presence of subarachnoid hemorrhage and the association of arterial aneurysms and arteriovenous malformations. As a matter of fact, in our three cases where we suspected the association "arterial aneurysm/arteriovenous malformation," we found one subarachnoid hemorrhage with hematomyelia and central softening (*"en crayon"*) and two patients with a clear fluid whose symptoms were explained in one by a central spinal softening and in the other by an intrasaccular thrombosis. In the five cases of solitary aneurysmal sacs, there were two subarachnoid hemorrhages and three ischemic episodes. This total of three cases out of eight approximates to the frequency of subarachnoid hemorrhage in arteriovenous malformations (41%).

The Draining Veins

The draining veins of the angiomas are always very large and very extensive; in certain cases, they extend over the whole length of the spinal cord. These dilated veins in certain cases take on a pseudoaneurysmal appearance, the size varying from that of a pea up to huge vascular masses (Figs. 13D, 15A, B). The draining veins are the dilated normal veins of the spinal cord (Fig. 16A). They therefore show the same features:

1. The anterior spinal vein runs on the anterior aspect of the cord behind the anterior spinal artery in the anterior median fissure. It drains intramedullary angiomas.
2. The posterior spinal vein runs centrally on the posterior aspect of the cord, without any accompanying artery. It drains the retromedullary angiomas. The anterior and posterior spinal veins are clearly seen in the lateral views whereas they are superimposed in the AP views. Sometimes in the dorsal region, they are duplicated and difficult to identify separately.

◀ Fig. 13. Spinal arterial and arteriovenous aneurysms. (A) True arterial aneurysm situated at the bifurcation of the descending branch of the artery of Adamkiewicz (the latter arises from the 11th *left* intercostal artery), (B) Same case. Subtraction. The arterial aneurysm can be seen without the draining veins, (C) Pseudoaneurysmal appearance of an angioma. Aneurysmal sac with an angiomatous mass and draining veins. This is an arteriovenous aneurysm, (D) Vascular sac of a spinal angioma, in a case of Rendu-Osler-Weber disease

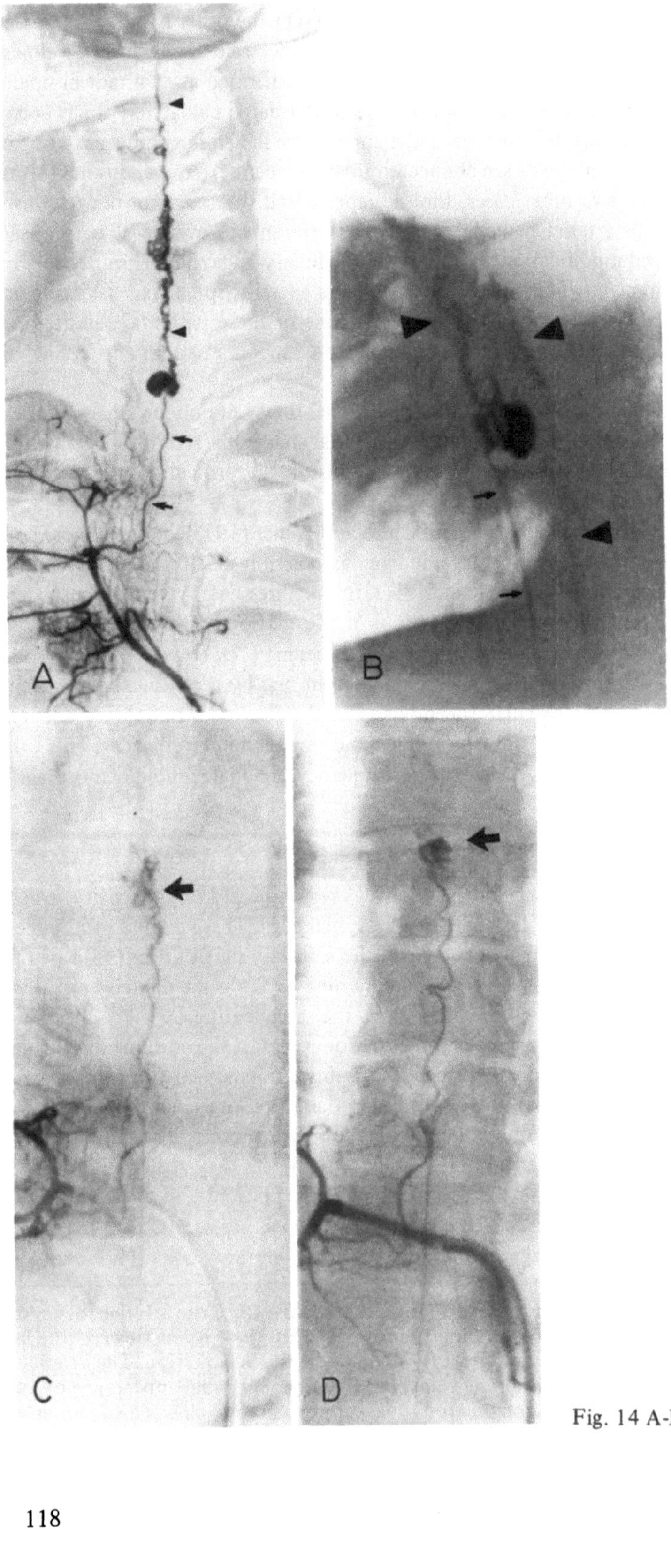

Fig. 14 A-D

3. It is not unusual to find a communication between the anterior and posterior spinal veins (Fig. 26C); thus, certain retromedullary angiomas are drained not only by the posterior, but also by the anterior spinal veins, and in contrast to the intramedullary angiomas, they can be drained by the anterior and posterior spinal veins. The communications are common in the dorsolumbar region. This communication is most frequently perispinal, but sometimes it is the venous channel, described by Suh and Alexander (1939), actually passing right through the cord and providing a communication between the anterior and posterior spinal veins.

Termination of the Anterior and Posterior Spinal Veins

These veins drain away in three directions: laterally through the radicular veins, inferiorly toward the sacral veins, and upward toward the mesencephalic veins. It is because of these veins, dilated by the angioma, that we have been able to follow and recognize in vivo the precise termination of the spinal veins.

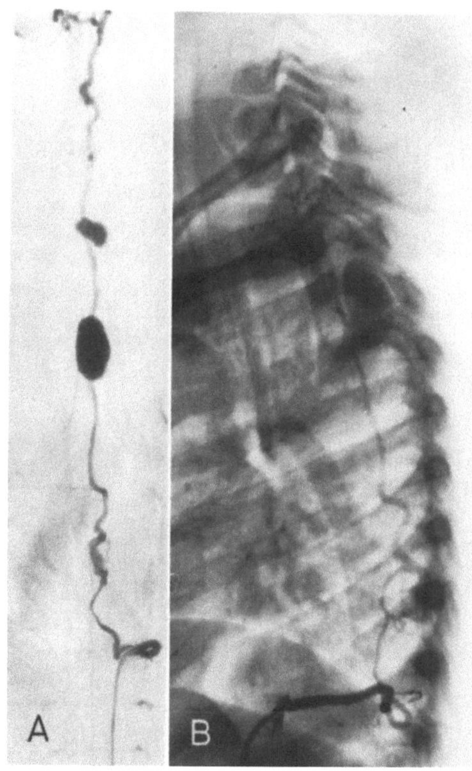

Fig. 15. Pseudoaneurysmal appearances found on the draining veins. (A) Dorsal angioma fed by the artery of Adamkiewicz (9th left intercostal artery). Two vascular sacs on an ascending draining vein, (B) Same case. Lateral view. The two vascular sacs are shown

◀ Fig. 14. Pseudoaneurysmal appearances with spinal angiomas. (A) Pseudoaneurysmal appearance, fed by an upper dorsal radiculomedullary artery (small arrows); draining veins leaving the upper pole of the aneurysmal sac (short arrows), (B) Same case. Lateral view. Intramedullary position of the aneurysmal sac between the anterior and posterior spinal veins (short arrows), (C) Dorsal intramedullary angioma fed by the ascending branch of the artery of Adamkiewicz (common trunk of 9th and 10th intercostal arteries). No operation, (D) Same case. Change in the appearance of the angioma into an aneurysmal sac (patient presented with an acute flaccid paraplegia)

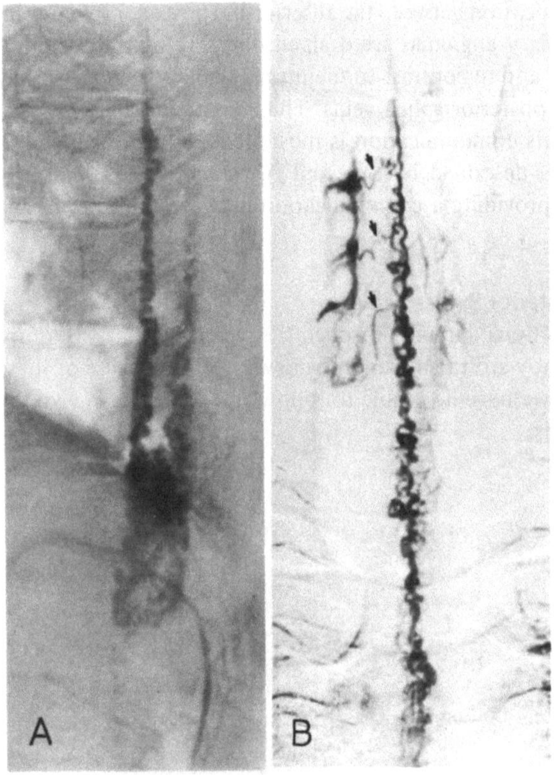

Fig. 16. Spinal veins in the angiomas. (A) Lateral. Anterior and posterior spinal veins in the dorsolumbar region (dorsolumbar angioma), (B) Radiculomedullary veins (arrows) between the spinal veins and the spinal venous plexuses

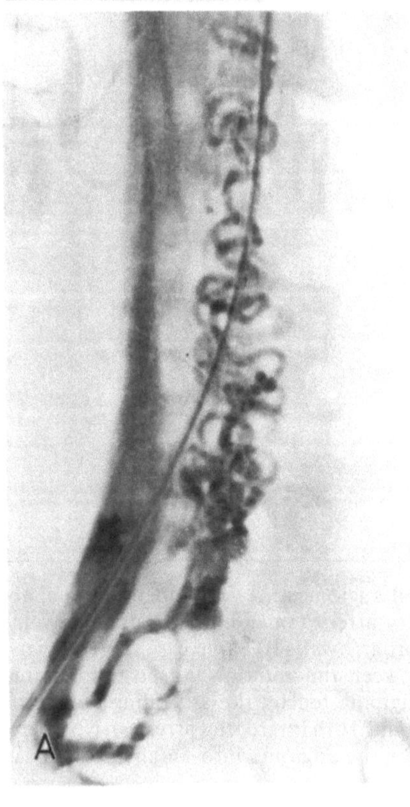

Fig. 17. Termination of the spinal draining veins. (A) Drainage downward by the sacral veins with opacification of the inferior vena cava, (B) Drainage toward the azygos vein from a dorsal angioma, (C) Drainage toward the spinal plexuses from a cervical angioma, (D) Intracerebral drainage from a cervical angioma

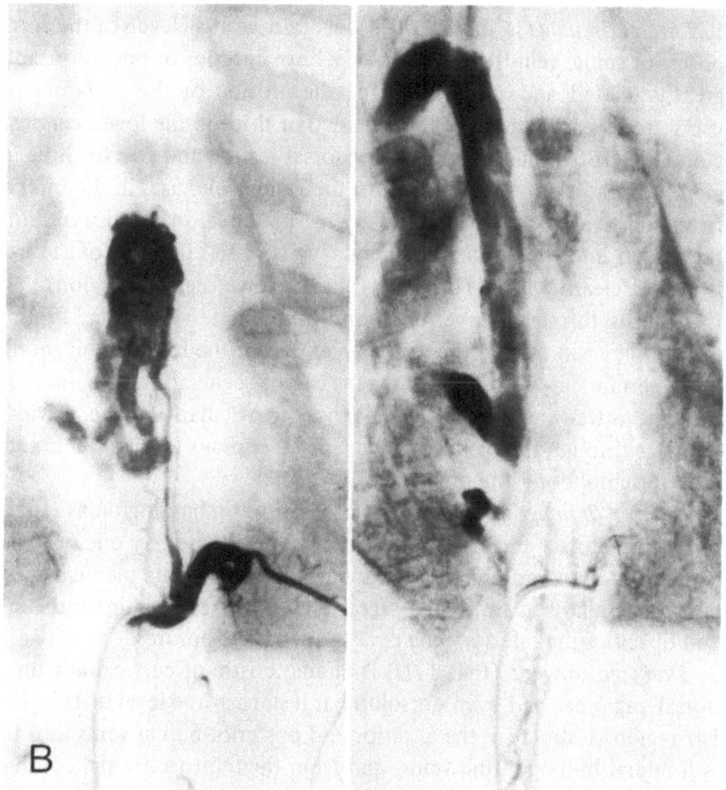

Fig. 17 B-D

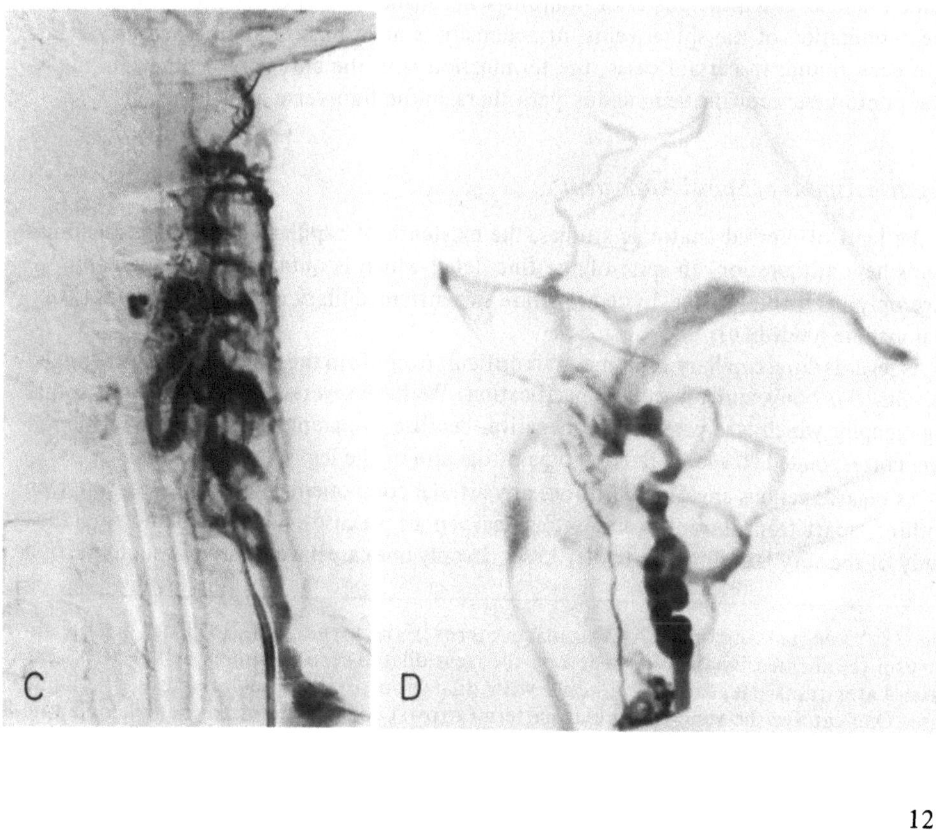

1. *Lateral drainage* is, in fact, the usual drainage at all levels of the cord; from the anterior or posterior spinal vein there comes off a huge anterior or posterior radicular vein, sometimes greatly dilated and responsible for the erosion of the vertebral pedicle. The radicular veins are few in number; one finds two or three in the lower cervical and upper dorsal region (Fig. 16B), one or two in the dorsal region, and two or three in the dorsolumbar region. The radicular veins drain into the venous plexuses in the intervertebral foramen and from there join up with the extraspinal plexuses. In the dorsal and dorsolumbar region, they drain into the azygos and hemiazygos, with dilatation of the arch of the azygos which is always clearly visible (Fig. 17B); in the lower cervical region, they communicate with the azygos through the vertebral and innominate veins (Fig. 17C); in the upper cervical region, they run toward the venous plexuses of the foramen magnum.

In certain cases, no radicular veins can be seen and the angiomas seem to drain directly into the intra- and extraspinal plexuses, particularly in the cervical region. This venous drainage through the plexuses is even more copious when a spinal angioma is superimposed on a vertebral bony ' ıgioma.

2. *Inferior drainage* is characteristic of dorsolumbar angiomas (Fig. 17A) but also of certain upper dorsal angiomas. This drainage is effected by one or several very dilated veins, sometimes by a veritable lumbosacral radicular venous plexus which runs down from the conus medullaris as far as the sacral region; there, it drains into the sacral and iliac veins and opacifies the inferior vena cava in the late exposures.

3. *Drainage upward* (Fig. 17D) is characteristic of cervical angiomas but also of certain dorsal angiomas and even dorsolumbar lesions at the level of L 2. The veins reach the bulbar region to drain by the anterior and posterior bulbar veins into the anterior, posterior, and lateral bulbopontine veins, and from them into a normal confluence, i.e., the petrous veins at the level of the inferior petrosal sinus. Certain anterior and lateral pontomesencephalic branches reach the posterior pontomesencephalic veins and the great vein of Galen. The termination of the spinal veins intracranially is most bizarre and numerous variants have been found. In certain cases, the termination is in the anterior, in others, in the lateral pontomesencephalic vein, and in yet others, in the transverse bulbar veins.

Negative Aspects of Spinal Angiography

In the light of morbid anatomic studies, the existence of capillary and venous angiomas seems beyond question. In spite of the fine detail which is obtained by angiography, we have only been able, so far, to demonstrate two intramedullary capillary angiomas (Foix-Alajouanine syndrome).

As regards dural capillary angiomas, it is difficult to confirm these because they are mixed up with the bony and muscular opacification. We have several times carried out spinal angiography which was pronounced negative, because of paraplegia, where the segmental level corresponded to a large flat angioma of the arm or the leg.

As regards venous angiomas (without any arterial component), here again we have seen nothing, apart from the intra- and extraspinal venous plexuses, in spite of a most detailed study of the very late films, up to 30 - 35 sec. In only one case have we seen a venous pattern

---

Fig. 18. "Venous" angioma. (A) Vascular patterns in the myelogram, (B) Huge arterial aneurysm (confirmed by histology) fed by the right dilated second lumbar artery, (C) Same case. Later films. Huge draining veins with dilatation of the spinal plexuses, (D) Same case. One can see the venous vascular pattern (arrows) corresponding to the myelographic appearances ▶

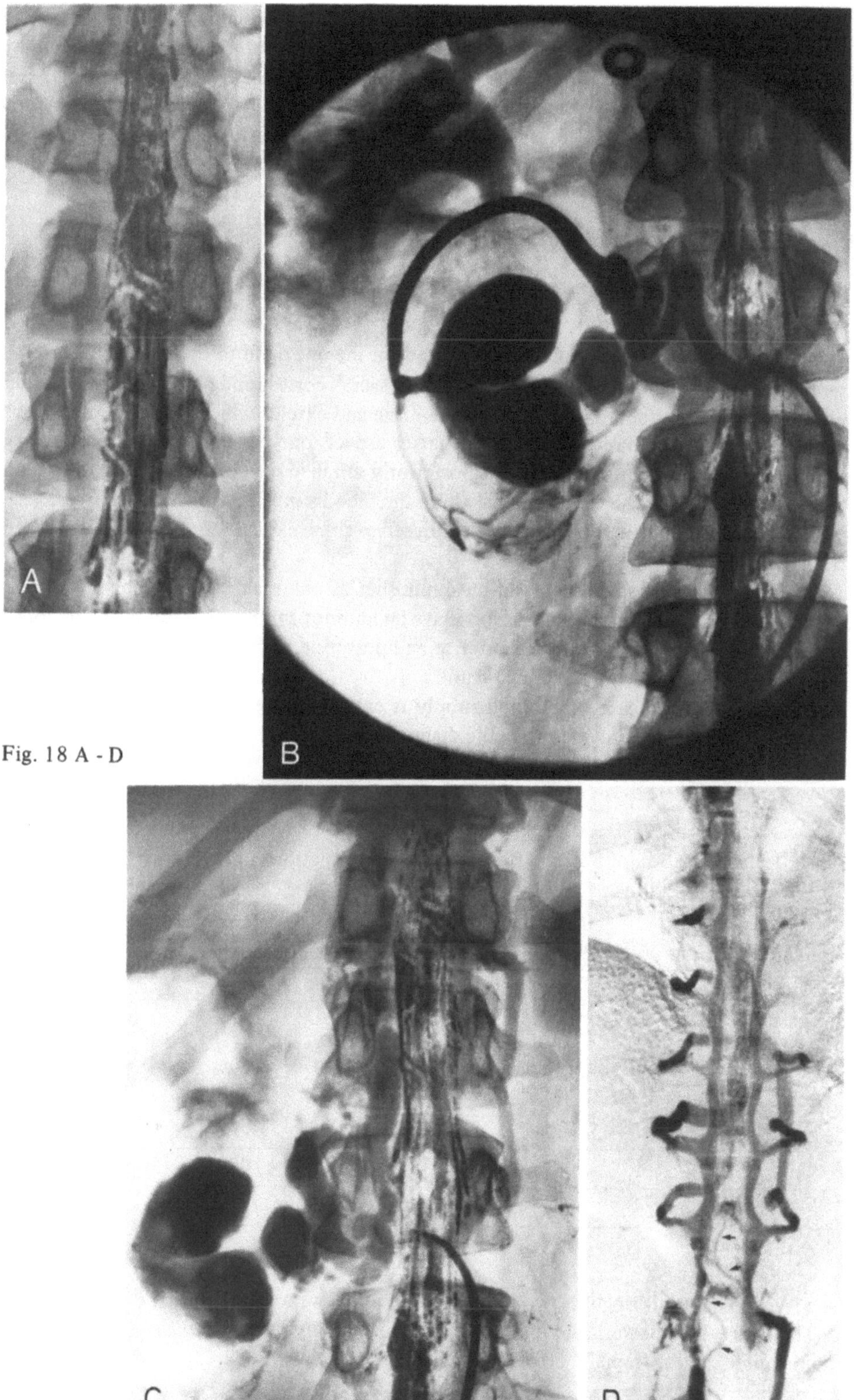

Fig. 18 A - D

corresponding to the vascular appearances shown in the myelogram. This was a case of a huge paravertebral aneurysm, filling from the second lumbar artery, which was drained by huge spinal plexuses (Fig. 18A, B, C, D); it is probable that this dilatation of these plexuses has involved the dilatation of a radiculomedullary vein. The technique of direct phlebography of the spinal veins has still to be achieved, but in several cases of phlebography by angiography we have seen normal veins.

The Classification*

The classification of spinal angiomas is related on the one hand to their anatomic level – cervical, upper and middorsal, and dorsolumbosacral corresponding to the three spinal vascular territories – and on the other to their size and extent, which is a function of their penetration of the spinal cord. From this latter aspect, one contrasts the intramedullary types with an anterior blood supply, the posteriorly supplied retromedullary, and the mixed types in the region of the cauda equina where the blood supply is from both sources.

The distribution as it appears in Table 1 deserves some explanation (statistics collected from 150 cases).

1. The percentage of spinal penetration diminishes as one reaches the conus medullaris. Diagrammatically, all the cervical lesions have an anterior supply, two-thirds of the dorsal types are supplied equally from the anterior and posterior, and only one-third of the lower lesions depends on the anterior spinal trunk.
2. In one-half of the cases, the blood supply is entirely posterior, and thus these lesions appear easily curable, provided that the diagnosis is made sufficiently early, which unfortunately is far from being the case.

Table 1. Classification of Spinal Arteriovenous Malformations in Relation to their Blood Supply

	Anterior or mixed	Posterior	Total	Percentage
Cervical (C 1 - D 1)	20	1	21	14%
Dorsal (D 2 - D 6)	21	12	33	22%
D/L/S (D 7 to cauda equina)	49	47	96	64%
Total	90	60	150	100%
%	60%	40%	100%	

One is thus able to distinguish two main types of arteriovenous malformations:

1. The type with a posterior blood supply: extramedullary, *retromedullary* (RAVM), subarachnoid, and extrapial 60/150 = 40%

*This section is by the courtesy of Dr. Michel Djindjian.

2. The type with an anterior or mixed blood supply (anterior or posterior); the proportion of these is 90/150 = 60%
   a) Partly or completely intramedullary: 84/90 = 93%
   b) Extramedullary: 6/90 = 7%
      3: AVM of conus and cauda equina
      1: AVM at L3 level
      1: AVM below the conus medullaris
      1: AVM at D 5

Classification of the Intramedullary Angiomas (IAVM)
(Based on 84 cases, of whom 28 had laminectomy).

Rapid serial spinal angiography (three films per second for 2 seconds) located over the angiomatous mass, with lateral views and image magnification, has recently enabled us to achieve a much better understanding of the vascular supply and drainage of the intramedullary arteriovenous malformations. On the basis of 84 cases, of which 28 were confirmed at operation, we have been able to divide these malformations into three types (Michel Djindjian, Thesis, Paris 1976. Investigation carried out at the Lariboisière Hospital, in collaboration with Prof. A. Rey and Prof. R. Houdart)[1] (Fig. 19).

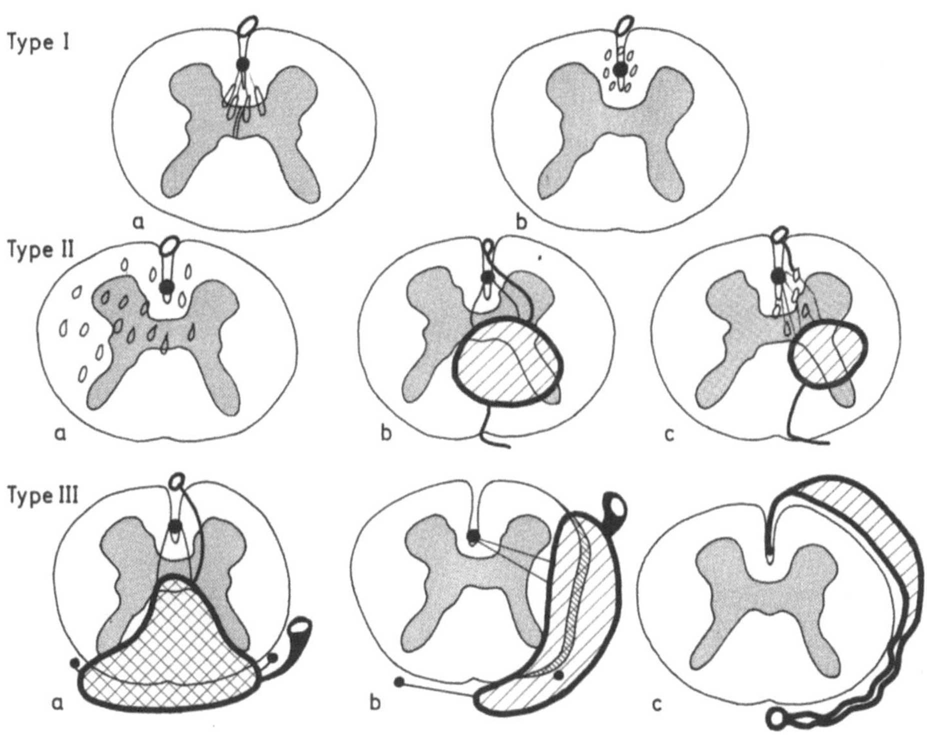

Fig. 19. Diagrams of the different types of intramedullary angiomas (Type I, II and III)

[1] Communication presented at the French Neurological Society: A. Rey, R. Djindjian, M. Djindjian, R. Houdart (June 1976). To appear in Revue Neurologique (Paris).

Type 1: *The spinal cord appears normal at laminectomy.* The angioma can only be recognized at arteriography.

Type *1a:* Intramedullary angioma fed by the sulcocommissural arteries. Operation – cure. Preservation of the trunk of the anterior spinal artery shown by control angiography (Fig. 20A, B).

Type *1b:* Diffuse angioma developed around the trunk of the anterior spinal artery. No plane of cleavage. Operation – contraindicated. (Fig. 21A, B).

Type 2: *At operation one finds a large swollen cord, suggestive of a tumor.*

Type *2a:* This proves to be a diffuse IAVM and thus operation is contraindicated (Fig. 22A).

Type *2b:* Pseudoaneurysmal type of IAVM. In the angiogram and at operation one sees an isolated aneurysmal sac. Total excision (Fig. 22 B,C).

Type *2c:* Pseudoaneurysmal type of IAVM associated with an angiomatous malformation (sac plus angioma). Partial excision. (Fig. 23A, B).

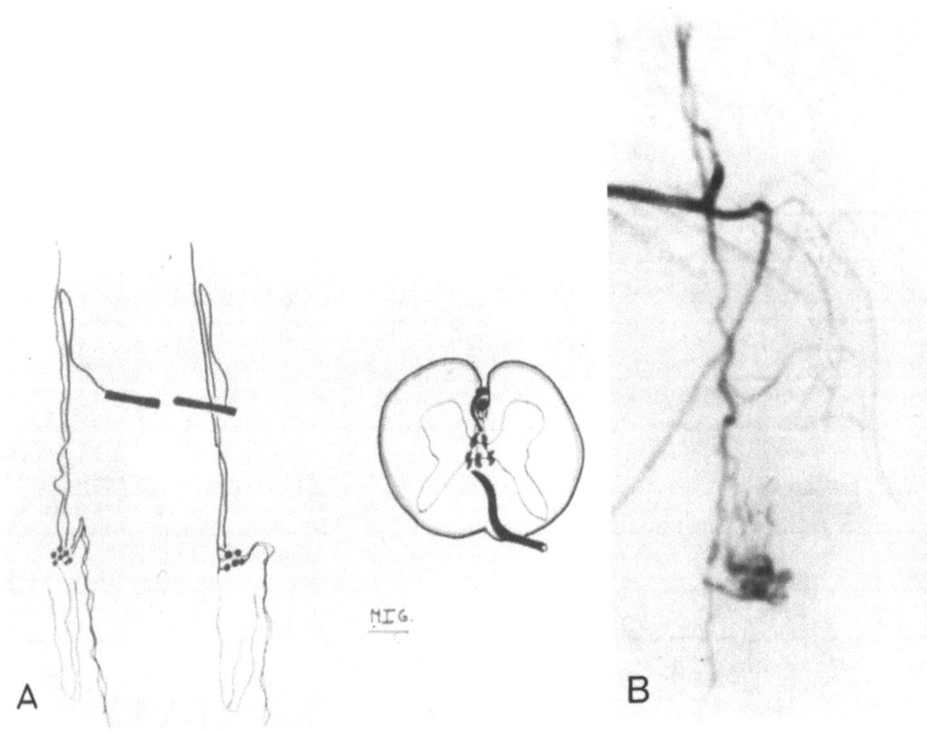

Fig. 20. Intramedullary arteriovenous malformations. Type 1a (Normal spinal cord at laminectomy). (A) Diagram of the malformation, (B) Lateral arteriogram. Intramedullary angioma fed by the artery of Adamkiewicz arising from the 10th right intercostal artery. Early exposures. The sulcocommisural arteries feeding the malformation are shown

Type 3: Mixed AVM. *Intramedullary angioma with large extramedullary vascular lakes.*

Type *3a:* AVM with a midline vascular lake, "an iceberg" (Fig. 24A, B).
Type *3b:* AVM with a laterally placed vascular lake (Fig. 25A, B).
Type *3c:* Anteriorly placed, purely extramedullary AVM (Fig. 26A, B, C, D).

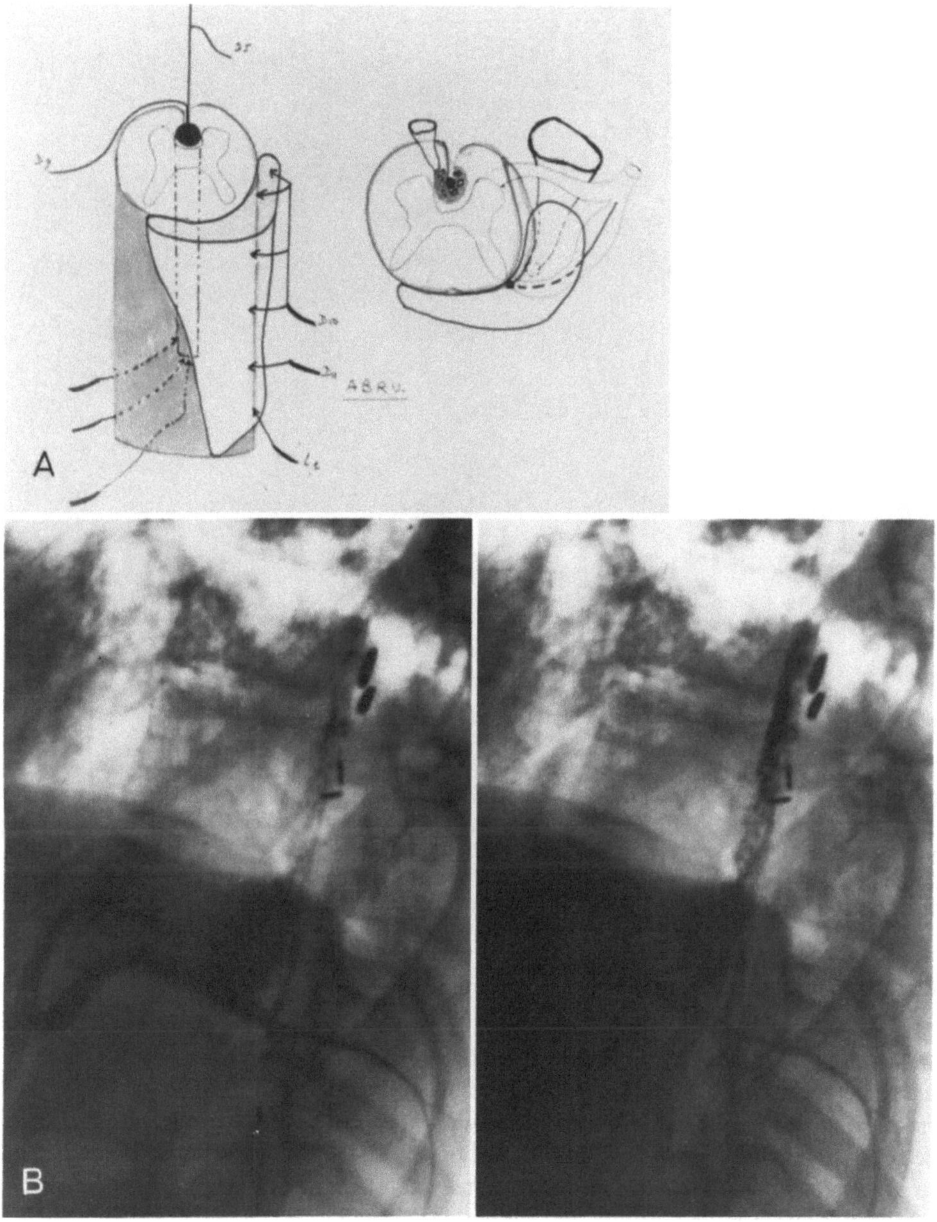

Fig. 21. Intramedullary arteriovenous malformations. Type 1b. (A) Diagram of the malformation, (B) Lateral arteriogram. Malformation occupying the whole thickness of the spinal cord. The retromedullary portion of the angioma was excised. Control (postoperative) angiogram. Some diffuse angiomatous tissue persists ensheathing the artery of Adamkiewicz. Contraindication to surgery

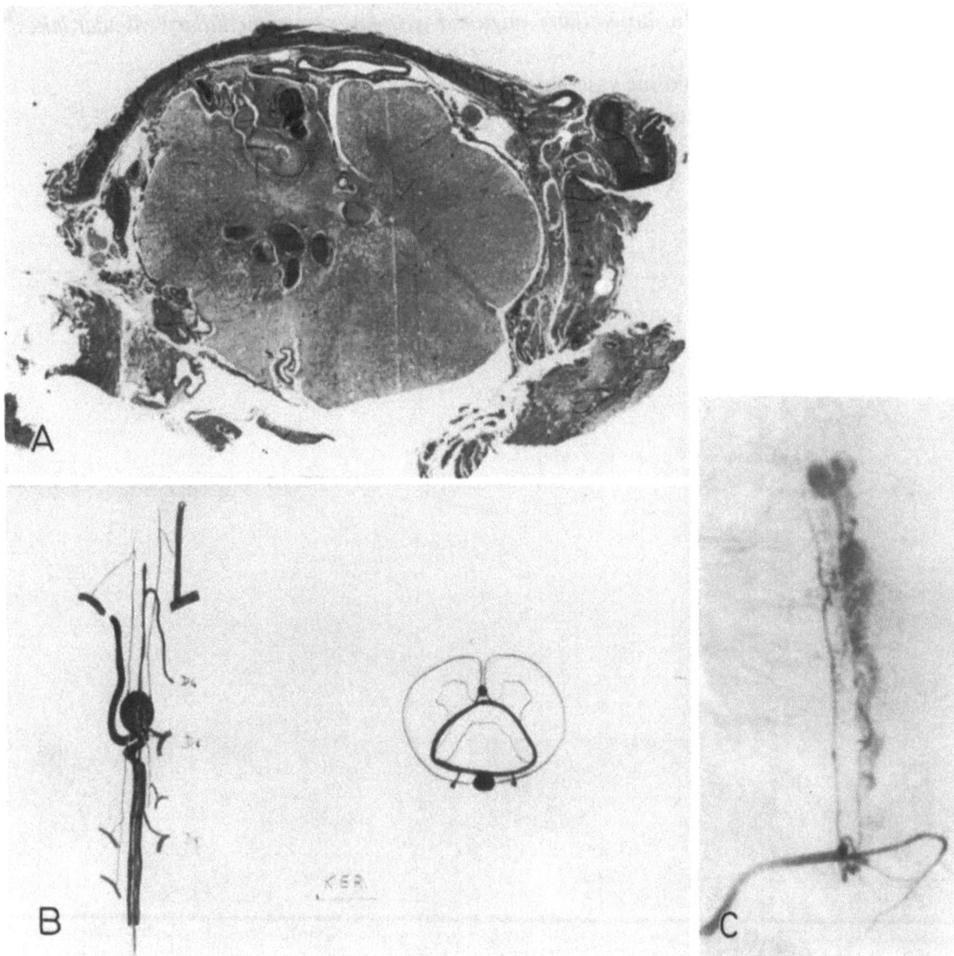

Fig. 22. Intramedullary arteriovenous malformation. Type 2a (Large cord found at operation). (A) Histologic section of a diffuse intramedullary angioma, (B) Diagram of IAVM type 2b (pure pseudoaneurysmal type without intramedullary angioma). (C) Lateral arteriogram of a medium-sized, dorsal, intramedullary angioma fed by the artery of Adamkiewicz. Vascular "lake" which is drained by a large retromedullary vein

Cervical Angiomas

There are 21 of these cases which are situated most frequently at the level of the cervical enlargement, and all our cases except for two are confined to the upper cervical segments. The feeding vessels originate from the vertebral artery and the costocervical trunk from the subclavian. All our cases with one exception showed anterior afferents. The pedicles are often numerous, frequently more than three in number; the efferents are very large, a function of the size of the malformation, and reach the venous system of the posterior fossa. They are often diagnosed early owing to the appearance of acute neurologic signs, or on the contrary, they may develop very slowly (six cases more than 10 years) because in these cases the ischemia is reduced in its effect by the richness and multiplicity of the arterial anastomoses. From the clinical point of view, any root involvement is minimal (three cases),

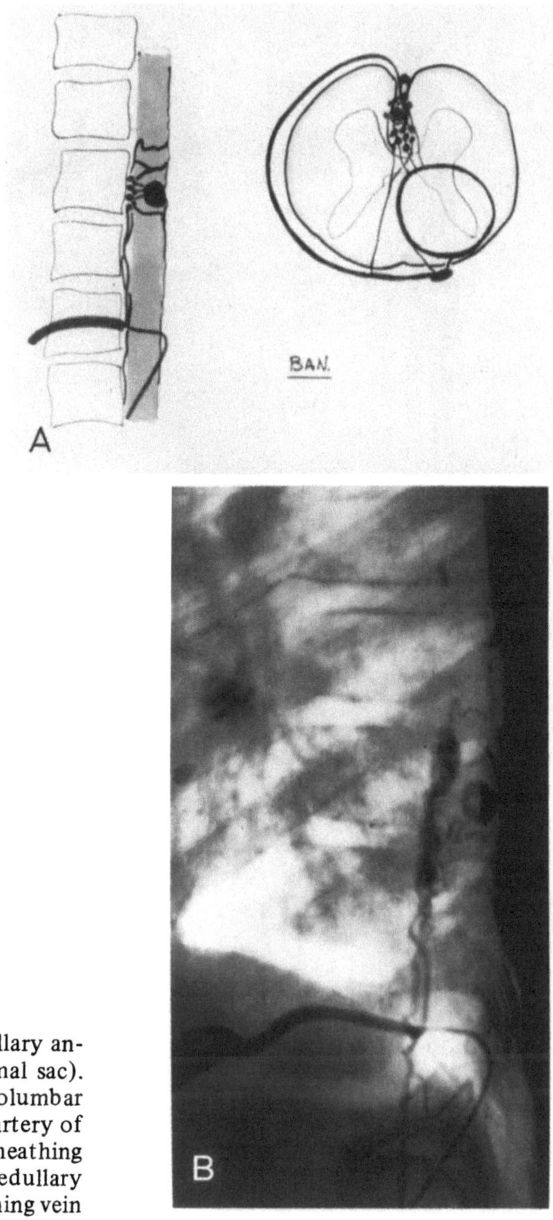

Fig. 23. IAVM. Type 2c (intramedullary angioma with intramedullary aneurysmal sac). (A) Diagram, (B) Arteriogram. Dorsolumbar intramedullary angioma fed by the artery of Adamkiewicz. Angiomatous mass ensheathing the artery of Adamkiewicz. Intramedullary aneurysmal sac. Retromedullary draining vein

always unilateral, and often purely subjective. By contrast, the cord symptoms are always serious, in accordance with the intramedullary penetration: five times a Brown-Séquard syndrome, five times a syringomyelic pattern, in two cases paraplegia, three times tetraplegia, and associated subarachnoid hemorrhage very frequently (thirteen cases).

Dorsal Angiomas

There are 33 of these cases which are situated at the level of the upper six or seven dorsal segments. They occupy a vascular territory between the cervical region which depends on

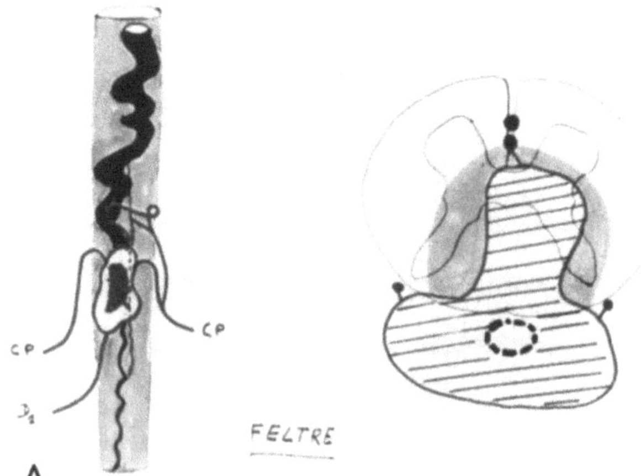

A

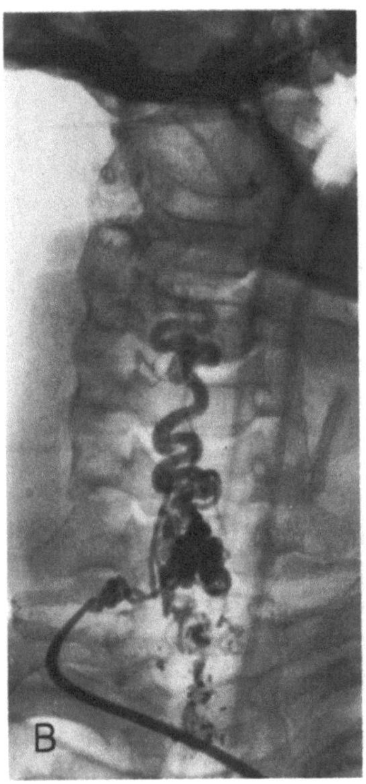

B

Fig. 24. IAVM. Type 3a (intramedullary angioma with large extramedullary vascular lakes). (A) Diagram (Intramedullary angioma with a median vascular lake mostly beneath the surface – "like an iceberg"), (B) Arteriogram. Cervical intramedullary angioma fed by the artery of the cervical enlargement coming off the costocervical trunk (R). Huge ascending draining veins

the subclavian system and the lower cord which depends on the artery of Adamkiewicz, which may reach as high as the sixth dorsal segment. The arteries originate from the dorsospinal branches of the first six or seven aortic intercostal arteries. In 21 cases, there was penetration of the spinal cord (two of three); the extent of the malformation is intermediate between those seen in the cervical and dorsolumbar regions, because of the smaller number of pedicles (two). The efferents drain sometimes toward the cranio-occipital junction, sometimes toward the caval/azygos system. These dorsal types often have an eloquent symptomatology which explains their early diagnosis; the frequency of subarachnoid bleeding is less here (nine cases).

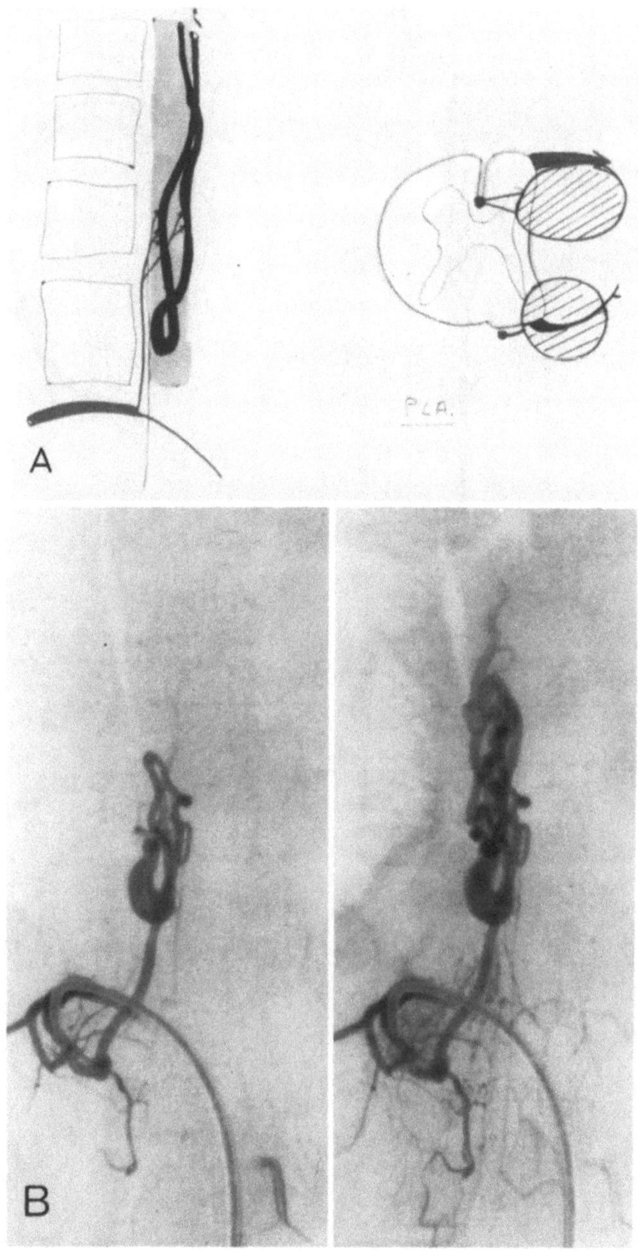

Fig. 25. IAVM. Type 3b (Intramedullary angioma with a lateral vascular lake). (A) Diagram, (B) Arteriogram. Angioma fed by the artery of Adamkiewicz arising from the 10th right intercostal artery. Vascular lake at the origin of the malformation

The possibility of producing symptoms at a distance is another characteristic: five cases showed themselves by a cauda equina syndrome, which was due to the diversion of the blood flow at the expense of the lumbar enlargement. This was seen in the lower malformations (D 6).

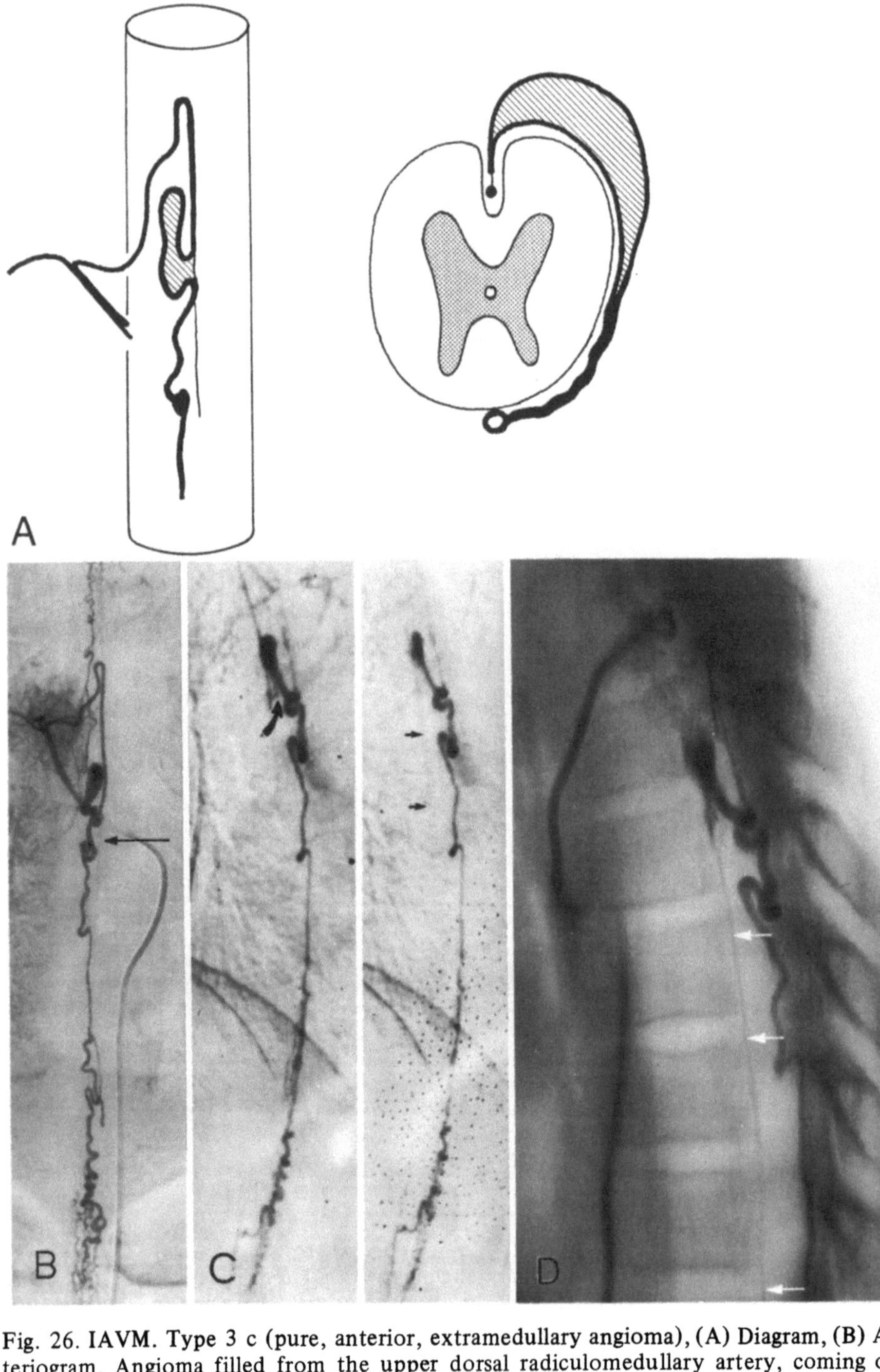

Fig. 26. IAVM. Type 3 c (pure, anterior, extramedullary angioma), (A) Diagram, (B) Arteriogram. Angioma filled from the upper dorsal radiculomedullary artery, coming off D 5 (R). Vascular lake on the descending branch which is seen to be very slender (arrow). This malformation continued right down to the conus medullaris, (C) Lateral view. One can see the point of origin of the vascular lake which arises from a sulcocommisural artery (curved arrow) and is continuous with a retromedullary malformation. One can see the trunk of the slender anterior spinal artery (arrows) and in the late films premedullary and retromedullary arteries which communicate, (D) Angiotomography. The malformation and the anterior spinal trunk can be seen more clearly (arrows)

Dorsolumbosacral Angiomas

There are 96 of these cases which developed in the lower dorsal segments of the cord, the conus medullaris, and the roots of the cauda equina (two cases), dependent on the vascular territory of the artery of Adamkiewicz.

The arteries originate from the lower intercostal and the upper lumbar arteries. The preponderance of posterior lesions at this level (47 cases) makes them a variety eminently suitable for treatment; the anterior afferent is consistently formed by the artery of Adamkiewicz. The malformation is small and usually unipedicular; as a rule, the separate draining veins reach the caval system and the azygos vein, although not constantly.

The clinical latency of angiomas in this situation is a characteristic fact, in contrast to the general pattern. One cannot avoid being struck by the fact that the malformations having a direct contribution from the artery of Adamkiewicz correspond to those cases which present early (average age 33 years), compared with age 51 for those cases which are exclusively posterior. This may be either because the vigor of the arterial flow favors hemorrhages or else the arterial steal is revealed sooner (the average age when diagnosed is 14 years) for those types fed by the artery of Adamkiewicz, as against 8 years in the mixed types. The clinical silence of the posterior types becomes apparent when one studies the location of angiomas in subjects older than 60 years (11 cases); they all actually correspond to those dorsolumbar types with an acutely developing clinical picture. The short period of evolution (28 years) is explained by the deprivation of blood and aggravated by the atherosclerosis which is always present and which is seen in the arteriograms. Virtually all the cases belonging to the posterior groups have developed in this progressive manner, with the exception of two cases corresponding to the mixed types, which have presented with successive episodes. The first symptoms of dorsolumbosacral aneurysms are caused by some root signs which are associated at a more advanced stage with a syndrome of cord damage. The therapeutic advantage which is conferred by the frequency of the posteriorly situated lesions is tempered by the severity of the neurologic state, at the stage when the diagnosis is made.

Pathologic Physiology of the Arteriovenous Malformations in the Light of the Angiographic Findings*

The pathologic interpretation of the spinal symptoms of the arteriovenous malformations is based on the comparison and integration of the clinical, arteriographic, surgical, and autopsy data. Being congenital, the arteriovenous malformations undergo a process of evolution which has been well shown by repeated arteriography. Because of the dynamic character of the circulation where the malformation is situated, the whole of it may undergo changes and modifications, which predominate on the venous side which becomes distended and may produce actual "varicose veins" (ectasias).

Four different mechanisms may occur, according to the intramedullary or extramedullary position of the malformation:

1. Medullary ischemia because of diversion of the blood flow
2. Hemorrhagic phenomena
3. Mechanical compression
4. Thromboses

---

*Section kindly contributed by Dr. Michel Djindjian.

The Retromedullary Types

The retromedullary types act entirely by a phenomenon of vascular steal; actually the absence of subarachnoid bleeding, except for our solitary case of cervical arteriovenous malformation, and the small size of these malformations confines their symptomatology to this sole factor.

Clinically, the remote symptoms are well-explained if one accepts this mechanism, e.g., cauda equina symptoms with the dorsal lesions (seven cases out of 12), and anterior spinal symptoms involving the posterior columns in certain dorsolumbar lesions. In the arteriograms, this steal is shown by direct signs, viz. the absence of filling of the anterior spinal trunk, which reappears after excision of the malformation, and also by indirect signs, such as filling of the arteries of the terminal network which disappear postoperatively.

The decompensation of these arteriovenous malformations, which proceeds sporadically in the majority of cases, argues in favor of repeated ischemic incidents. The advanced age of the patients, the obvious signs of atherosclerosis, and the remarkable asymptomatic tolerance right up to their delayed presentation are all in favor of a *mixed ischemia,* where on top of the effects of the vascular diversion is added the fall in the blood flow to the cord, occasioned by atheromatous stenosis of the intercostal and lumbar vessels. The pure circulatory diversion explains the presentation much earlier (3rd decade) of those types, sometimes much larger (two or three pedicles), sometimes quite small in size, but attached to an artery of Lazorthes (branch of a common anterior and posterior spinal).

The phenomena of *thrombosis* are exceptional and never constitute a process of clinical cure, because they coexist with a clinical aggravation and are, therefore, not demonstrable on the arteriographs (two cases). On the other hand, venous thromboses are a frequent finding at operation, but they only involve some of the venous efferents, and the concept of venous softening in the retromedullary types is rather unlikely.

The absence of subarachnoid hemorrhage in the retromedullary arteriovenous malformations (one case in 60) may be explained as much by the small size of these malformations as by their attachment to the posterior spinal system which is at a low pressure and where the perfusion is further lowered by the atheromatous ischemia.

The Types With Anterior or Mixed Feeders

Vascular Diversion

The phenomena of vascular diversion also play quite an important part. The arguments in favor of this factor are clinical, operative, and above all arteriographic; embolization and its radiologic verification provide in this way a true experimental confirmation.

The development by successive "strokes" showing partial remissions is typical of an acute circulatory insufficiency, all the more so as they can be quite isolated without any hemorrhagic episodes. The operative findings at laminectomy, which show the malformation surrounded by an area of softening are confirmation of this. The disparity in level between the site of the malformations and their symptoms is also explained by the vascular steal, in particular with the dorsal types which do not have a very precise individual blood supply; there were five cauda equina syndromes and four tetraplegias in 21 cases.

With intramedullary arteriovenous malformations, the difference in their clinical manifestations and their ultimate gravity is related to their anatomic site and can be explained by the richness or otherwise of the blood supply of the region. The good tolerance of the cervical types and to a lesser degree of the dorsolumbar types, as compared to those dorsal lesions with a mediocre blood supply, is characteristic of this phenomenon.

The pre- and postoperative arteriographs produce additional arguments in favor of this ischemic process by virtue of the circulatory changes which they show; these are direct and indirect, as in the case of the retromedullary arteriovenous malformations.

Hemorrhagic Manifestations

Subarachnoid hemorrhage is common in the intramedullary arteriovenous malformations (41%), rarely as a pure bleed, but most often associated with focal root signs and rarely with massive neurologic signs (10%). This "pure" character explains the rarity of hematomyelia which we have only encountered in two cases, one at autopsy which showed a clear fluid and one operative finding, out of 28 radical explorations, but in this case the symptoms were explained more by the localized central softening (*"en crayon"*) which surrounded the malformation. We think that the neurologic signs associated with subarachnoid hemorrhage, which are in close agreement with the operation findings, result from the phenomena of softening, which very likely follow an early arterial spasm of the arterial feeders of the malformation resulting from the hemorrhage. Among the other manifestations related to the subarachnoid bleeding, in the relapsing cases we would stress the possibility of hydrocephalus, which may require a shunt.

Mechanical Factors

These represent a more important cause of symptoms than had been previously thought. It is a constant feature of the pseudotumoral arteriovenous malformations, whether they be intramedullary or partly extramedullary, particularly in the setting of the syndrome of Rendu-Osler-Weber, where the manifestations always appear terrifying. Further arguments in favor of an associated mechanical cause are: the marked dissociation of albumin and cells, the block on myelography, the operative findings of a large cord with a dysplasic sac or backward displacement with tilting of the cord, and the fact that disappearance of the arteriovenous shunt does not prevent the aggravation of the neurologic state.

Thrombotic Phenomena

Thrombotic phenomena in the venous efferents with a resulting rise in the pressure proximally seem to merit separate consideration for the understanding of certain symptoms of the Brown-Séquard type, or of syringomyelia, where the operative findings are neither those of a hematomyelia or a softening, but rather a partial thrombosis of the intramedullary dysplasic cavities. They would explain the arteriographic changes in certain malformations followed up after an interval of several years, where the changes would seem to be more the result of thrombotic phenomena than the result of hemodynamic development of the lesion.

The physiologic and pathologic phenomena of the arteriovenous malformations explain the necessity of an early diagnosis and an operation as radical as possible, whenever the

Table 2. Physiopathology of the arteriovenous malformations

	IAVM	RAVM
Vascular diversion	++++	++++ Atheroma
Subarachnoid hemorrhage	++	-
Mechanical compression	++	-
Thrombosis	+	+

malformation leads itself to such a course. Each ischemic episode leaves behind neurologic sequelae which hinder a return to normal. Even if the shunting of the blood is the most important factor, this alone cannot represent the only factor responsible, and it seems that one should attribute a much more important place to the mechanical and thrombotic factors than hitherto. And if the threat of ischemia dominates the management of the case, embolization which is the ideal treatment of the vascular "steal" has shown its limitations with regard to expanding lesions which, whether they be intra- or extra-medullary, require a surgical decompression (Table 2).

Therapeutic Aspects
Operative Classic and Microsurgical Treatment

Operative Treatment of Spinal Angiomas

Hans Werner Pia

The operative treatment of spinal angiomas owes a lot to the crucial impulses toward improved diagnosis provided by selective spinal angiography and the technical advances resulting from microsurgery. Indications and operations have been extended, so that even intramedullary angiomas have become accessible. In spite of these improvements, there are many questions about indications and special operative procedures which remain obscure or debatable. A radical excision may be impossible on account of site, extent, complications of an already existing cord lesion, or for other reasons. Subtotal removals and other incomplete operative measures are debatable or are too little known, both in respect to their significance or to possible dangers to the cord. During recent years, intra-angiographic, intravascular embolization opened up an additional way of eliminating or influencing angiomas. Further problems have thus been posed regarding the indications and treatment, although for the present, the situation remains in a state of flux.

A special difficulty is provided by the small number of spinal angiomas and hence the limited experience of most neurosurgeons. This shows itself in the individual technical, diagnostic, and therapeutic possibilities and hence the practical procedures, so that a range of subjective criteria and conclusions make the judgement more difficult. The starting point of this contribution is our own experience. As far as possible, it will be compared with the work of other authors, with the aim of adapting the indications and therapeutic procedures to our present knowledge.

Historic Preamble

The story of the operative treatment of spinal angiomas mirrors the current reality, at the same time recalling the courage, the enterprise, and the limitations, but also the remarkable technical skill of the pioneers in this field.

Fedor Krause on the 10th October, 1910, operated on a 34-year-old man with a 7-year tumor history, with a spinal paralysis of 4 years duration. After a laminectomy of D 9- 12 and opening of the tense dura, he found an appearance similar to that in the case of a previously operated racemose venous angioma in the Rolandic region. Here also there was a neoformation with very distended thin-walled dark violet vessels, which ran in serpiginous tangles (Fig. 1). As also in this case no pulsation could be observed, it was regarded as an "angioma venosum racemosum." There was no question of its extirpation as the massive pedicles and numerous convolutions were penetrating directly into the cord. He contented himself with numerous ligatures and purse string sutures. There was no improvement. The patient died 3 months later as a result of a transverse lesion with paraplegia. The autopsy

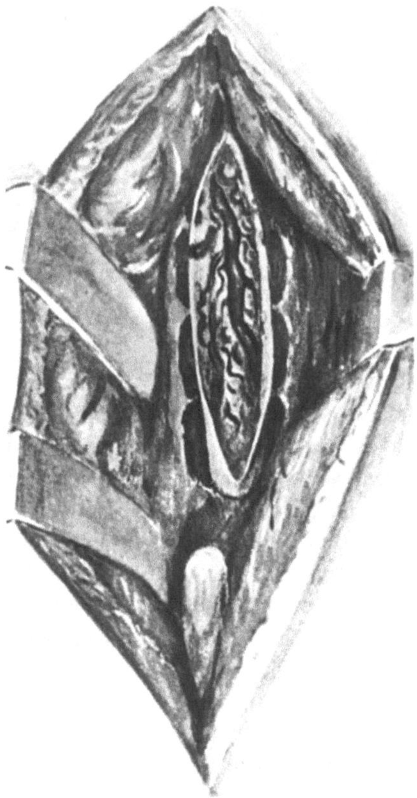

Fig. 1. Case of Krause (1910). Dorsal racemose angioma of the thoracolumbar spinal cord

showed greatly distended veins, increased vascularity, and thickened tissues surrounding the cord. The venous congestion was more marked dorsally than ventrally. The cord was shrunken. The cross-section showed only remnants of normal cord tissue, the main mass being formed of greyish-red tissue with numerous pathologic vessels. The remaining parts were softened, more particularly the posterior columns. Nowadays one would regard this as an extra-intramedullary arteriovenous angioma.

Charles Elsberg (1916) reported on five cases with pathologic changes in the dorsal spinal veins, which in one case were very tortuous. Partial exclusion led to a definite improvement and in one case to recovery.

Georg Perthes described in 1927 the first verified arteriovenous cirsoid angioma, which he had totally excised in 1921 (Fig. 2). This had also been the first occasion that one had been demonstrated by myelography. It was formed by a cluster of blue-colored vessels. After passing a ligature around the lower end and intentionally releasing his hold on the upper stump, a fierce arterial hemorrhage occurred. The angioma had no connections with the spinal cord. After four ligatures, it could be freed from the pia by blunt dissection and was completely removed from the subarachnoid space. The patient who had previously been paralyzed became mobile again. In the period which followed, individual case reports on operations appeared, but mostly with less than satisfactory results. More frequently palliative measures continued, in order to avoid any direct attack on the angioma (see Yasargil). An important milestone was the first full account of the spinal angiomas by Wyburn-Mason (1943). The number of successful radical and subtotal resections increased, the results became better and revealed their superiority.

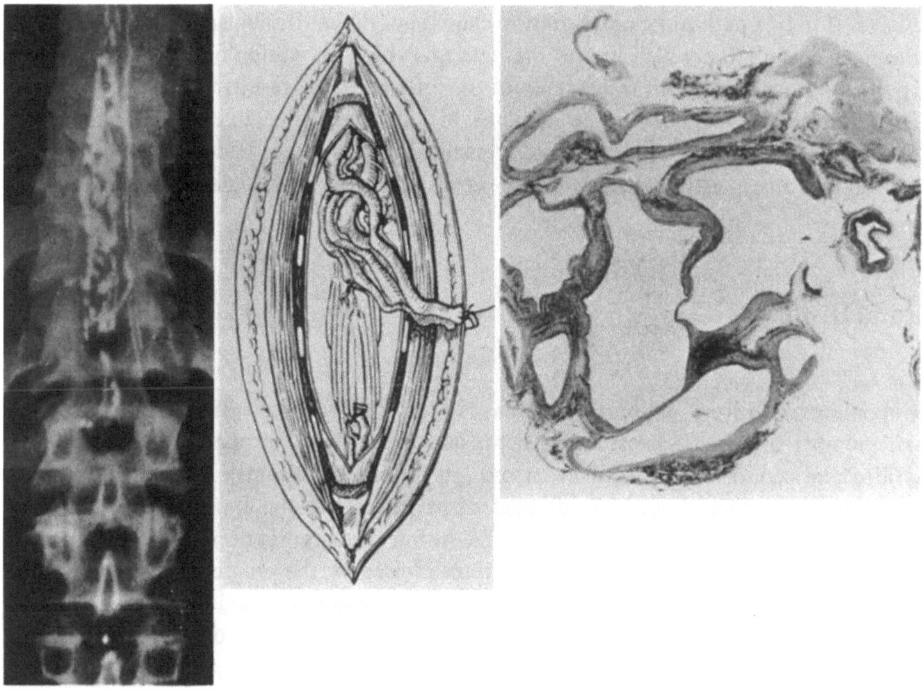

Fig. 2. Case of Perthes (1921). Dorsal arteriovenous angioma. Myelographic evidence, operation field and histologic appearances

Table 1. Prognosis of spinal angiomas up to 1962 (N = 235) (after Yasargil)

	Improved	Unchanged	Worse	Total
Radiation	2	18	16	36
Decompression	18	37	41	96
Post. rhizotomy	2	1	1	4
Coagulation – ligation	20	17	22	59
Partial or total extirpation	24	8	8	40

Yasargil summarized the material up to 1962 (Table 1), (Elsberg, 1916; Häckel, 1929; Echols and Holcombe, 1941; Wyburn-Mason, 1943; Scoville, 1948; Trupp and Sachs, 1948; Basset et al., 1949; Nittner and Tönnis, 1950; Klug, 1958; Verbiest and Calliauw, 1960; Svien and Baker, 1961; Guidetti and Silipo, 1961; Umbach, 1962). A critical analysis of this material allows one to draw the following conclusions:

1. *Radiotherapy* of spinal angiomas is ineffective.
2. *Decompression* by laminectomy including four cases of dorsal rhizotomy (Puusepp, 1939) and six cases with division of the denticulate ligaments (Teng and Shapiro, 1958) can lead to some improvement in a certain proportion of cases: 20% improved, 37% remained unaffected, and 42% deteriorated.
3. *Ligation and coagulation of vessels* evidently had better results than decompression. Out of 59 patients, 20 (34%) were better, 17 (29%) were unchanged, and 22 (37%)

worse. If only a part of the deterioration can be put down to the damage caused by the unipolar coagulation which was all that was available, one could say that it is essentially the method itself which is the cause of the unsatisfactory results.

4. *Partial and total excision* of the angioma had the most favorable results. Out of 40 cases, 24 were improved and eight each remained unchanged or became worse.

In the light of this, a critical analysis of the present-day position should be sought.

Natural History

The spontaneous history of spinal angiomas is essentially well-known due to the preponderant number of late diagnoses and patients not operated on. *Spontaneous cures* are not described and cannot be expected in cirsoid arteriovenous angiomas. The progress of the complaints proves that about 10% of angioma patients, with the appearance of the first symptoms or very soon afterward, and 50% within 3 years develop severe spinal cord damage (Aminoff and Logue, 1974). In the remaining cases, the progress may be slower or their condition remains static. Altogether the latter group is small, for in the series of Aminoff and Logue (1974) only 9% were without deficits or showed no progression. Of 11 cervical angiomas of Yasargil, the deficits in five remained unchanged for 4 - 22 years, and five progressively deteriorated. In our own material, only a few cases were symptom-free or slightly disabled. Half of the patients were unable to walk. A serious event, which can appear at any stage, is the onset of spinal apoplexy. A comparative investigation by M. Djindjian (q.v.) on dorsal and intramedullary angiomas with reference to their location confirmed that a definite arrest of progress did not occur and only a trivial proportion (five out of 90 intramedullary angiomas) remained without significant impairment.

Even if an exact assessment of the natural history is not possible in any individual cases, the severe and irreversible cord damage which is to be expected sooner (50%) or later, forces one to an early diagnosis and if at all possible to an early operation, i.e., to total excision.

Pathology and Pathogenesis

Arteriovenous Shunt

As in the cerebral arteriovenous angiomas, the most important and constant pathologic and pathogenetic factor, even with the large spinal subarachnoid arteriovenous angiomas, is the local impairment of circulation, resulting from the arteriovenous shunt, viz., the *spinal steal syndrome.* The ability of the spinal cord to compensate is variable and is apparently directly dependant on the normal arterial blood supply; for this reason it seems to be particularly large in cerebral angiomas.

As a further factor it may be noted that, as a rule, there are persistent segmental arteries, i.e., additional arteries, involved in the supply to the angiomas (Kunc and Bret, 1969). Although the angioma has its own pathologic circulation and its exclusion does not impair the circulation of the cord, there can be no doubt regarding direct connections between angioma and cord circulation through the radicular and the large spinal arteries. This applies particularly to the ventral and intramedullary angiomas which receive their supply partly or almost entirely from the normal main arteries, i.e., the arteria radicularis magna (Adamkiewicz) and the large artery of the cervical enlargement. The interruption of these arteries always causes severe cord deficits.

Corresponding to the experiences with cerebral angiomas, at least those with large shunts, the isolated occlusion of the feeders is not only insufficient, due to the rapid dilatation of neighboring arteries, but it is dangerous for the circulation of the cord either immediately or remotely. Without having any effect on the angioma, the nourishment of the cord is made worse; the power of compensation diminishes or disappears and there is an *accentuation of the spinal steal syndrome.*

So far, during operation, we have never noted any change in the volume of the angioma or any blue coloration of the blood as a result of closing off the feeding vessel which had been either demonstrated in the angiogram or by direct inspection. A most impressive example (Fig. 3A, B, C) is a patient with an extensive extramedullary and intramedullary angioma of the dorsal and lumbar cord, which had a large ventral efferent, draining into the deep cerebral veins. As there had been over a period of years a progressive transverse cord lesion, it was decided to follow the suggestion of Djindjian for the treatment of painful spasms. Accordingly, seven radicular arteries which had been identified by angiography were occluded by embolization. The angioma remained unfilled. Control angiography 2 weeks later showed the angioma to be as extensive as before, but now it was fed by the dilated arteria radicularis magna (Adamkiewicz). Its embolization once more produced occlusion of the angioma with removal of the spasticity but a deterioration in the slight residual power. We do not know if the embolization is now permanent; at least it is not unreasonable to have some doubts about this. Such a procedure should not be undertaken in the absence of neurologic deficits, as it can only be achieved at the cost of a transverse lesion.

The significance of the steal syndrome for the subpial capillary angiomas cannot be assessed. In spite of their very small size, the danger for the cord can be regarded as even greater on account of their direct involvement in the cord blood supply and their possible extension into the cord itself.

General circulatory disturbances associated with advancing age seem to be one of the possible additional pathogenetic factors determining preferential onset of the illness in older subjects, i.e., it is a decompensation. An observation of our own, in a patient of 62, allows one to recognize interrelationships of this sort. Due to a rapidly advancing incomplete paraplegia, the subpial angioma was exposed and the associated, moderately strong arachnoid thickening was removed. The angioma itself was not tackled. After a slight but definite improvement, 6 months later the patient developed an acute transverse lesion in association with a heart infarct, from the effects of which she finally died.

The result of the constant reduction in the circulation is initially a functional lesion but later an irreversible *myelomalacia.* How great the possibilities of compensation can be is shown when definite localized softening is noted at operation. Thus, a 17-year-old girl who had a complete monoparesis of a leg, recovered postoperatively without any residual impairment, in spite of the definite evidence of softening in the posterior columns. Aminoff et al. (1974) discussed venous congestion as a possible explanation of the chronic progressive cases. They assume that the rise in pressure in the veins in the spinal cord as a result of the shunt can by venous congestion lead to stagnation and a subsequent disturbance of the circulation. This assumption cannot so far be supported by observations at operations, as no visible increase in volume or particular congestion exists; the characteristic findings are atrophy and pallor of the cord.

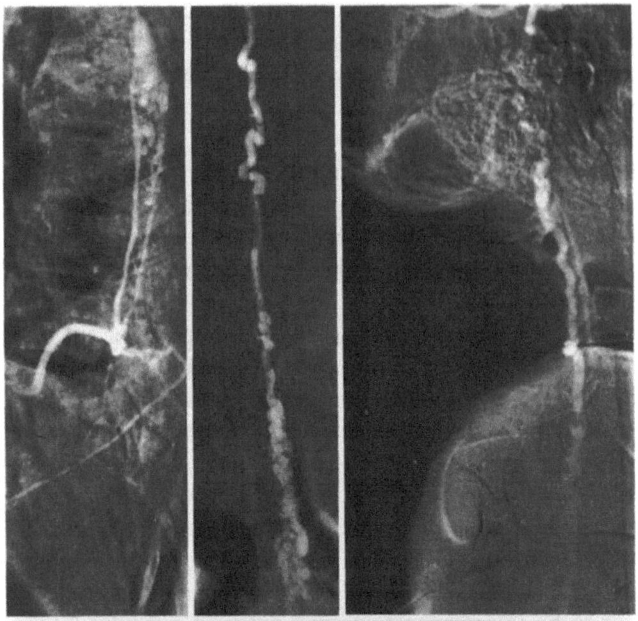

Fig. 3A

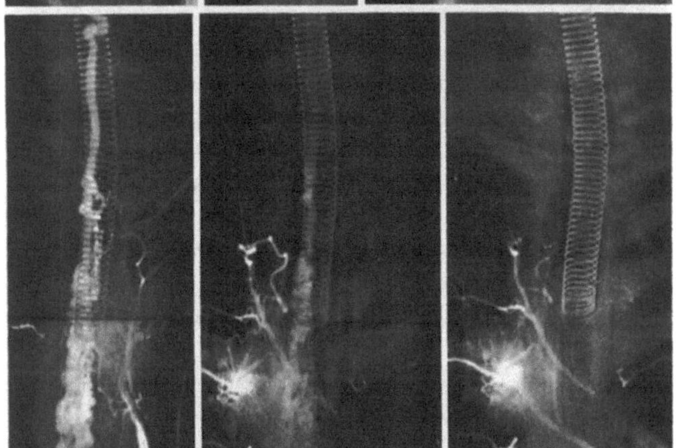

Fig. 3B

Fig. 3. (A) Large extramedullary/intramedullary arteriovenous angioma in thoracic and lumbar region with drainage into the deep cerebral veins, (B) Condition after embolization of seven radicular arteries

Rupture of the malformed vessels in 50% of our typical arteriovenous and "mixed" angiomas, and 30% of our capillary angiomas, represents an important pathogenetic factor in acute and even more so in chronic cord damage. The *resultant arachnoiditis,* which is accentuated with each further bleed, leads to a progressive narrowing and restriction of the cord and hence to compression. According to our experience, it is arachnoiditis which

Fig. 3C

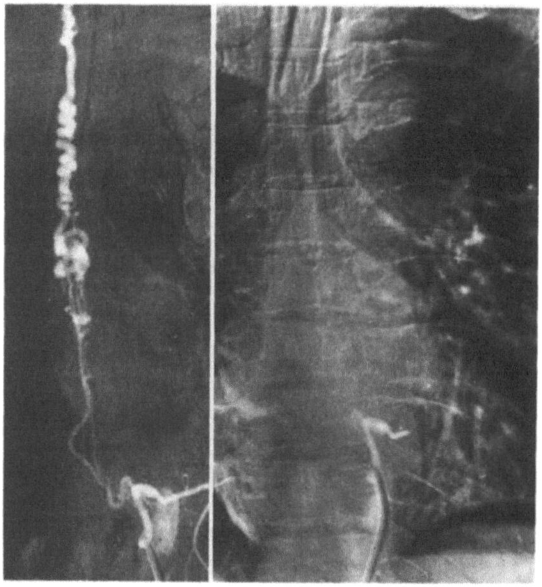

Fig. 3. (C) After 2 weeks, the angioma can again be seen, fed by the now dilated *arteria radicularis magna* (Adamkiewicz.) After further embolization, the angioma can no longer be seen

is the main cause of *spinal cord compression.* The *compressive effect of the angioma* is evidently overestimated; this observation also coincides with the experiences in cerebral arteriovenous angiomas.

A genuine physical compression of the cord is quite unusual and is only seen with particularly large, circumscribed angioma nodules. The customary unobstructed CSF pathway even in extensive uncomplicated angiomas is a further pointer in support of our own idea. Compression damage exists with space-occupying hematomas, with intramedullary and subdural hematomas, with the uncommon extradural hematomas, and also with pathologic fractures in vertebro-extradural angiomas. With extradural angiomas, particularly the cavernomas, compression is evidently of the greatest significance in the pathogenesis. The factor of compression is trivial or can be ignored altogether with angiomas in the region of the cauda equina and the lumbosacral roots. Compression does not explain the predominantly apoplectiform and intermittent course often seen in extradural angiomas, with a fluctuation of the spinal signs and symptoms. The conclusion is obvious, that differently acting circulatory disturbances can exist and exert their effects with or without a shunt. It is not known in what way the already discussed predisposing and exciting factors intervene in the events of the illness, whether it is through an increased congestion of the angioma, i.e., compression, or through a generalized or local disturbance of circulation.

It is undisputed that the arteriovenous shunt, and in nearly all cases the simultaneous primary or secondary compression, are significant factors in the pathogenesis, and they determine the appropriate treatment, viz., interruption of the shunt and removal of the compression.

Operative Treatment

Experience in the treatment of cerebral arteriovenous cirsoid angiomas over about 40 years has unreservedly confirmed total excision of the angioma as the procedure of choice. It alone can effectively and permanently eliminate the shunt, the compression, and the danger of hemorrhage. The same principles apply to the spinal arteriovenous angiomas. Other questions concern how this goal is to be attained, and what should be done, or left undone, in lesions which are inaccessible.

Total Extirpation

The synopsis (Table 1) makes it clear that total or partial removal of the angioma is clearly preferable to any palliative measures. We will consider the relative merits in the section on prognosis. The actual *operative technique* has not really changed and resembles the classic procedure first undertaken by Perthes (1927). *Microsurgical technique* is responsible for two important advances, the magnification itself and the range of specially adapted instruments which have been developed.Thus, the relationships of the angioma to the leptomeninges, particularly to the pia, and to the small and smallest collaterals going to the pia and cord, are better seen or indeed become actually visible for the first time!

The general traumatic effect of traction or pressure becomes slighter and injuries to the vessels can be avoided. The second improvement is the use of *bipolar coagulation*. Its advantages are so well-known that I will not go into them further. However, at the same time, it is necessary to indicate some of its dangers, which the technical advances may conceal. It can make the risk seem slight when operating on a damaged spinal cord, as the manipulation seems so gentle. This also applies as much to an excessive use of the bipolar coagulation as to a too precise and sharp time-consuming dissection. Permanent local heat damage and microtraumatization can adversely affect a previously damaged cord, in which, as is well-known, all structures are carriers of important functions. The decision to do less and whether to abandon this or that particular action is often more important and more difficult than the contrary. The removal of a spinal angioma is a particularly complicated intervention, fraught with risk, and demands a delicate touch and considerable experience. Any excessive or too intensive detail must be paid for with additional morbidity. In comparison, the removal of an uncomplicated, cerebral angioma from a less eloquent part of the brain is easy and free from risk.

Dorsal subarachnoid arteriovenous angiomas form the largest group in the operative series. *Laminectomy* should expose the whole of the angioma. This rarely involves removing more than four to six laminae.

The opening of the *dura* rarely causes difficulties as adhesions are the exception. The intervention begins with the removal of the *arachnoid*. In early cases without arachnopathy, it can be split in the midline and, like the dura, be held aside with sling sutures. In late cases scarring and adhesions of every intensity and extent are the rule, involving the angioma vessels, and here and there also the pia mater. The stronger the scars and adhesions are, so much more complicated becomes the operation. In general, this can be the most difficult part of the operation. What is required is, if possible, the complete untangling and decompression of the cord by separation and removal of the arachnoid from the angioma itself and also laterally from the roots and radicular arteries. The excision in toto, starting either above

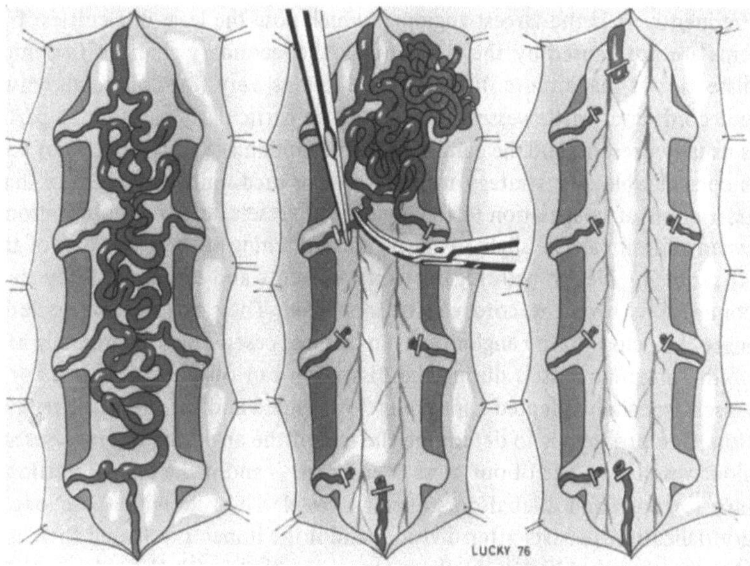

Fig. 4. Excision of a dorsal subarachnoid anteriovenous angioma

or below, has the advantage that one can lift up the arachnoid and stretch it slightly, so that the adhesions become easily visible and, according to its strength, each one can be divided by blunt or sharp dissection, with or without the bipolar coagulation. Particular care is called for in older subjects with fragile angioma vessels.

The removal of the angioma (Fig. 4) follows the same principles. The demand that one should begin by occluding the feeding vessels is not always practical or appropriate. This applies particularly to the dorsolateral or predominantly lateral angiomas, where the bulk of the lesion lies between the roots and radicular arteries, or intensive scarring makes the general view more difficult. The prerequisite for interrupting an arterial afferent is the establishment of its exclusive role in supplying the angioma. In each case, the occlusion of the vessel should take place as close to the angioma as possible. It is not always easy to decide if one is dealing with an afferent or an efferent vessel, but in general, the latter are larger and have thinner walls. The occlusion of a draining vessel is almost always uneventful. In spite of this, it is advisable to avoid particularly large vessels in the initial stages. We recommend small special clips. Whether one coagulates at the same time is of secondary importance. Their closure is easily effected. Small circumscribed angiomas can usually be treated by immediate occlusion of the feeders, and this is usually undertaken by us. I regard the advantages of this primary occlusion as doubtful, as in no case so far have I seen a reduction of the arterialization or of the volume. In this context, one should ask whether the demand for greater amounts of blood from the normal cord circulation during the extirpation is dangerous and is one of the causes of postoperative deterioration. These facts should always be kept in mind and each case judged solely on its merits. One starts the *extirpation of the angioma* in relation to the main drainage at the lower or upper pole. With a predominantly lateral and cranial drainage this is the lower pole. This or the polar vessel is occluded, the stump is lifted up with slight tension, and the line of demarcation between angioma and pia is defined. In uncomplicated cases, there are no adhesions so that with gentle lifting and division of the afferents and efferents, the angioma is mobilized in a short time and after interruption of the cranial portion can be removed in toto.

Frequently it is the largest angiomas which pose the least difficulties. The technical problems are not caused by the size, but by the secondary changes. In complicated cases, the dissection is made more difficult by adhesions, very fine collaterals between angioma, pia and cord, and brittle vessels. One has to be particularly careful as a partial cord softening is usually present, and the danger of increased damage to the posterior and lateral columns is considerable. My strategy in these cases is predominantly blunt or sharp dissection and restriction of coagulation to the dividing of vessels, and the mobilization of the more flattened adhesions. The slight lifting up and stretching of the freed part of the angioma solves all problems ideally with regard to its afferents and efferents. They are easily visible and connections with the cord can be identified. They can then be occluded at the correct place, i.e., close to the angioma. Even in these cases, I also regard a clip as suitable. Rupture of the angioma vessels during the dissection can cause difficulties. For large thin-walled vessels, specially adapted clips are recommended and for the small vessels bipolar coagulation. One problem is to determine the *end* of the angioma, if it involves an extensive anomalous vessel – in one of our cases over 25 cm – and if the cranial portion consists of a solitary tortuous and dilated dorsomedian vessel. The rule with these long vessels is that the arterialization persists after division, and if the lumen is released there is arterial bleeding. One assumes that higher up there are connections with the arterial system and that this explains the reversal of the blood flow. Only in one case was there an immediate blue coloration. In the early days, I used to mobilize the vessel gradually and at a later stage thrombose it by coagulation. Nowadays I dispense with each of these measures and occlude the vessel, on the assumption that by removing the shunt thrombosis takes place later. This procedure holds good solely for large efferents which are lying outside the actual angioma.

Subpial Capillary Angiomas

The removal of associated or solitary subpial capillary angiomas is contraindicated. They are partly in the subarachnoid space, and even under strong magnification one cannot determine with the necessary accuracy whether or not the cord is involved. Unrewarding experiences in two cases with apparent clear demarcation between angioma and cord circulation suggest a general policy of masterly inactivity.

The closure of the dura does not present any problem. An enlargement of the dural sac by means of a 5–10 mm strip of *lyophilized dura* is recommended in all cases of incomplete removal, palliative procedures, or exploratory operations. The majority of total extirpations are in the strict sense of the word *partial removals.*

The mobilization and removal of the prominent nodule or glomus can be more complicated than a total extirpation on account of hemostasis in the remaining portion. Therefore, one should always strive to do a total extirpation in order to avoid hemorrhage, increase in volume of the angioma, and back pressure with its consequent increased compression. The partial removal of dorsal angiomas is certainly more dangerous to the cord than total extirpation.

Intramedullary Angiomas

Originally the removal of these lesions was regarded as too risky. It is only in recent years that operations have been undertaken using microsurgical techniques and encouraged by favorable experiences with intramedullary tumors. We are indebted to Yasargil et al. (1975)

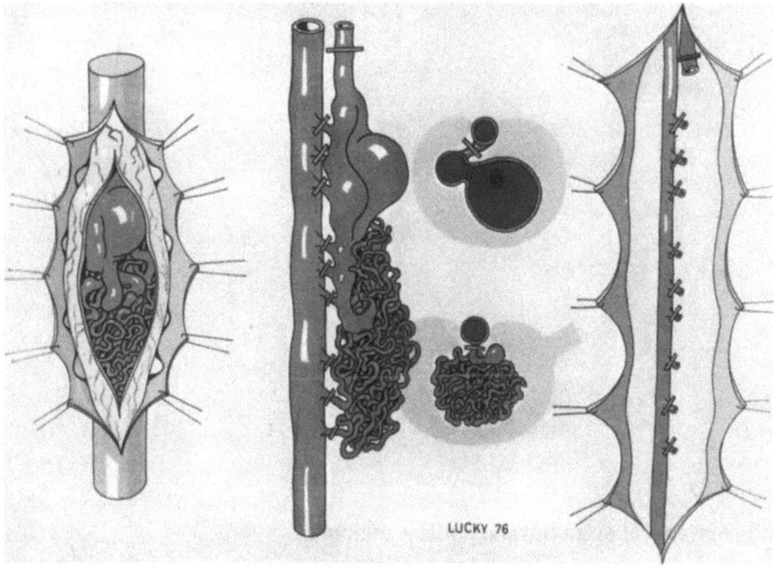

Fig. 5. Cervical intramedullary angioma with varix; supplied by branches of the anterior spinal artery. Total extirpation (Case 2 of Yasargil)

for the largest published series of one intramedullary and nine extraintramedullary angiomas. Our experience is limited to four cases. The technique corresponds to that used in intramedullary tumors. The cord is opened on its dorsal aspect, exactly in the midline, and the angioma exposed. The procedure is facilitated by widening the opening by the use of fine traction sutures on the pia. Yasargil describes in detail the bipolar technique, using the finest dissecting forceps. He regards it as particularly important that the coagulation shall *always* be used intermittently, i.e., a continuous "on" and "off", and that all the feeders directly on to the angioma are carefully occluded by stages. His "case 2" with a solitary intramedullary angioma and a varix from C 4–C 7 that was supplied exclusively by branches of the anterior spinal artery (Fig. 5) exemplifies quite convincingly the tremendous technical advances. Every neurosurgeon who would operate on intramedullary angiomas must see the impressive film of this operation and the patient before and after.

Contrary to the myelographic and angiographic findings, the majority (nine out of 11) of the cervical angiomas proved to be extramedullary and intramedullary in position, six times dorsal and dorsolateral, twice lateral, and once ventrolateral. The vascular supply was very prominent in all the cases as shown by angiography. According to the position of the angioma, the feeding vessels may come from the anterior and posterior spinal, posterior inferior cerebellar, numerous radicular arteries, and also sometimes the thyreocervical and costocervical arteries.

In one of our cases with an extraintramedullary dorsolateroventral angioma C4–C6 on the left, the main supply, according to the normal angiogram, was from the greatly dilated C 5 radicular artery on the right and two smaller ones on the left, but on the macroangiogram, seven afferents were shown and at operation at least ten were identified. Hence follows the necessity for a most painstaking definition of the extramedullary portion of any vessel and then its occlusion only if it is quite clear that it is exclusively supplying the angioma. The intramedullary portion is removed together with the extramedullary portion in one piece. The greatest care is called for during the dissection and the division of the

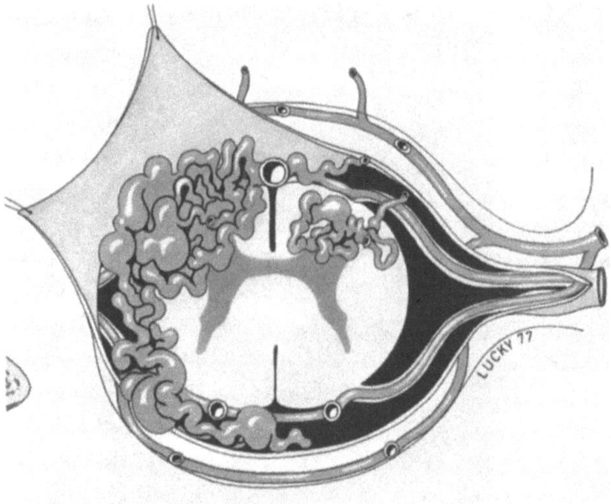

Fig. 6. Cervical extra-intramedullary angioma

feeders from the anterior spinal artery. The ligation of the largest draining veins, lateral or ventral, is left to the last.

Our own experiences are too meager for us to make any significant contribution to the technique. Apart from the lateral extramedullary and intramedullary angiomas with dorsal and ventral extensions, we have operated on three solitary intramedullary angiomas, two of them with localized intramedullary hemorrhage. The removal of the intramedullary angiomas, using the intramedullary tumor technique already described, was accomplished reasonably well as all the angiomas were clearly demarcated from the cord substance by a definite membrane, so that they could be taken out without any trauma. Moreover, the thrombosing and shrivelling of the angioma vessels, as recommended by Yasargil, proves to be very useful. When the intramedullary procedure is completed, the two halves of the cord are loosely approximated by tying the pial traction sutures.

Extra- and intramedullary angiomas ("mixed type") are found predominantly in the cervical and thoracolumbar region (Fig. 6). The cervical ones have already been discussed when referring to Yasargil's experiences. Houdart et al. (1974) saw this type in one-quarter of their patients. We have only had four cases ourselves. In two of our own cases, we removed the large dorsal portion and even under the microscope did not see any intramedullary part. The cord was not strikingly abnormal, in fact it appeared slightly atrophic. One patient has remained well for 6 years, and in the other, the intramedullary portion was removed at a second session. Houdart emphasizes the absent or only slight attachments between the dorsal and intramedullary portions and recommends partial extirpation, leaving the intramedullary part alone. After three total extirpations, I would now advocate early operation, as that alone guarantees some degree of useful function in the cord.

Ventral Angiomas

Solitary angiomas are unusual. Their total removal is regarded as impractible. Houdart (1974) in a case with paraplegia exposed the angioma by commissural myelotomy and was able to remove it fairly well. Further developments in this area cannot be foreseen at present.

Extradural Angiomas

On account of their predominantly ventral location, the total removal of extradural angiomas can be difficult or impossible. With cavernomas and other venous angiomas, bipolar coagulation is a definite advantage, as the angioma can quite easily be encouraged to thrombose completely. Arteriovenous angiomas require the same procedure as described for the intradural angiomas. The danger from bleeding is significantly greater, but the securing of hemostasis on the other hand is much less dangerous, as the cord is not directly involved. With combined ("mixed") vertebroextradural angiomas, we have confined ourselves to the removal of that part of the angioma in the vertebral canal and merely removed the laminae which are involved. We have not seen any recurrences and second operations have not been necessary.

Global Angiomas and Extraintradural Angiomas

Global and extraintradural angiomas make particular demands. The greatest problem was hemostasis of the angioma in the subcutaneous tissues and in the musculature. Regarding this, I would refer to the clinical history in the Chapter on "Symptomatology" (Case 1 p. 50) and also to Fig. 7.

According to our own experiences, the mobilization and separation of the individual parts of the angioma, especially between the muscles and extradural space, is sufficient. No direct connection seems to exist between the extradural and intradural angiomas. The main task is the removal of the shunt and the compression, which is first of all undertaken intradurally and then extradurally.

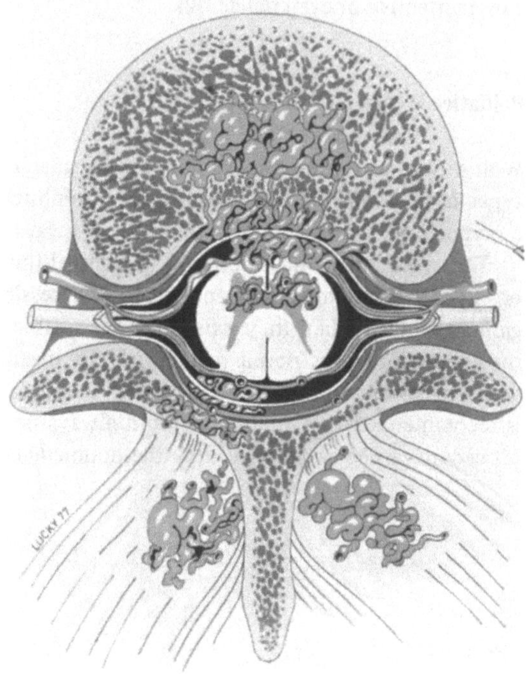

Fig. 7. Global arteriovenous angioma

Houdart et al. (1966) and Ommaya et al. (1969) discussed the selective intradural ligation of the feeders as demonstrated by angiography. They had the idea that in this way they could achieve a reduction in the size of the angioma and a removal of the local pressure effects. Houdart again reported in 1974 on his experiences with ligation in inoperable cases such as the "mixed type" angiomas, and he reported that there was a reduction in volume of the angioma shown in the angiogram. Our own experiences are described in the Section on "Pathology" and they coincide with those of Yasargil (see "Intramedullary Angiomas"). In my opinion, it runs counter to all experience that extensive angiomas with a large shunt volume, and this means the angiomas which are inaccessible to operation, can be effectively influenced by ligature of the feeders. The "suction" of the shunt or the "blood attraction" (Bier) is so great that the smallest efferents become dilated in a short time and again supply the angioma. How rapidly these processes which are stimulated by the shunt can come about, is confirmed by operative findings; they coincide exactly with what happens in cerebral angiomas.

The circumstances seem to be fundamentally different in those angiomas which arise from a solitary arterial stem. Taylor (1964) reported on four such patients, with improvement in three. Blood pressure measurement above and below a temporary clip showed a fall in the blood pressure from 70 mm Hg to 10 - 15 mm Hg. He combined the ligature with a partial extirpation. Chatterjee (1967) reported on similar experiences.

Transthoracic ligation of vessels in the region of the intercostal arteries (Houdart et al. 1966) is now only of historical significance. The same principle of shutting off the feeders was employed by Newton and Adams (1968) in a ventral angioma. "The feeding vessels were selectively cannulated under closed circuit television fluoroscopy and then *embolized* to effect occlusion." The patient is reported to have tolerated the procedure well and shown improvement of the neurological deficit.

In spite of positive single observations and postangiographic controls, the question must remain open at least until some verified late results are reported. My own experience suggests that occlusion of feeders – except in solitary arteriovenous fistulas – is, in the long run, ineffective or even dangerous.

Palliative Measures

With subpial arteriovenous capillary angiomas and in individual cases of other extracerebral types of angiomas, direct measures are prohibited, even partial resections. The finding of a complete or partial block in the CSF pathways indicates the possible lines of treatment.

The causes of the obstruction of the spinal fluid pathways are almost always an adhesive or cystic arachnoiditis, and only rarely inaccessible extramedullary or intramedullary angioma nodules. When they exist, it is reasonable to carry out a microsurgical excision of the adherent or constricting membranes. By means of the laminectomy and the associated widening of the dural sac with lyophilized dura, a good decompression can be achieved. It is recommended that the dura should always be closed. The decompressive effect of the procedure can be easily proved by the double Queckenstedt test.

Prognosis

Intradural Angiomas

The prognosis after direct operation or indirect measures (embolization) is not easy to assess at the present time, as the details in the literature are inaccurate or insufficient, are completely lacking, or are concerned only with early results.

Since Yasargil's collected statistics up to 1962 (Table 1), smaller and also larger series have been presented from such centers as Giessen, Paris, Washington, and Zürich, some of which have been reported elsewhere. The following results have been reported.

TE = total excision
PE = partial excision)

Tönnis' material (Bischof and Schettler, 1967)

16 cases 8 TE or PE: Pain and sensation better
Motor function unchanged
Deaths: 2
8 decompressions: no significant change

Kunc and Bret (1969)

9 cases 7 TE: 3 very good, 3 good, 1 poor
1 PE: good
4 walk without assistance, 2 with orthopedic appliances

Houdart et al. (1966)

50 cases: Operation in 29, no operation in 21

19 TE:	Dorsal
	4 with slight impairment, normal
	8 paraparetic, slight improvement
	7 paraplegic, no improvement
9 PE:	Ligations included
2 PE:	Normal
2 PE+Lig.:	1 good, 1 fair
6 Ligation:	2 almost cured (2-4 years)
	3 improved
	1 worse

Yasargil (1971)

43 cases: Microsurgical

	No.	Very good	Good	Fair	Poor	+
TE	13	7	6	–	–	–
PE	10	–	3	4	3	–
Decompression	10	–	2	–	6	2
None	10	–	5	1	3	1
Total	43	7	16	5	12	3

Ley (1973)

12 cases: Microsurgical

4 TE:	All worse postoperatively – after that improvement in 4
4 PE:	Marked improvement 2, doubtful 1, death 1
4:	No operation

Profeta et al. (1974)

8 cases:
2 TE: 2 good
Decompression: 2 good, 2 poor
No operation: 2

Yasargil (1975) (cervical intramedullary and extraintramedullary angiomas)

11 cases: Microsurgical
11 TE: 3 very good, 2 good, 4 fair, 2 bad

Bailey and Sperl (1969)

For comparison: out of 23 laminectomies in cervical angiomas,there were 5 deaths and 16 showed no improvement. Four cases with ligation of feeders improved.

The above results show the superiority of total extirpation, particularly in the series of Kunc and Bret (1969) and of Yasargil (1971). This is particularly true for the totally extirpated cervical angiomas. They confirm quite emphatically the possibilities and advances of microsurgery. On the other hand, the number of partial resections and palliative interventions is very large. This is partly because it includes interventions dating back over a long period (Bischof and Schettler, 1967; and partly also Profeta et al.,1974).

One must not ignore the mortality. Out of 97 patients operated on, eight died. Further, postoperative deterioration is as a rule temporary; as in all the cases of Ley (1973) and two of Yasargil's (1975) cervical cases. In order to assess the results, we should introduce a *system of grading* according to clinical state and risk, as has been customary for a long time with aneurysms. Our own suggestion is derived from the grading of aneurysms.

Grade I : No deficits (very good)
Grade II : Slight deficits, no restriction of mobility (good)
Grade III : Moderately severe deficits, mobility restricted,but possible without assistance (moderate)
Grade IV : Severe deficits, mobility greatly restricted, only partial with help (poor)
Grade V : Para- or tetraplegia, unable to stand or walk, dependant and in need of care.

The classification allows one at the same time to determine postoperative progress in either direction better than previously. Two cases illustrate the difficulties of any sort of grading.

Our own experiences go back over 20 years and started with a woman *now aged 52* (NM 2257/56) who 4 years before admission experienced an onset of episodic, long tract pain in both lower limbs and later a feeling of weakness. It was striking that soon after the start of the illness, she always had these episodes during menstruation and the feeling of weakness progressed to a paraparesis which each time improved in a few days and then completely recovered. By the 3rd year, although the paralysis remained partial, it was advancing slowly. By the 4th year, the patient was unable to walk but there was always a deterioration and improvement during her menstrual periods. The diagnosis for 3 years was multiple sclerosis! A peculiar, threefold partial block – suspicious of an angioma – between D 8 and D 11 led to an operation. The 8 cm long angioma was removed. For 20 years, Mrs. M. has done her housework and she gets around fairly well with crutches and supports. The menstrual exacerbations were abolished at once. Preoperatively grade IV, but in spite of definite improvement, the postoperative grade remains IV; nevertheless, a satisfactory result.

My second case, Mr. E.L.,then aged 50 (3596/58), came 2 years later, referred from a neurology clinic with a previous history of 8 years, started apparently with a spinal hemorrhage, after which a remitting course ensued. Fundi thought to show bitemporal pallor, intention tremor, absent abdominal reflexes, and an amyotrophic paraparesis allowed the earlier diagnosis of multiple sclerosis to stand for 5 years. On account of a raised CSF protein on two occasions (60 and 80 mg%), I asked that he should be referred for myelograpy. A similar finding to that in Mrs. M. led to operation and total excision of a grape-like solitary angioma. The neuropathologist reported it as an arteriovenous angioma, but in my opinion it was a cavernoma. On admission, he was grade V and postoperatively showed only very slow improvement; 1 year later he was able to stand and walk with sticks and was provided with a mechanized wheelchair. After 10 years there was no change; postoperative grade IV/V. For the patient, on the other hand, it represented a really decisive improvement with once more an almost normal existence. For the rest, neither patient has any postoperative posterior column deficit whatsoever, in spite of unipolar coagulation!

Our own material shows the relationship between prognosis and previous damage (Table 2). In grades I and II there was no morbidity, but grade III showed improvements up to normal (in two) and only minimal damage (in seven). One death and three severely disabled indicate unfavorable prognosis and greater risks. In grades IV and V "very good" and "good" results can be expected only exceptionally. The rule is slight improvement or an unaltered condition, rarely slight deterioration. The fatalities fall into this group, from which follows the pathogenetic significance of the spinal cord damage. If we consider the two cases described, we see that statistics can be misleading. Even in grades IV and V the results are better than they appear, if the arrest of the disease or slight improvement and walking with help instead of being bedridden are taken as the criteria.

The significance of age (Table 3) is apparent. Nine out of twelve patients over 60 fall into grades IV and V; three died and four remained unchanged or improved slightly. Surprisingly, one patient became fit again, a unique case with recovery from grade V to grade I.

Table 2. Prognosis of intradural angiomas (grade of disability)

Preoperative grade	No.	Postoperative grade I	II	III	IV	V	Death
I	3	3	–	–	–	–	–
II	4	4	–	–	–	–	–
III	16	2	7	3	3	–	1
IV	8	–	1	3	3	1	–
V	29	1	–	2	12	10	4
Total	60	10	8	8	18	11	5

Table 3. Prognosis of intradural angiomas (patients over 60 years of age)

Grade	No.	I	II	III	IV	V	Death
I	–	–	–	–	–	–	–
II	–	–	–	–	–	–	–
III	3	–	2	–	1	–	–
IV	1	–	–	–	–	1	–
V	8	1	–	–	2	2	3
Total	12	1	2	–	3	3	3

D.A., 74464, aged 67. Subpial capillary angioma with arachnoiditis rapidly progressing to a transverse lesion, 2 weeks inability to stand or walk, partial block on L.P. Removal of the arachnoid and decompression D 10–D 12. Rapid recovery, still living after 5 years and shows no abnormality.

The influence of the angioma type on the prognosis (Table 4) is much less apparent. About 40% of the subarachnoid and 30% of the subpial arteriovenous angiomas became good or very good; around 50 (30%) showed a slight improvement or no effect, the remainder were worse or died. With one exception, the deaths occurred among the subpial angiomas (three) and one global angioma.

The significance of the type of operative procedure (Table 5) is again particularly emphasized and our own experiences confirm this. Out of 23 total and eight partial extirpations, 13 and three, respectively, were favorably affected. A slight improvement was shown by five and one, respectively. Three remained unchanged and of each group two were worse. From the group of subtotal excisions, two died. The results are significantly less favorable after decompression and this includes the majority of the subpial angiomas. Out of 25, eight were definitely improved, but 12 were slightly or scarcely improved, two were worse, and three died. Late deterioration after months or years was seen on two

Table 4. Prognosis of intradural angiomas (type of angioma)

	No.	Normal	Markedly improved	Slightly improved	No change	Made worse	Death
Subarachnoid arteriovenous a.	30	6	8	7	5	3	1
Subpial capill. arteriovenous a.	23	3	6	3	5	3	2
Intramedullary a.	9	2	1	1	3	1	(1)
Intramedullary h.	4	–	–	1	2	–	(1)
Global a.	7	2	–	3	1	–	1
Angioma and angioblastoma	7	1	–	3	3	–	–

Table 5. Prognosis of intradural angiomas (type of operation)

	No.	Normal	Markedly improved	Slightly improved	No change	Made worse	Death
Total extirpation	23	5	8	5	3	2	–
Partial extirpation	8	2	1	1	–	2	2
Decom-pression	25	2	6	4	8	2	3
No treatment	4	1	–	–	–	3	–
	60	10	15	10	11	9	5

Table 6. Operative deaths of intradural angiomas

	Name	Case No.	Age	Grade	Level	Type of a.	Operation	Cause and time of death
1	E.S.	204/58	61	V	Thor.-lumb.	Subarachnoid subpial. hemorrhages	Decompression	Pulmon. embolus 3 weeks
2	L.D.	475/63	67	V	Thor.	Subpial	Decompression	Cardiac Failure 2 weeks
3	K.H.H.	421/64	62	V	Thor.-lumb.	Global a.	Decompression	Pulmon. embolus 6 weeks
4	L.Sch.	712/65	39	V	Cervic.-thor.	Intramed. a and hematoma	TE	Pulmon. embolus 3 weeks
5	T.v.Sch.	28/70	38	III	Thor.-lumb.	Extraintramed. a.	PE	Sepsis 3 weeks

occasions, once after a cardiac infarct and the other with influenza had an acute onset of a transverse lesion.

In spite of the bad grading at the outset, the prognosis is unexpectedly good, if measured by the ability to stand or walk. The number of the bedridden had definitely diminished. Eighteen patients remained dependant and in need of care, including one recent post-operative case; 14 achieved a limited ability to stand and walk with orthopedic appliances, of whom two are postoperative deteriorations. Eight remained slightly disabled and were able to follow their work. Fifteen had no motor deficits. Finally, the fatalities were informative (Table 6). Case 5 was already convalescing and in good general condition when, within a couple of days, she developed an acute sepsis, immediately before her transfer to her home, which had already been organized. As for the remaining four patients, the decisive factors were age (three), the complete or nearly complete paraplegia, the inoperable angioma type and/or complications (two hemorrhages and one intramedullary hematoma), on top of which the normally risk-free intervention came and contributed to the formation of the fatal pulmonary embolus (three) or the heart failure (one). By a more careful selection, the possibilities of modern intensive care, and perhaps also a still more careful operative technique, we have not lost any more patients in this group since 1965. Our last death was the patient with sepsis. We can thus take note of some significant points which affect the prognosis.

1. The previous damage to the spinal cord and the degree of the myelomalacia
2. The age
3. The type of angioma
4. The operative procedure. The latter is decisively determined by points one to three. Radical excision has the best results since it is possible in the favorable cases.
5. Damage during the operation is possible; it is predominately influenced by points 1–3, but also depends on personal experience.

Extradural Angiomas

The prognosis of extradural angiomas is significantly more favorable than that of the intradural angiomas. Radical removal leads to good permanent results (Guthkelch, 1948; Bergstrand et al., 1963; Pia and Vogelsang, 1965). Our personal contribution to the clarification of extradural angiomas (1965 - 1975) has featured, beside the solitary angiomas, complex (or mixed) angioma types, among which are vertebral, extraintradural, and global angiomas. This classification is important for the differentiation of the vertebral and also the extradural angiomas on therapeutic and prognostic grounds. Solitary vertebral angiomas produce no neurologic deficits. These arise only when there is involvement of the extradural space, when they must be regarded as vertebroextradural angiomas, i.e., cavernous-venous angiomas. Solitary extradural angiomas can indeed also represent these types; however, they are frequently also arteriovenous cirsoid angiomas.

The relationship between prognosis and preoperative disability is confirmed (Table 7). As the previous damage to the cord increases, there is a linear relationship with the deterioration. In grades I and II, recoveries are regular; from grade III, they are less common but even so they remain astonishingly high – 12 of 13 in grade III, seven out of 12 in grade IV, and three out of ten in grade V. Even in grade V four out of ten patients had become one or two grades better. The two deaths were in grade V. Postoperative deterioration has not been observed.

The significance of age (Table 8) is equally apparent as with the intradural angiomas. Seven out of 11 patients, altogether 22 of 46, fell into grade IV and V, including both fatalities. Both completely paralyzed patients died in each case after 4 weeks from pulmonary infarct and cor pulmonale, respectively, at ages 62 and 72 years, a venous and an arteriovenous angioma, respectively. On the other hand, with extradural angiomas in older men, the prognosis cannot be considered unfavorable, if six out of 11 can achieve a "very good" or "good" postoperative condition.

Table 7. Prognosis of extradural angiomas

Preoperative grade	No.	Postoperative grade I	II	III	IV	V	Death
I	2	2	–	–	–	–	–
II	9	8	1	–	–	–	–
III	13	9	3	1	–	–	–
IV	12	2	5	3	2	–	–
V	10	1	2	1	3	1	2
Total	46	22	11	5	5	1	2

Table 8. Prognosis of extradural angiomas (patients over 60 years of age)

Grade	No.	I	II	III	IV	V	Death
I	–	–	–	–	–	–	–
II	1	1	–	–	–	–	–
III	3	1	2	–	–	–	–
IV	4	1	1	2	–	–	–
V	3	–	–	–	1	–	2
Total	11	3	3	2	1	–	2

Table 9. Prognosis of extradural angiomas (type of angioma)

	No.		I	II	III	IV	V	Death
Isolated a.	30	Preop.	2	5	10	6	7	–
		Postop.	14	8	3	2	1	2
Vertebro-extradural a.	16	Preop.	2	4	3	6	1	–
		Postop.	8	3	2	3	–	–

Table 10. Prognosis of extradural angiomas (type of operation)

	No.	Normal	Markedly improved	Slightly improved	No change	Death
Total extirpation	21	10	6	2	2	1
Partial extirpation	24	12	5	3	3	1
Radiotherapy	1	–	–	–	1	–
Total	46	22	11	5	6	2

The influence of the angioma type (Table 9) seems to be less important. Of ten moderately and 14 severely disabled solitary angiomas, two and three, respectively, remained virtually unaffected and these included two deaths. With the vertebroextradural angiomas, the results were similar (viz., a surprising improvement). A further classification into cavernous and venous, as well as arteriovenous cirsoid aneurysms, did not lead to any obvious conclusions.

In the statistics of Bergstrand et al. (1964) with 13 typical vertebroextradural angiomas ("vertebral angiomas compressing the spinal cord"), eight were completely improved, four significantly improved, and one unchanged. This state of affairs continued unchanged for 1–18 years (average duration 7 years).

Our two *extradural hematomas* were only slightly improved; one learned to walk with crutches and the other with less assistance. Pathologic vertebral fractures do not present a very threatening complication. Two were operated on in grade III and improved to grades I and II, respectively; one patient refused operation and was irradiated without any benefit.

Any significance with regard to the *radical nature* of the operation is not apparent (Table 10). One can regard as a reason the marked compression and its easy relief. Adequate or total excisions with or without coagulation are indeed very vascular but relatively safe and are thus practicable in the rarer arteriovenous angiomas. For all that, recurrences are unusual, but local and root pains are more frequent. One patient after 8 months of good health developed an acute transverse lesion without our having the chance to see him, and eight complained about pains of varying frequency and intensity. In no case was a second operation required.

Indications

Circulatory disturbances, arteriovenous shunt, and rupture with bleeding and compression are the pathogenetic factors which on their own or in combination are the indications for treatment. The dangers of apoplectiform (acute) or progressive damage to the cord are considerable at any stage of the illness and are unrelated to its duration or the long periods of freedom from any clinical symptoms. Consequently, an expectant attitude or neglecting to treat the possible cause of the trouble is indefensible. There is no exception to these *fundamental and absolute indications for treatment*, as spontaneous cures of spinal angiomas do not occur and all experience shows that one can rule out a permanent capacity for compensation.

The second important point is the timing of the treatment. It should be done as soon as possible, preferably at a stage when any deficits are reversible. Therefore, treatment must take place before the stage of irreversible cord damage as a result of myelomalacia or at least when it has just started. In general, the cord lesion is determined by the disturbance of the circulation and the changes which they provoke, rather than by any real element of compression. The danger is particularly great when a spinal apoplexy, with or without a subarachnoid hemorrhage,has occurred. Relapses and secondary arachnoiditis (arachnopathy) are the cause of diminishing compensation and tolerance.

One must keep in mind the relative sizes of cord and angioma. The angioma is frequently many times larger than the cord, and it is for this reason that early diagnosis and treatment is of much more importance than in cerebral angiomas. All relevant data, including the onset, age, course, exacerbations, and clinical findings, must be taken into consideration, and on the slightest suspicion, angiography must be performed without waiting for any unequivocal clinical picture. The iatrogenic morbidity from faulty interpretation and missed diagnosis is very great and nowhere near comparable to the morbidity of radical treatment. One of our principal tasks is to improve the early diagnosis, to contribute to neurologic knowledge, and to widen the field of awareness among clinicians generally. This is the prerequisite for *correct* and timely *early* treatment. The hitherto customary *late* and *too late* treatment is, in spite of the unexpectedly good results, unsatisfactory and disappointing.

Special Indications

Extradural Angiomas

Vertebral angiomas only come under treatment in exceptional cases where there is a pathologic fracture of the vertebra. Accompanying radiculospinal symptoms or signs indicate an extension into the extradural space. Such *vertebroextradural angiomas* pose neither diagnostic nor therapeutic problems. Decompression and exclusion of the angioma are risk-free and always indicated. Radiation therapy is useless. The same indications apply to the *solitary extradural angiomas*. Their clinical recognition is difficult. Apart from the nonacute lumbosacral angiomas, they have symptoms very much like the intradural angiomas, and there is almost always a complete or partial obstruction of the CSF pathways. Once a space-occupying lesion is confirmed, operation is indicated. No special diagnostic procedure is called for and the diagnosis is confirmed by the operative appearance; the damage resulting from the pressure and impaired circulation is removed. There are no special contraindications.

Intradural Angiomas

Dorsal subarachnoid arteriovenous angiomas come into the category of those treatable by extirpation. As with the similar cerebral arteriovenous angiomas, it is total excision alone that guarantees the efficient and permanent removal of the circulatory disturbances and pressure. In all late cases (up to now the normal situation), it cannot be replaced by any other method, as this alone can remove the compression, the strangulating adhesions and scars, and rarely a hematoma. Ligation of the feeders, as a treatment directed at the cause, is restricted to the few cases of uncomplicated arteriovenous fistulas ("single coiled type"). According to experiences to date, it is in these cases that intravascular embolization is equally effective and saves an operation. In the cases of extensive arteriovenous angiomas, the exclusive use of embolization is not recommended, as the steal syndrome is increased or at least the risk of this is very great. A combined procedure is a possibility and may facilitate the operative intervention. A final verdict cannot be given at the present time.

Subpial capillary arteriovenous angiomas, even with an extradural extension, are not accessible to direct extirpation, as they are always involved in the blood supply of the cord or encroach on the cord. Due to their size, it does not appear possible to demonstrate them by angiography. The symptoms and myelography confirm the partial obstruction of the fluid pathways and thus the indication for operation. Decompression is effective, if it follows the general lines for the treatment of adhesions and cystic arachnoiditis, viz., microsurgical resection of the membranes and if need be, enlargement of the dural sac with lyophilized dura.

Intramedullary angiomas regarded for a long time as "inoperable" have become accessible as a result of microsurgical technique. The experiences in cervical angiomas, particularly those of Yasargil (1975), are so encouraging that the indications can legitimately be widened. The particular experience of the operator is obviously a factor to be taken into account. The same point of view applies to the numerically more frequent extraintramedullary angiomas ("mixed type" of the Paris workers). The unusual vascular supply and the tight plexus of vessels as verified at operation (Yasargil, 1975; Pia, 1976) excludes embolization or comparable ligation of vessels as an effective radical procedure. Partial extirpations of the easily accessible extramedullary portions of the angioma are possible, but it remains to be seen if they have any lasting effect. Partial procedures on intramedullary angiomas are dangerous. I personally believe that doing nothing in these cases is better than tying the feeders. In any case, there is no firm evidence, and we need to have long-term observation on "ligated patients".

Ventral angiomas are unusual. Up to the present, they are not accessible by direct or indirect measures. An embolization of the anterior spinal system is contraindicated and exposure by myelotomy in the absence of neurologic symptoms is scarcely defensible (see Houdart's case). In spite of recent technical advances, I regard them as inoperable.

Global angiomas with diffuse involvement of the subcutaneous tissues, muscles, bone, and extradural and intradural space make particular demands which cannot always be overcome. Isolation of the vasculature and decompression are possible as palliative measures; to some extent direct measures are possible.

Compressing hematomas because of the acute risk require immediate diagnosis and treatment. The limited general and personal experience with the intramedullary hematomas does not permit any definite statement concerning indications and contraindications. However, it is certain that not only extradural and subdural hematomas but also in certain cases even intramedullary hematomas can be successfully treated, i.e., with improvement in their symptoms.

Contraindications

Acute apoplectiform complete transverse lesions (with paraplegia) represent an absolute contraindication. In contrast to spinal tumors, the compressing lesion is not the decisive factor. I have already mentioned a possible indication with intramedullary hematomas.

A *complete paraplegia or tetraplegia* in the *elderly* should only exceptionally be operated upon because of the high general risk, but above all the risk of emboli. I repeat: the only paraplegic patient with almost complete recovery comes into the group over age 60. It is not the calendar age which determines the indication but the patient's general condition irrespective of his actual recorded age. There are certainly *contraindications* with regard to site and extent, but in general these have to be decided on their merits. The rapid development which is still taking place is in no way concluded, so that even for the border area subjective impressions dominate too much, and that is why further experience must be reported.

The *operative morbidity* and a *certain mortality* cannot be denied. I believe I have proved that this is essentially the result of the previous damage and is only indirectly determined by the operation itself. In certain cases, the intervention can also be regarded as the "last straw." When measured against the decisive improvement of the majority of similarly disabled patients unable to walk, to a stage of personal independence, I am prepared to take the risk. As long as late and terminal cases come to us, there is no alternative; the only genuine alternative is early diagnosis and early treatment.

Final Personal Considerations

The foregoing results of a 20-year endeavor concerning the recognition and treatment of spinal angiomas derive from close cooperation with interested neurosurgeons and neuroradiologists the world over, the stimulus being provided by their results. The improvement is evident and has been advanced decisively by microsurgical technique. In the meantime, we cannot boast about any satisfactory results. Further progress is possible. The prerequisites are improvements in early diagnosis and treatment. The former is possible if the clinical picture and course becomes generally known, so that when there is any suspicion, the specialist department which has at its disposal the relevant diagnostic possibilities and experience will be called in. With regard to treatment, I am convinced that the cerebrospinal angiomas represent a diagnostic, morphologic and etiologic entity and that they can only be treated successfully and permanently by total extirpation. Even in recent years, the technical possibilities have improved and the indications have been widened.

The risk of operative morbidity and mortality carries no weight. Embolization has secured some therapeutic significance as a primary, secondary, and exclusive measure. Indications and contraindications are not yet sufficiently clarified. Personally, after considering the long-term results of embolization of cerebral angiomas, I am convinced of the superiority of total extirpation, even for the future.

Surgical Treatment of Intramedullary and Anterior Spinal Angiomas

A. Rey, Michel Djindjian, René Djindjian, and R. Houdart

Intramedullary spinal angiomas fed solely or partly by the anterior spinal system have been considered for many years to be not amenable to surgical treatment. Only posterior retromedullary angiomas were operated upon and totally removed. Anterior spinal malformations were sometimes attacked indirectly by intradural ligature of an anterior feeding vessel, especially in the cervical area. However, these surgical attempts were only palliative treatment. Percutaneous embolization was a useful complement to surgery but was not always possible and could not achieve a radical cure for anterior spinal malformations.

The natural history of anterior spinal angiomas shows clearly that the neurologic status becomes rapidly impaired in young adults or children. On average, severe paraplegia occurs rather rapidly after the first clinical manifestation, within 4–6 years in the dorsal and dorsolumbar region, within 10 years or more in the cervical region. This disastrous pattern of events led us to a more active surgical attitude from December, 1973. With the help of microsurgical techniques, removal of anterior spinal angiomas was achieved in 24 cases with pre- and postoperative angiography in the majority of cases.

Preoperative spinal angiography is the most outstanding contribution to the success of the operation. It is essential for the surgeon to determine with accuracy before operation the volume and level of the malformation, its situation within the cord, its feeding arteries, and its draining veins in order to formulate an appropriate plan for surgical attack.

Radiologic Localization

Radiologic studies allow us to classify the anterior spinal arteriovenous malformations on the basis of angiographic and operative findings. In this way, four distinct groups can be identified.

Group I : The malformation is totally intramedullary, deeply situated in the vicinity of the anterior spinal artery, and fed by sulcal arteries. In the lateral views, the angioma is completely separated from the anterior spinal artery.

Group II : The malformation is totally intramedullary and composed of two separate parts: a group I angioma and a pouch which may be totally thrombosed. In some cases, the anterior spinal artery in group I or II may be surrounded by angiomatous vessels coming from the cord in the anterior sulcus (two cases in group I, one case in group II).

Group III : The malformation is partly intramedullary and visible on the dorsal or posterolateral aspect of the cord. Arterial supply comes both from the anterior and posterior arterial systems.

Group IV: The malformation is totally extramedullary and located usually in the cauda equina region.

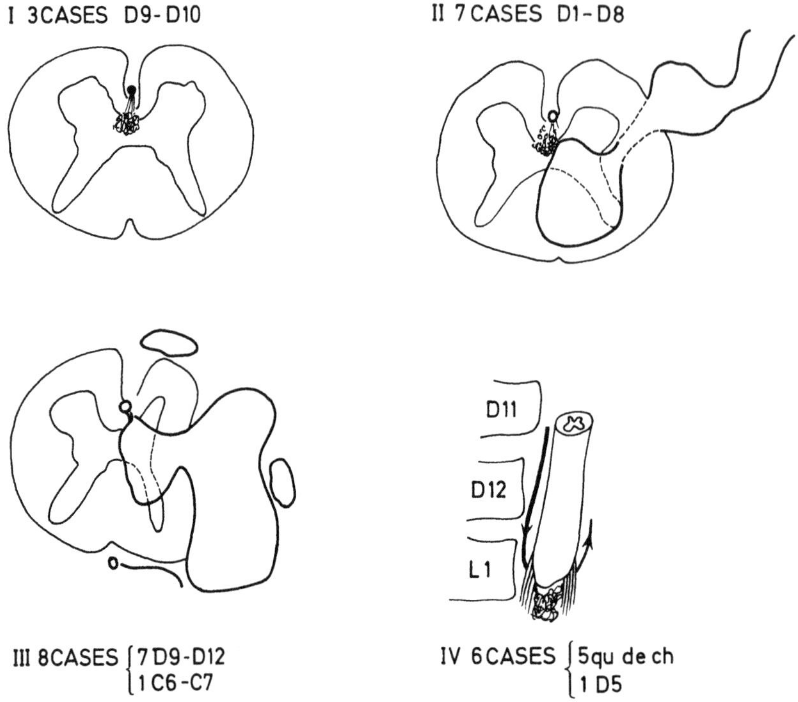

Fig. 1. Location of anterior spinal angiomas in the spinal cord

For each of these groups, a posterior retromedullary angioma can be associated with the anterior malformation according to different patterns. The anterior and posterior parts may be totally independent or may be connected through large venous channels on the lateral aspect of the cord. In our series, the situation of anterior spinal angiomas is as follows (Fig. 1).

Group I : (three cases) situated at the level D 9 - D 10
Group II : (seven cases) between D 1 and D 8
Group III : (eight cases) mainly between D 9 and D 12, except one case in the cervical region (C 6–C 7)
Group IV : (six cases) were situated in the cauda equina adherent to the filum terminale and the conus medullaris. In this latter group, one malformation was at the level of D 5

The location of these malformations within the cord provides the clue for the surgical approach which should be adopted. Posterior commissural myelotomy in groups I and II, dissection close to the margin of the malformation in group III, and direct extramedullary approach in group IV.

Clinical Cases

Groups I, II, III, and IV will be illustrated by the following cases.

Group I : (case DEC., No. 15, Fig. 2)
F. 20 years old, sudden onset of paraplegia.
Neurologic deficit cleared partially within 3 days.

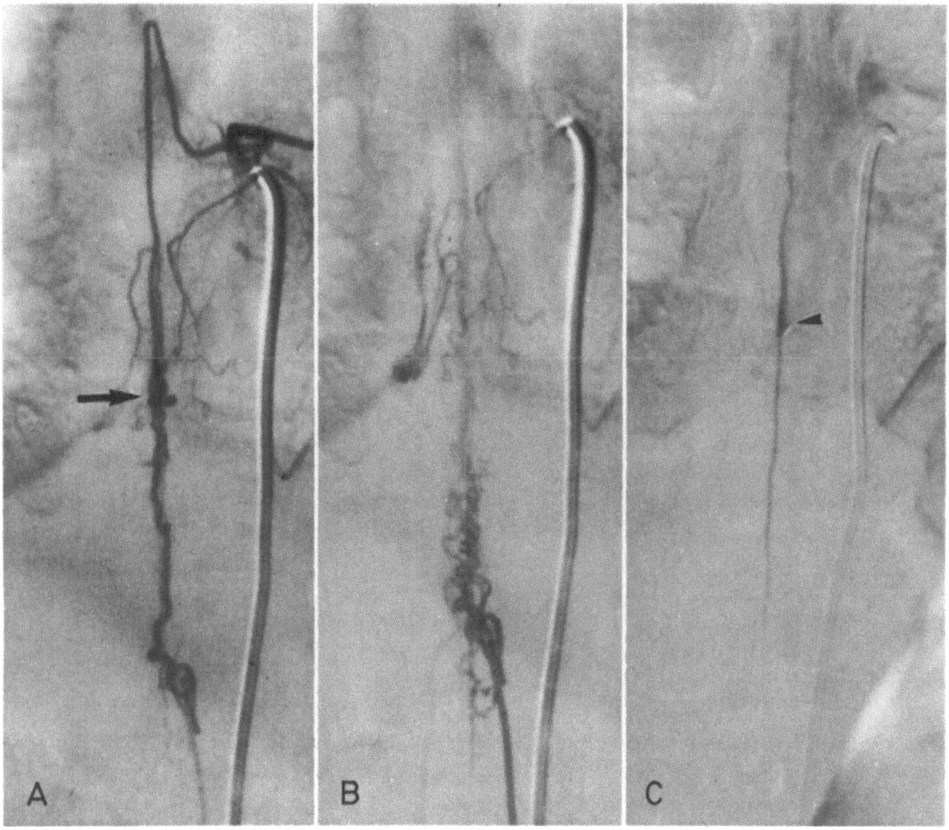

Fig. 2. (A) Preoperative angiogram, AP view, (B) preoperative angiogram, AP view (later phase), (C) postoperative angiogram, AP view, clip at the side of the former malformation

She could walk with a slight spasticity in the left leg. Neurologic examination demonstrated left Brown- Séquard syndrome. Previous history was free of neurologic symptoms. Spinal angiography showed a small angioma at the T 9 level, fed by sulcal arteries arising from the anterior spinal artery. Surgical removal was performed through posterior commissural myelotomy (12/3/76). Postoperative course was uneventful. Control angiography showed disappearance of the angiomatous vessels and preservation of the anterior spinal artery which remained fully patent. This patient returned to work (secretary) 3 months after operation.

Group II : (case BAN No. 17)

Young boy, 9 years old. First subarachnoid hemorrhage with sudden onset of a right Brown-Séquard syndrome. This patient was walking without aid in spite of marked spasticity and a motor deficit in the right lower limb. Spinal angiography demonstrated a group II malformation at the T 8 level (Fig. 3). Operation through a posterior commissural myelotomy allowed removal of the partially thrombosed intramedullary pouch (12/10/75). Small angiomatous vessels which were not within the cord but around the anterior spinal artery in the anterior sulcus were left in place. There was no postoperative deterioration. Control angiography showed radical removal of the intramedullary pouch and filling of some angiomatous vessels around the anterior spinal axis.

Group III : (case GUB, No. 19)

F. 18 years old, first episode of subarachnoid bleeding with low back pain and sciatica in 1973. Recurrence 1 year later. Myelography with Dimer was performed. Huge tortuous ves-

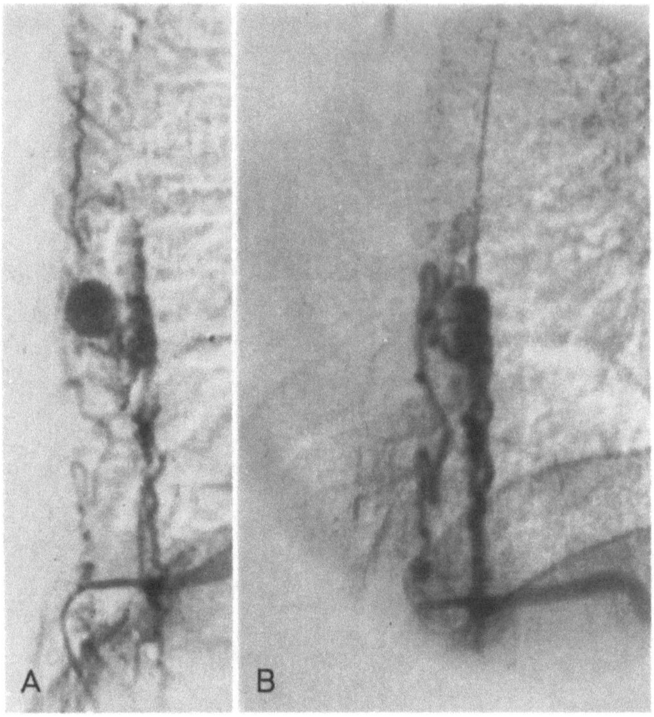

Fig. 3. (A) Preoperative angiograms, lateral view, (B) postoperative angiogram, lateral view

sels were visible within the dural sac in the lumbar region. The patient was transferred to our department. Preoperative neurologic examination revealed slight motor and sensory impairment in the territory of L 5 on the right side. Spinal angiography revealed a huge arteriovenous malformation fed by Adamkiewicz artery and a posterolateral afferent. Total surgical removal was achieved in two stages (24/10/75 – 18/11/75). Control angiography shows no residual abnormal filling. The patient has resumed her previous occupation as a student.

She has minimal deficit from operation: foot drop and hemihypoesthesia of the right perianal region without any sphincter disturbances. However, she complains of loss of sensation on the right side of the vagina.

Group IV : (case BIA No. 22, Fig 4)

F. 13 years old, first episode of meningeal hemorrhage, symptom-free before operation. Angiography showed a spinal malformation, fed by Adamkiewicz artery. The main part of the malformation was at L 2 level.

Total removal was possible with a two-stage procedure. Even in the cauda equina, beneath the conus medullaris, the removal of such an embedded malformation within a small spinal canal may be a tedious and time-consuming procedure, even for a surgeon trained in microsurgery and surgery of spinal cord angiomas. The postoperative result was very satisfactory with no worsening of the neurologic status and total removal demonstrated by control angiography.

Cervical Angiomas

We only had the opportunity to operate on one case in the cervical region (case FEL, No. 6, Fig. 5).

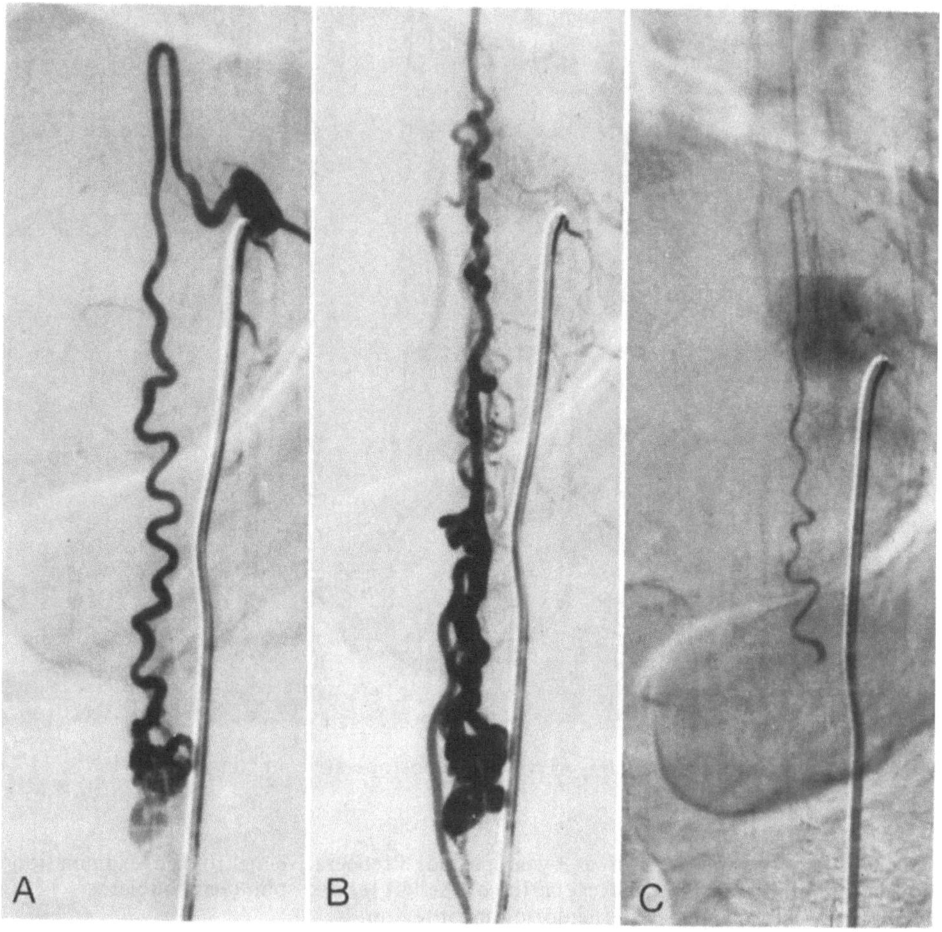

Fig. 4. (A, B) Preoperative angiograms, AP view (early and late phases), (C) postoperative angiogram, AP view

M. 30 years old. At the age of 11, he experienced a total but transient paraplegia. For 15 years he was free of symptoms and could work. Progressive neurologic disability occurred and led to a clinical picture of cervical syringomyelia with severe spastic paraplegia and motor weakness of the upper extremities. Angiography showed a group III arteriovenous malformation.

Total removal (23/04/76) was possible and control angiography satisfactory. Postoperative improvement occurred dramatically in the early postoperative period mainly in the upper extremities. He is now in a rehabilitation center and can walk with aid.

Pseudoectasic Malformations: Role of Trauma

Case COU, No. 10 illustrates this problem (Fig. 6).

This man, 37 years old, first experienced marked paraparesis at the age of 22, when he was a paratrooper. This episode took place immediately after landing during a parachute exercise. No fracture of the vertebral column was demonstrated at the time. Fifteen years later, he

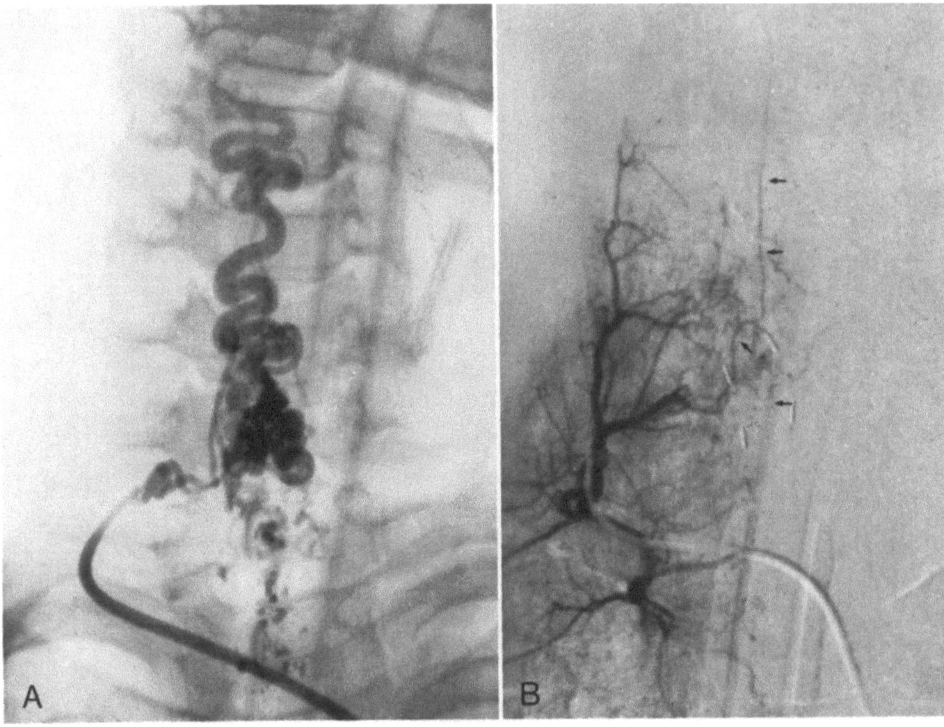

Fig. 5. (A) Preoperative angiogram, AP view, (B) postoperative angiogram, AP view

became slowly paraplegic over a 3-year period. Preoperative neurologic examination showed total deficit of the right leg, partial of the left leg and sphincter troubles.
Myelography showed a block in the dorsolumbar region.
Spinal angiography demonstrated a huge malformation which mainly consisted of a large arteriovenous fistula between the artery of Adamkiewicz and a big pouch situated anterior to the conus medullaris. Venous drainage is impressive with a tortuous draining vein retro- and premedullary going to the extradural venous spinal plexus. This lesion was treated by direct attack. (Jan. 1977).
The neck of the fistula was approached through a myelotomy, 3 cm long in the lowest part of the conus medullaris and was closed by a straight Heifetz clip. Postoperative course was uneventful. Control angiography no longer shows the fistula nor the huge venous drainage. This patient was operated only 3 months ago and is still in a rehabilitation center.

Results

Preoperative Neurologic Status

Level, age at time of operation, time elapsed since the first clinical symptom of the disease, and episodes of subarachnoid hemorrhage are summarized in Table 1. Five patients had a total paraplegia and were operated on early in this series. Four patients had severe spastic paraparesis and were bedridden before operation. Five patients had moderate paraplegia but could not walk before operation, mainly because of proximal deficit. Ten patients

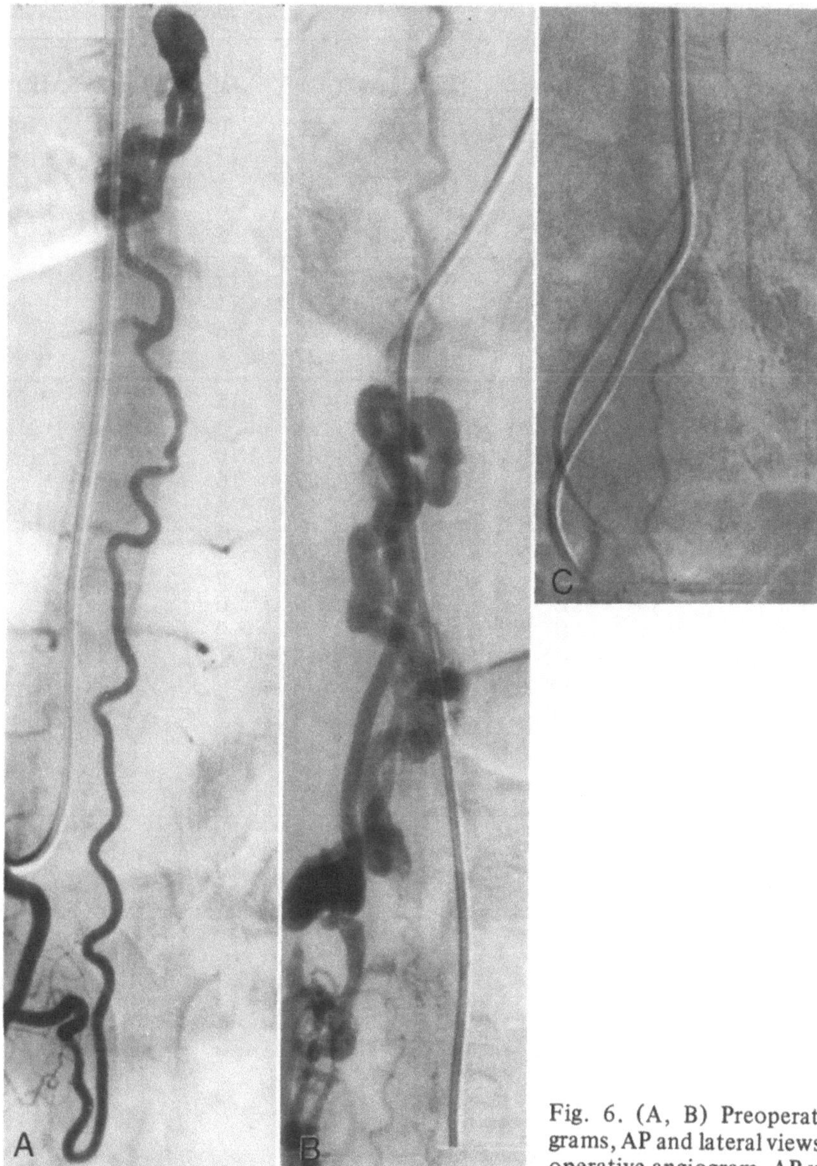

Fig. 6. (A, B) Preoperative angiograms, AP and lateral views, (C) postoperative angiogram, AP view

had slight neurologic impairment or were symptom-free before surgery. Patients with minimal deficit are young. Diagnosis was made at the first neurologic disturbance except for five who experienced an episode of subarachnoid hemorrhage or regressive paraparesis some years earlier (1–9 years); groups III and IV angiomas are frequent in these patients. Patients with marked neurologic disability are older and had several episodes of bleeding, paraparesis, or paraplegia before operation. In these patients, groups I or II angiomas are very frequent. Subarachnoid hemorrhage is a very characteristic feature of anterior spinal angiomas and is present in the course of the disease in 13 out of 24 cases (over 50%).

Table 1. Clinical picture

	Case No.	Group[a]	Level	Age[b]	1st symptom[c]	SAH[d]
Total paraplegia	1	I	T 9	10	0	
	2	II	T 3	28	17	+
	3	II	T 3	37	3	+
	4	II	T 3	10	6	+
	5	IV	T 12 - L 1	54	5	+
Severe paraplegia	6	III	C 6	30	19	
	7	II	T 6	21	11	
	8	II	T 6	26	6	+
	9	II	T 8	27	8	+
Moderate paraplegia	10	IV	T 8 - T 12	37	15	
	11	III	T 9 - T 12	18	2	+
	12	III	T 9 - T 12	45	10	+
	13	III	T 9 - T 11	27	16	+
	14	IV	I 3	36	4	+
Slight deficit, no deficit	15	I	T 9	20	0	+
	16	I	T 9 - T 12	16	9	+
	17	II	T 8	9	0	+
	18	III	T 12	12	0	+
	19	III	T 12	18	1	+
	20	IV	L 1	38	0	+
	21	IV	T 5	13	9	+
	22	IV	L 2	13	0	+
	23	III	T 8 - T 9	36	1	+
	24	III	T 9 - T 12	35	1	

[a] Group classification, see Fig. 1.
[b] Age at operation.
[c] First symptom means number of years elapsed from the first symptom of the disease to operation.
[d] Subarachnoid hemorrhage.

Postoperative Neurologic Status – Surgical Results

Pre- and postoperative spinal angiography is absolutely necessary to assess the surgical result after direct attack on anterior spinal malformations (Table 2). We were able to perform this pre- and postoperative control in 21 cases. Total removal of the malformation was achieved in 17 cases. In four cases, the malformation was removed only subtotally. Small angiomatous vessels surrounding the anterior spinal artery were still visible on control angiography. In our opinion, these angiomas situated not only within the cord but also in the anterior median sulcus around the anterior spinal artery cannot be removed completely. The small part surrounding the anterior spinal artery must be left in place to avoid undue postoperative deficit. Three cases had no postoperative angiography. Surgical removal has been probably total in one case, subtotal in two other cases. No permanent worsening of the preoperative neurologic status was observed in any cases. However, the surgical result is chiefly related to the preoperative neurologic impairement:

Table 2. Surgical treatment (24 cases)

	Case no.	Group	Level	Preop. status[a]	Postop status[a]	Control angiography	Total removal	Subtot. removal
Total paraplegia	1	I	T 9	0	0	+		+
	2	II	T 3	0	0	+	+	
	3	II	T 3	0	0	+	+	
	4	II	T 3	0	0	+	+	
	5	IV	T 12 - L 1	0	0			
Severe paraplegia	6	III	C 6	2	3	+	+	
	7	II	T 6	1	1	+	+	
	8	II	T 6	2	3			
	9	II	T 8	3	3			
Moderate paraplegia	10	IV	T 8 - T 12	3	3	+	+	
	11	III	T 9 - T 12	3	5	+	+	
	12	III	T 9 - T 12	3	4	+	+	
	13	III	T 9 - T 11	3	4	+	+	
	14	IV	L 3	3	5	+	+	
Slight deficit, no deficit	15	I	T 9	5	5	+	+	
	16	I	T 9 - T 12	5	4	+		+
	17	II	T 8	4	4	+		+
	18	III	T 12	4	5	+	+	
	19	III	T 12	5	5	+	+	
	20	IV	L 1	5	5	+	+	
	21	IV	T 5	5	5	+	+	
	22	IV	L 2	5	5	+	+	
	23	III	T 8 - T 9	5	5	+	+	
	24	III	T 9 - T 12	5	5	+		+

[a] 0: no movement,
1, 2: slight distal movements, walking impossible,
3: moderate deficit, walking possible with aid,
4: slight deficit, walking possible with aid for long distances,
5: no deficit.

1. Patients with complete paraplegia got no benefit from the surgical procedure.
2. Those with severe deficit were improved in three cases and unchanged in one; three of these patients who were bedridden before operation can walk now with crutches and have a spastic and pendular gait.
3. Patients with moderate paraplegia can walk without aid for short distances and with aid (one or two sticks) for longer distances.
4. Patients with slight deficit or without preoperative deficit had no postoperative worsening except in two instances (case 13 and case 18).

In case 13, total deficit of the right leg followed operation instead of a slight deficit of the same leg preoperatively. Happily, this deficit subsided within 3 weeks. It is undoubtedly related to excessive dissection around the spinal artery in the anterior sulcus. For that reason, we do not advise attempting removal of such angiomatous vessels closely adherent around the anterior spinal artery itself. In case 18, a definite deficit in the territory of L 5, and hemihypoesthesia from S 1 to S 5 occurred following operation and must be attributed to unavoidable section of rootlets passing through the malformation.

These 24 patients have been operated within the last 3 years (Dec. '73 - Dec. '76). Results of operation demonstrate that surgical attack is especially indicated in patients free of symptoms or with slight neurologic deficit. In fact, neurologic recovery depends mainly upon preoperative neurologic disability. This is the main argument for operating on such patients early in the natural course of the disease before serious and irreversible lesions of the cord occur. In this respect one must emphasize once more the necessity for early diagnosis and treatment.

Operative Treatment of Spinal Angioblastomas

M.G. Yasargil, R.W. Fiedeler, and Th.P. Rankin

Historical Review

The first report in the literature of the disorder that has come to be known as von Hippel-Lindau's Disease (multiple angiomatosis of retina, CNS, and viscera) was published by Hughlings Jackson in 1872 (Jackson, 1872). In 1879 Panas and Rémy published the first anatomical description of the retinal lesion (Panas and Rémy, 1879), although this is usually incorrectly attributed to Fuchs (Fuchs, 1882). Collins described the histology in 1894 and also noted the familial character of the disease (Collins, 1894). In 1904 von Hippel, unaware of Collins' work, published the article which has caused his name to be associated with the retinal lesion, and in 1911 he concluded that the primary retinal lesion was a hemangioblastoma (von Hippel, 1904; 1911). In 1926 Lindau first described the association of cystic angiomas of the cerebellum with the "angiomatosis retinae" of von Hippel; Lindau further noted that both were associated with visceral tumors and cysts (Lindau, 1926). He also described 4 cases of spinal cord angioma associated with cerebellar tumor (Lindau, 1931). Cushing and Bailey in 1928 defined these neoplasms as hemangioblastomas and distinguished them from arterio-venous malformations (Cushing and Bailey, 1928). In 1929 Möller proved the genetic character of the disease (Möller, 1929). Roussy and Oberling in 1931 suggested the name angioreticuloma for these tumors; the term is synonymous with hemangioblastoma (Roussy and Oberling, 1930; Melmon and Rosen, 1964; Minckler, 1971). In 1943 Wyburn-Mason published his excellent monograph describing the 47 cases of spinal hemangioblastoma in the world literature at the time (Wyburn-Mason, 1943). His monograph remains the classic work on the subject. Another excellent monograph was published in 1975 by Hurth et al. (1975) [in French].

Definition

Von Hippel-Lindau's Disease is a heredo-familial disease, transmitted by an autosomal dominant gene with incomplete penetrance (Levin, 1936; Otenasek and Silver, 1961; Thomas and Burnside, 1961; Craig and Horrax, 1949; Perlmutter et al., 1950; Palmer 1972; Christoferson et al., 1961; Möller, 1929; Silver, 1954), and characterized by vascular tumors of the retina and of the central nervous system, most commonly cerebellum but also spinal cord, cerebrum, and brain stem; and by visceral lesions including cysts, adenomata, and angiomata of the adrenals; cysts and tumors of the kidneys; cysts of pancreas, lung, and liver, cysts of the epididymis and cystadenomata of the ovaries; vascular skin nevi; anomalies of diploic vessels; and enlargement and tortuosity of the veins of the mesentery and stomach wall (Minckler, 1971; Houdart and Djindjian, 1974; Melmon and Rosen, 1964; Wyburn-Mason, 1943; von Hippel, 1911, 1904; Lindau, 1931; Craig et al., 1941; Kinney and Fitzgerald, 1947). However, since the complete syndrome is exceedingly rare, we agree with Houdart and Djindjian (Houdart and Djindjian, 1974) that the term von Hippel-Lindau's Disease should be used to refer to all forms of hemangioblastoma, single or multiple, with or without visceral lesion, in which a familial character can be demonstrated. As Kendall and Russell (1966) suggest, the association of spinal and cerebellar hemangioblastoma is also sufficient to establish the diagnosis, and the same should of course hold true for the combination of central nervous system and retinal lesions. Spinal hemangioblastoma is a benign neoplasm, as defined by Lindau and Cushing and Bailey. It may occur intramedullary or extradurally. Its histology has been well described (Rubinstein, 1970; Kinney and Fitzgerald, 1947; Craig et al., 1941; Houdart and Djindjian, 1974; Perlmutter et al., 1950; Huk and Klinger, 1973; Minckler, 1971; Casteigne et al., 1968; Sloof et al., 1964; Russell, 1932). Very briefly, it is a mixed tumor composed of thin-walled blood vessels of varying caliber, separated by a variable amount of stromal cells, the "pseudoxanthoma" cells containing fat. There is an abundant network of reticulin fibers but no glial or neural elements. The histologic picture of hemangioblastomas is strikingly similar to that of angioblastic meningiomas and renal clear cell carcinoma. Grossly the tumor may have a yellowish, orange, or deep red color. It is almost always well circumscribed although there is no capsule (Cramer and Kinsey, 1952; Rubinstein, 1970); it may be partly cystic and may be associated with pial varices. It is to be distinguished, according to the classification of Bergstrand et al. (1965) from vascular malformation, angioma cavernosum and angioma racemosum.

Epidemiology

Primary spinal cord neoplasms are rare, having at autopsy, an incidence of approximately 1 in 10,000 (Sloof et al., 1964) (2 to 3% of primary spinal cord neoplasms are hemangioblastomas). Our review of the available world literature including our own, revealed a total of 111 intramedullary spinal hemangioblastomas, 61 of which were male, 39 female and the remainder undesignated (Schultze, 1912; Roman, 1913; Wyburn-Mason, 1943; Sloof et al., 1964; Otenasek and Silver, 1961; Bardal et al., 1973; Illingworth, 1967; Kinney and Fitzgerald, 1947; Langlois et al., 1964; Huk and Klinger, 1973; Paillas et al., 1968; Herdt et al., 1972; Kendall and Russell, 1966; Palmer, 1972; Bannerjee and Hunt, 1972; Guidetti and Fortuna, 1967; Krishnan and Smith, 1961; Bettaieb, 1964; Bergstrand et al., 1965; Sakhai, 1966; Lepoire et al., 1969; Pecker, 1971; Krayenbühl and Yasargil, 1963; Cassinari and Bernasconi, 1961; Wright, 1969; Saito, 1971; Black and Farber 1943). The age at time of evaluation ranged from 9 to 62 years (Illingworth, 1967; Wyburn-Mason 1943; Black and Farber, and our cases), with mean age of 36.9 years.

Symptoms

The natural history of the disease is that of a typical intramedullary tumor producing spinal cord compression, progressing to paraplegia or tetraplegia. The advance is usually fairly slow with an average duration of about 3 years between the onset of symptoms and the time of definitive neurological evaluation (mean 34.2 months for 65 cases). Symptoms of cord compression are more prominent and more rapidly progressive with extradural hemangioblastomas, having an average duration of 9.2 months according to Wyburn-Mason and 6 months according to Iizuka (Wyburn-Mason, 1943; Iizuka, 1970). Hemangioblastomas are located primarily in the posterior spinal cord (Kinney and Fitzgerald, 1947; Zülch, 1956; David et al., 1968; Melmon and Rosen, 1964); however the first symptom is usually pain rather than sensory loss. They may be found anywhere in the cord, but the preponderance is in the cervical and thoracic regions (55 out of 65 in our review). However, the first symptoms involve the upper or lower extremities equally frequently, and remission of symptoms early in the clinical course is common (Bergstrand et al., 1965; Sakhai, 1966; Schultze, 1912). Simultaneous posterior fossa and spinal lesions are quite common; 22 out of 65 cases clinically, 5 out of 9 autopsy cases in our review (Sloof et al., 1964; Kinney and Fitzgerald, 1947; Kendall and Russell, 1966; Guidetti and Fortuna, 1967; Bergstrand et al., 1965), and 8 out of 12 in our clinical series (cases number 1, 2 and 3 being bulbar and spinal; and cases number 4, 5, 6, 7 and 8 being cerebellar and spinal). With a simultaneous posterior fossa and spinal lesion, the initial symptoms are usually those of increased intracranial pressure. However the combination of symptoms increases the reliance on neuroradiologic techniques. It is noteworthy that subarachnoid hemorrhage in the unoperated case is extremely rare, but is not uncommon after operation, for example our case number 5.

The retinal lesion is typically peripheral with a tortuous dilated vein and artery leading to a hemangioblastoma, which may be obscured by exudate or gliosis (Silver, 1954; Craig et al., 1941). It is present in approximately 33% of cases of spinal hemangioblastoma and is often bilateral (22/65 clinically; 4/9 autopsy; and in our clinical series 3/12). Retinal symptoms usually precede spinal symptoms, but are a far less common presenting complaint than pain. Because of the common association, careful ophthalmological examination is mandatory once a spinal lesion has been diagnosed. Photocoagulation is effective for the majority of early retinal lesions, whereas the untreated lesion progresses inevitably leading to blindness of the affected eye.

Syrinx is present in approximately 70% of cases, pial varices in roughly 40%, root involvement in about 15%, visceral involvement in about 30% but is usually asymptomatic. It is noteworthy that pheochromocytoma, although generally felt to be rare (Illingworth, 1967; Nibbelink et al., 1969), was present bilaterally in two of our cases number 4 and 5. We would emphasize that the presence of hypertension with hemangioblastoma indicates the need to look for a pheochromocytoma.

Clinically, von Hippel-Lindau's Disease is present in approximately 50% of the reported cases of spinal hemangioblastoma, but it is likely that closer examination would reveal an even higher incidence (Kinney and Fitzgerald, 1947; Huk and Klinger, 1973; Levin, 1936). In view of the genetic character of the disease, once a diagnosis of von Hippel-Lindau's disease has been made, screening and long term follow-up of the patient's relatives is mandatory.

The association of polycythemia with cerebellar hemangioblastoma is well established (Carpenter et al., 1943; Melmon and Rosen, 1964; Minckler, 1971; Waldmann et al., 1971) and Cramer estimates it to be present in 9% of cases (Cramer and Kinsey, 1952). It is probable that a similar figure would be reached in association with spinal angiomas.

Radiology

Plain x-rays are almost never diagnostic but are suggestive in roughly half the cases. Kyphoscoliosis is not uncommon (Paillas et al., 1968), and typically there may be spinal canal widening or pedicle erosion.

Myelography was positive in all 43 cases where adequate information was available. There was a partial or complete block in 32 of these. Myelography should be done in both supine and prone positions to assure adequate visualization and is only occasionally diagnostic of spinal hemangioblastoma. If there are associated pial varices this shows typical wormlike defects in the contrast column, and if cord widening is also present this usually indicates a diagnosis of hemangioblastoma rather than AVM. Hemangioblastomas without varices are indistinguishable from other intramedullary tumors.

Lumbar CSF with intramedullary hemangioblastoma is usually xanthochromic and the Pandy is almost always positive. Average protein in 33 cases reviewed was 466 mg% with a cell count of 5 or 6 cells/mm^3. Cisternal CSF protein averaged 96 mg% with 3 cells/mm^3, a weakly positive Pandy, and frequent xanthochromia. With extradural hemangioblastomas, there is always a block, usually complete, and the lumbar CSF protein averages 254 mg% with only occasional xanthochromia (Wyburn-Mason, 1943).

The characteristic angiographic picture of hemangioblastoma is a well circumscribed dense homogeneous blush without evidence of individual vessels. The blush lasts from the early arterial through to the late venous phase, and there is neither an early draining vein nor dilatation of the AICA, PICA or vertebral arteries. Early draining veins or dilated arteries strongly suggest AVM rather than hemangioblastoma (see case number 2).

The method of choice is selective angiography by transfemoral route with catheterization of the arteries of the spinal cord as developed by Djindjian (Djindjian et al., 1971, 1970; Houdart and Djindjian, 1974), particularly with the use of subtraction technique. The association of spinal hemangioblastoma with cerebellar and visceral lesions of von Hippel-Lindau's disease, particularly renal clear cell carcinoma, make it imperative that these lesions be searched for angiographically once a spinal lesion has been demonstrated. Similarly, the entire spinal cord should be examined radiologically to rule out multiple hemangioblastomas.

Surgical Review

As early as 1912, Schultze was able, with success, to remove totally an intramedullary hemangioblastoma (Schultze, 1912). However, the results of surgery for this lesion have, in the past, been generally discouraging. Our review of the available world literature indicates that, of the 35 intramedullary cases operated (excluding our present cases) there has been surgical death in no less than 12, and there have been only 15 total removals (Sloof et al., 1964; Schultze, 1912; Roman, 1913; Otenasek and Silver 1961; Bardal et al., 1973; Guidetti and Fortuna, 1967; Kinney and Fitzgerald, 1947; Krishnan and Smith, 1961; Herdt et al., 1972; Kendall and Russell, 1966; Palmer, 1972; Minckler, 1971; Bettaieb, 1964; Bergstrand et al., 1965; Sakhai, 1966). This has led to such pessimistic statements as Melmon in 1964:

"the surgical treatment of spinal cord hemangioblastomas is hazardous, albeit successful on rare occasions" (Melmon and Rosen, 1964).
Krishnan and Smith 1961:
"before attempting to excise an intradural angioma, the possibility that an intramedullary hemangioma may also be present should be considered: operation is contraindicated if this is confirmed" (Krishnan and Smith, 1961).
And Bannerjee and Hunt, as recently as 1972:
"total removal of such a lesion (intramedullary hemangioblastoma) was not feasible and an attempt would probably have impaired the patient's ability considerably" (Bannerjee and Hunt, 1972).

It must be remembered that hemangioblastomas are true neoplasms which progress inexorably to a catastrophic clinical situation if left untreated. Radiation therapy has not been demonstrated to be of significant value (Kendall and Russell, 1966; Shephard, 1953; Wyburn-Mason, 1943; Dynes and Snedal, 1960; Sloof et al., 1964; Palmer, 1972; Bannerjee and Hunt, 1972; Bardal et al., 1973; Odom, 1962; Silver, 1954). Likewise, simple decompressive laminectomy or partial removal is only palliative therapy. It is felt that, with the use of the operating microscope and bipolar cautery, and employment of the microsurgical technique complete, safe, and successful extirpation of these tumors is possible (Yasargil et al., 1976).

Case Reports

Case No. 1

A 41-year-old man with ataxia, headache and vomiting underwent a suboccipital craniotomy in July 1965 and was found to have what was considered to be an inoperable cerebellar angioma. Despite multiple shunts by October 1969 the patient had developed nystagmus, multiple right-sided cranial nerve palsies, left-sided hemiparesis, marked ataxia of the trunk and left extremities in addition to papilledema.

Cerebral angiography at that time demonstrated a hemangioblastoma of the cerebellum extending down to C 3.

In November 1967 the patient underwent a bilateral suboccipital craniotomy and laminectomy of C 1 to C 3. An orange-sized right cerebellar hemangioblastoma with extension into the fourth ventricle was removed. The extramedullary cervical angioma was coagulated.

Postoperatively the patient was left with only ataxia and some nystagmus. Eleven months later the patient died of unrelated cardiac disease. Autopsy revealed a left cerebellar hemangioblastoma and cystic pancreas and kidney.

Case No. 2

A 27-year-old man presented with ataxia, blurred vision, occipital headache and neck pain of six months duration. Because of these difficulties a ventriculoatrial shunt was inserted at another hospital. In February of 1973 the patient had a left hemiparesis, ataxia, and nystagmus.

Cerebral angiography showed what was felt to be a hemangioblastoma with involvement of the fourth ventricle (Fig. 1).

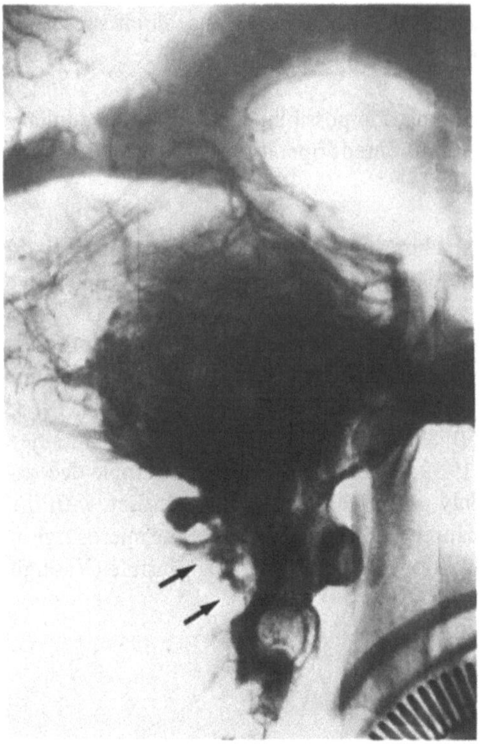

Fig. 1. (Case 2) Vertebral angiography with ventriculography showing subtentorial vascular staining with caudal extension into cervical cord (Black arrows)

At operation in February 1973 a hemangioblastoma, filling the fourth ventricle and cisterna magna with intramedullary cervical extension to C 3 was found and completely removed.

Postoperatively the patient had good use of all four extremities and was able to walk with assistance. He did, however, have bilateral paralysis of the 9th, 10th and 12th cranial nerves. Eighteen months later the patient died of a bulbar lesion.

Case No. 3

A 44-year-old woman had suffered from headache for years. In 1969 she was found to have a left hemiparesis, left hemiataxia, and papilledema. After nonlocalizing contrast studies she underwent multiple shunting procedures because of moderate hydrocephalus. In February 1974 the patient re-evaluated and found to have a left hemiparesis, left hemihypesthesia and hemiataxia.

Cerebral angiography demonstrated a very vascular lemon-sized tumor at the level of the foramen magnum (Fig. 2, 3 and 4).

At operation, after a suboccipital craniotomy and laminectomy to C 3, a hemangioblastoma was found, filling the fourth ventricle and cisterna magna with intramedullary extension to C 3. The tumor was completely removed.

At three year follow-up the patient was free of neurological deficit, leading a normal life and working full time.

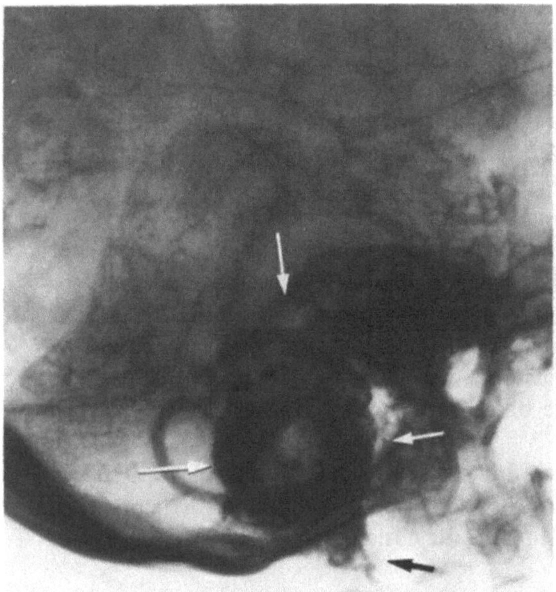

Fig. 2

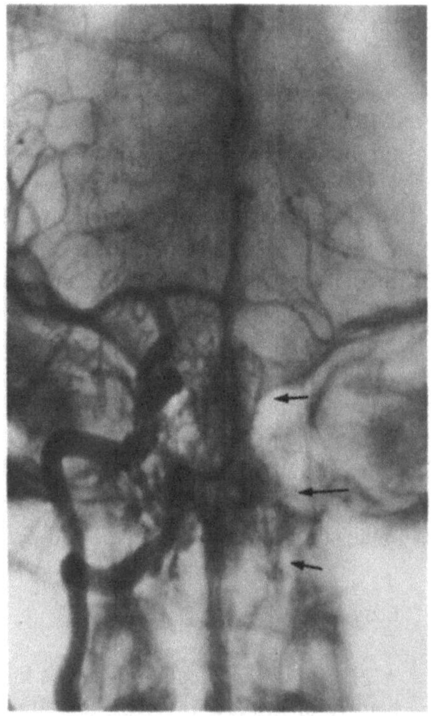

Fig. 3

Fig. 2. (Case 3) Vertebral angiogram showing a large very vascular tumor at the level of foramen magnum (arrows)

Fig. 3. (Case 3) Carotid and vertebral injection showing midline posterior fossa vascular staining

Fig. 4. (Case 3) Vertebral angiogram A-P projection demonstrating the vascular staining (Black arrows). Basilar artery (white arrows)

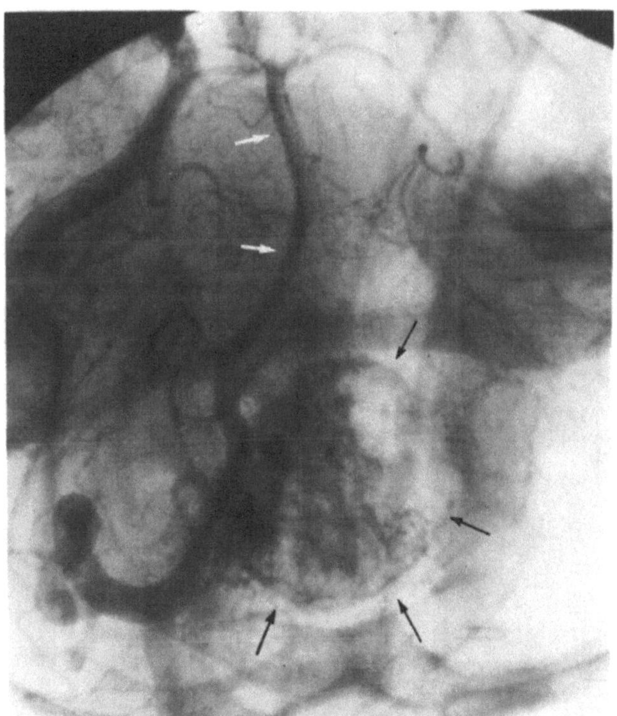

Fig. 4

Case No. 4

A 38-year-old man had had for 8 months a right hemiparesis, gait difficulties and headache. By the time he was examined he had bilateral rotatory nystagmus, right sided hemiparesis, hyporeflexia, sensory loss and ataxia. A left retinal angioma was also detected.

Bilateral carotid angiography was negative. Cervical myelography showed a vascular pattern of contrast displacement at C 1 and widening of the cervical cord.

In April 1970 a laminectomy from C 1 to C 7 was performed. After coagulating a thick tortuous vessel from C 1 to C 2 and two laterally placed arteries, as well as numerous feeding vessels, a 4 x 1 cm cystic intramedullary hemangioblastoma from C 2 to C 5 was totally extirpated. Because of severe ataxia,vertebral angiography was performed in June 1970 which showed a left cerebellar hemangioblastoma which was totally removed at that time. Subsequently the patient has undergone bilateral removal of pheochromocytomas and photocoagulation of the left retina.

At six year follow-up there was bilateral vibratory loss from C 4 distally. He was also experiencing intractable right shoulder pain. His paresis and ataxia had greatly improved allowing him to care for himself and perform domestic duties.

Case No. 5

A 22-year-old medical student was initially admitted in March 1969 because of a one year history of headache, vertigo and ataxia. At that time bilateral cerebellar hemangioblastomas were removed (Fig. 5). In June 1974 two more small extramedullary hemangioblasto-

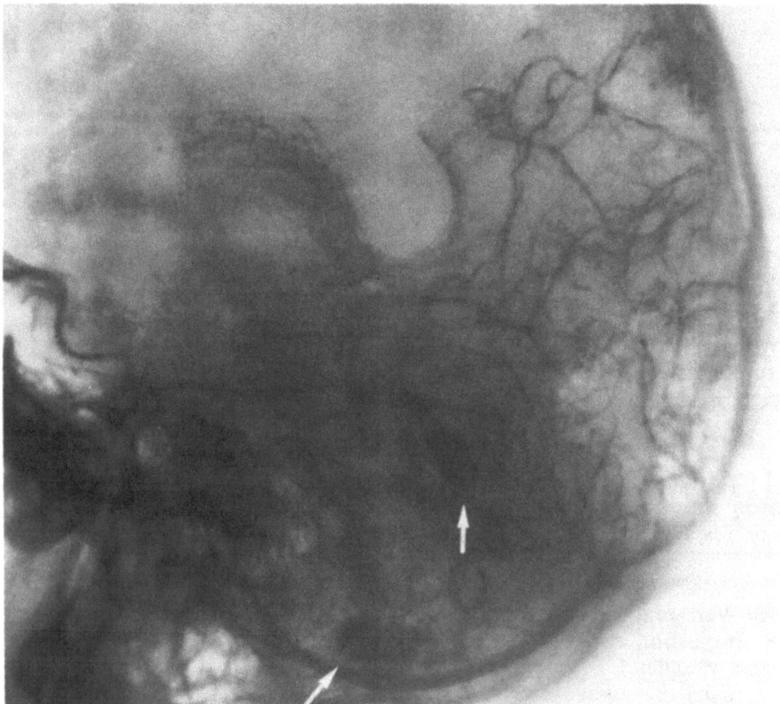

Fig. 5. (Case 5) Vertebral angiogram showing two stains localizing bilateral cerebellar hemangioblastomas (arrows)

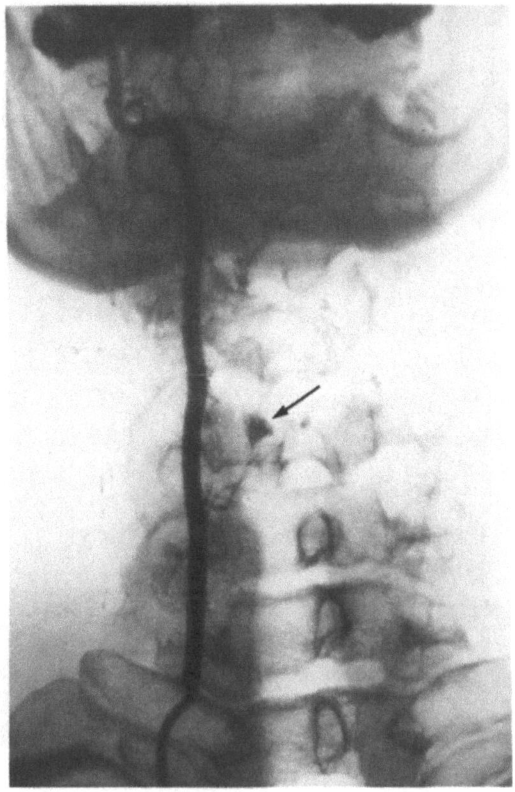

Fig. 6. (Case 5) Right vertebral angiogram showing a small intramedullary nodule at level of C_5 (arrow). Note the pathological vessels demarcating the cranial pole of the tumor

mas of the calamus scriptorius were removed. The patient was also shunted at that time. Subsequently, however, he developed a progressive weakness of his left arm.

This patient had a left renal pheochromocytoma removed. His sister died at the age of 27 with an ocular tumor and his mother died of renal carcinoma.

Vertebral angiography in June 1974 revealed a small vascular malformation at the level of C 5 (Fig. 6).

In July 1974 a laminectomy from C 2 – C 7 revealed a swollen, yellowish spinal cord from C 2 – C 6 with an evident tumor nodule. Feeding vessels along the spinal roots of C 4 and C 5 were coagulated and sectioned. The intramedullary hemangioblastoma was freed circumferentially and completely removed. Care was taken to spare a large dilated vein draining into the anterior spinal vein.

Two years after his last operation the patient has a Brown-Séquard syndrome with the paresis on the left. The patient has now completed his medical studies but will require treatment in the future for a retinal angioma.

Case No. 6

A 49-year-old woman was seen in October 1974 after an 18 year history of visual loss because of retinal angiomas. In 1957 a left hemiparesis was detected and cerebellar explorations were carried out in another hospital in 1958 and again in 1969. The diagnosis of hemangioblastoma was made on both occasions but the tumor was not removed. In Febru-

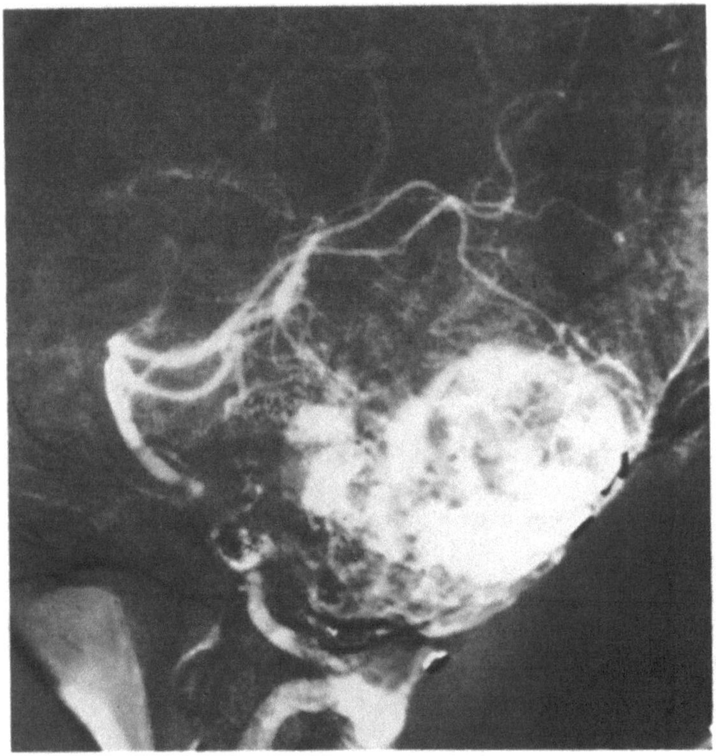

Fig. 7

Fig. 8

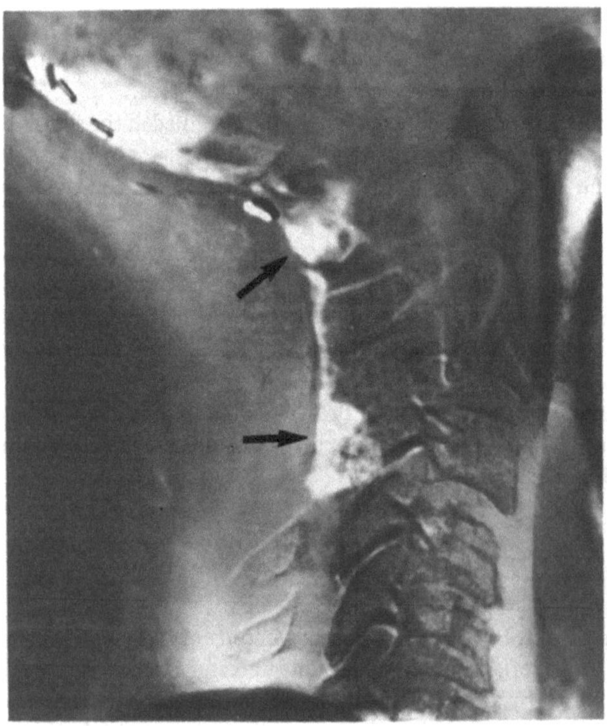

Fig. 7. (Case 6) Vertebral angiography demonstrates four angiomas of the posterior fossa

Fig. 8. (Case 6) Vertebral angiography shows a tumor stain at the levels of the foramen magnum and of the intramedullary cord at C3 - C4

ary 1974 headache and vomiting developed which were transiently improved by a ventriculoperitoneal shunt in August 1974. By October 1974 she had become tetraparetic with marked ataxia and profound sensory deficit in all four extremities. Vertebral angiography showed four angiomas of the posterior fossa with a nodule at the level of the foramen magnum and an additional extra- and intramedullary nodule at C 3 – C 4 (Fig. 7 and 8).

In October of 1974 after suboccipital craniotomy and laminectomy of C 1 – C 4 four cerebellar hemangioblastomas were removed totally. A 3 cm long intramedullary nodule was likewise completely extirpated along with two small extramedullary hemangioblastomas located at the origin of the sensory roots of C 1 and C 2.

Motor performance and ataxia were significantly improved one and a half years later enabling the patient to walk unassisted.

Case No. 7

A 30-year-old woman had experienced a transient left hemiparesis 3 years prior to admission. One year later she underwent a laminectomy from T 6 – T 12 after becoming paraparetic. An intramedullary hemangioblastoma was subtotally excised at another institution at that time. After improving, she subsequently developed a progressive paraparesis, incontinence of bowel and bladder and pain in the left arm. On examination in March 1974 the patient had a triplegia sparing the right arm, and a retinal angioma. She had a sister with retinal angiomas and her father had a hypernephroma.

Plain X-ray films of spine showed radiolucencies in the laminae of C4 and C5. Myelography demonstrated an incomplete block from T 4 to T 7. Vertebral angiography revealed

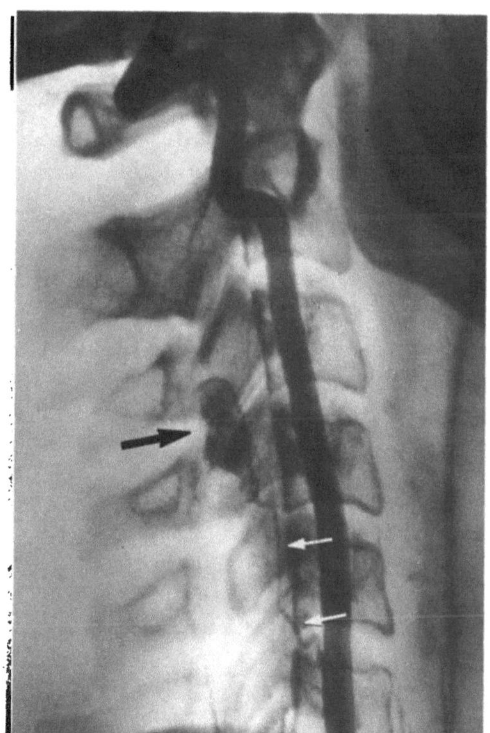

Fig. 9. (Case 7) Left vertebral angiography shows an intramedullary stain at level of C3-C4 (arrow). Note also the feeding vessels (white arrows)

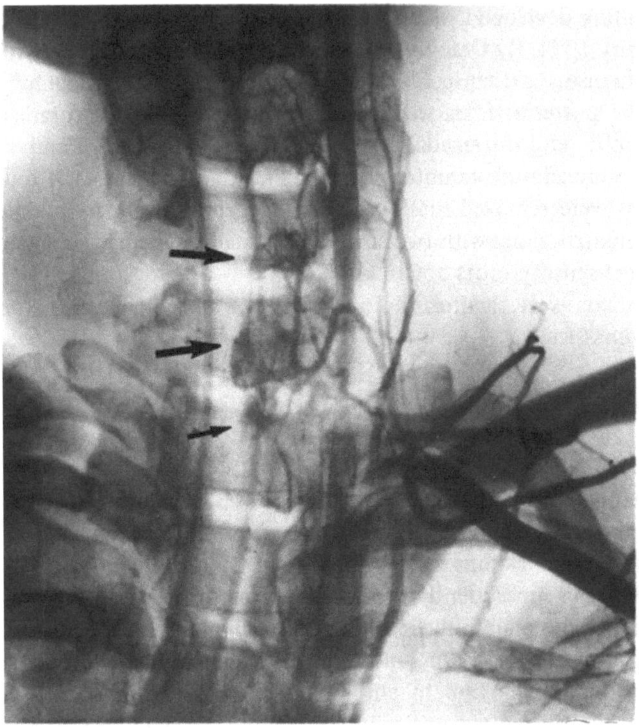

Fig. 10. (Case 7) Vertebral angiogram showing vascular stains at C6-C7 (arrows)

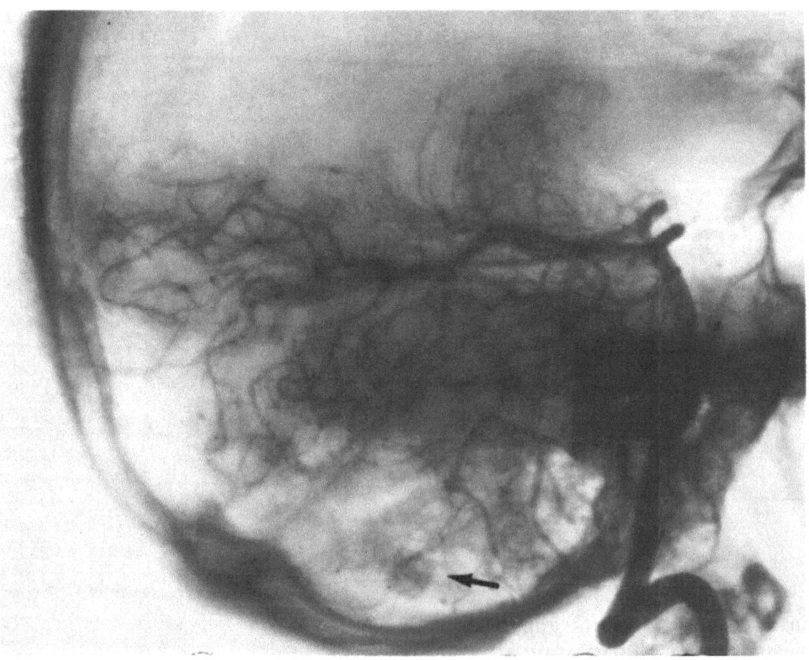

Fig. 11. (Case 7) Vertebral angiogram shows cerebellar hemangioblastoma (arrow)

cerebellar tumor and intramedullary spinal tumors at C 3 – C 4 and C 6 – T 1 (Figs. 9, 10 and 11).

In March of 1974 a left suboccipital craniotomy and C 1 – T 1 laminectomy were performed. Two intramedullary hemangioblastomas and surrounding pathologic vessels were completely removed from C 3 – C 4 and C 6 – T 1. These were both supplied by branches of the anterior spinal artery. The left cerebellar hemangioblastoma was then totally removed.

Four months after surgery the patient was able to walk with a stick and had only a mild weakness of the left arm. Pain in the left arm and urinary incontinence persisted.

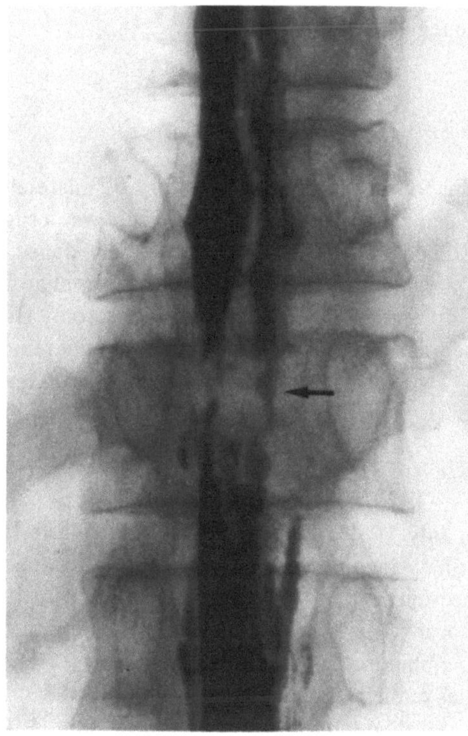

Fig. 12. (Case 8) Pantopaque myelogram shows a globular defect at the T11 - T12 level (arrow)

Case No. 8

After a 10 year history of low back pain this 62-year-old male experienced an acute exacerbation six weeks prior to being admitted. Three weeks later the patient developed a marked psycho-organic brain syndrome. In April 1974 vertebral angiography demonstrated hydrocephalus and a ventriculoperitoneal shunt was inserted. A small cerebellar hemangioblastoma was not visualized at that time.

Subsequent myelography demonstrated a vascular defect in the contrast medium at T 11 – T 12 (Fig. 12).

After a laminectomy from T 9 to L 1, two intra- and extramedullary hemangioblastomas were totally removed.

In October of 1975 the patient was neurologically completely normal. The cerebellar exploration is pending. The patient has returned to full-time employment.

Case No. 9

In this 25-year-old man, right arm weakness had followed pain in the neck and right shoulder for eleven months. On examination there was mild tetraparesis. An uncle was known to have an arteriovenous malformation of the spinal cord.

Myelography was suggestive of an intramedullary lesion from C 3 to C 7.

In February 1973, after a laminectomy from C 2 to C 7, a 3 cm long intramedullary hemangioblastoma was encountered 1 mm below the dorsal cord surface from C 3 to C 5. After two small ventral vessels were coagulated, the tumor was totally removed in one piece. A syrinx was opened at C 3.

Three years postoperatively the man has no neurologic deficit and is fully employed. He regularly enjoys skiing.

Case No. 10

This 9-year-old girl had a history of bilateral chest pain for six months. Examination revealed a paresis of the left leg. There was a suggestion of a bilateral T 7 sensory level.

Plain spine X-ray films showed a widened canal from T 3 to T 8. Myelography demonstrated a block at T 3 with multiple vascular defects (Fig. 13).

In March of 1975, after a laminectomy from T 3 to T 8, a 5 cm long multicystic intramedullary hemangioblastoma was totally removed.

Two years after operation, examination revealed no neurologic deficit.

Case No. 11

In July 1969 a 23-year-old man was transferred to this clinic with an eight year history of urinary incontinence and pain in the low back. Earlier that year he had undergone a laminectomy from T 11 to L 3 at another institution. A cystic tumor was found but not removed. There was no improvement despite a course of postoperative radiation therapy. Examination at the time of admission revealed bilateral mild sensory defects of all modalities in the legs and a paraparesis.

Myelography demonstrated a block at L 1 – L 2. At operation in July 1969 the previously made incision from T 11 to L 3 was reopened. A midline yellowish pulsating mass of many small vessels was noted. While the mass was being inspected a small vessel ruptured producing a hemorrhage from within the spinal cord substance at T 12 that was brought under control only with considerable difficulty. It was decided to close and postpone further intervention until spinal angiography could be obtained.

Selective spinal angiography subsequently demonstrated a tumor with the characteristics of a hemangioblastoma at T 12 – L 1 (Fig. 14 is Fig. 7 in Sept. 1976, Surgical Neurology). One year after the abortive operation the patient's examination was unchanged. He refused any further treatment.

Case No. 12

In February 1973 a 59-year-old man was transferred to this clinic with an eleven year history of low back and left leg pain. He had subsequently developed left leg weakness as well as urinary and fecal incontinence. On examination he had sensory loss of all modali-

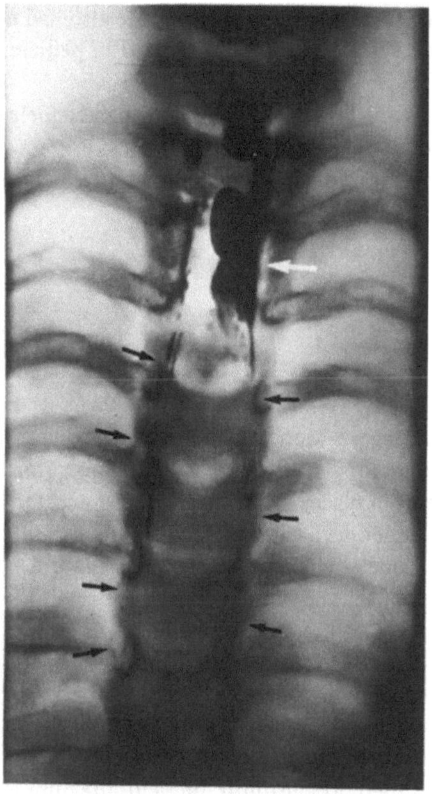

Fig. 13

◀

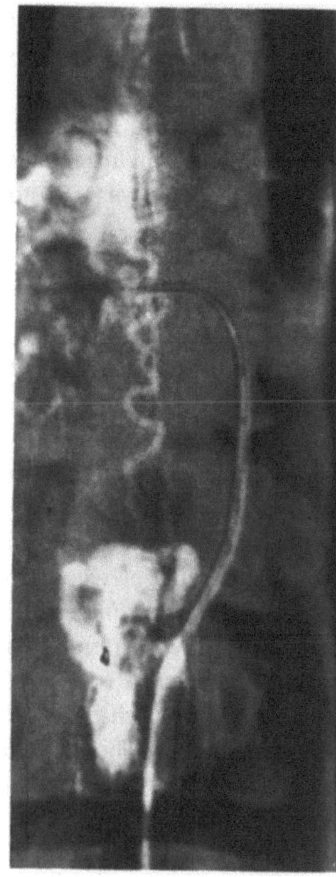

Fig. 14

▶

Fig. 13 (Case 10) Pantopaque myelogram of the thoracic region demonstrates an intramedullary type of deficit in addition to vascular loops (white arrow) and enlargement of spinal canal (black arrows)

Fig. 14. (Case 11) Selective spinal angiography shows an intramedullary vascular stain at the level of T12-L1 along with feeding vessels

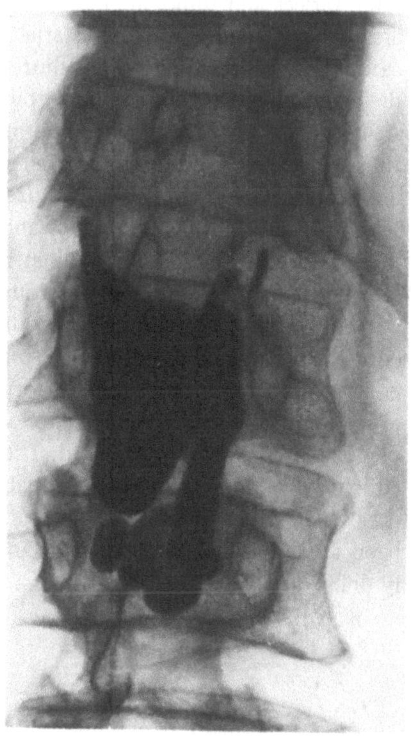

Fig. 15. (Case 12) Pantopaque myelogram shows a block at the level of T12

ties in both legs and moderate weakness and marked ataxia of the left leg. He also had a flaccid anus. Plain X-ray films of the spine revealed a slight erosion of the left T12 pedicle.

Myelography demonstrated a block at T 12 (Fig. 15).

At operation in February 1973, laminectomy from T 11 to L 2 revealed an extremely vascular extra- and intramedullary hemangioblastoma. It was totally removed.

Examination 3 years postoperatively revealed no neurologic deficit. The patient is working full time.

Microneurosurgical Technique

For cervical lesions, the patient is placed in the sitting position, which has been shown to be useful in reducing venous bleeding and allowing blood to flow clear of the operating field. It is essential to have a central venous catheter in place, and an experienced anesthesiologist capable of recognizing air embolus. A doppler device is a valuable adjunct in this regard. A longitudinal midline skin incision is made, the paravertebral musculature is freed from the posterior spinous processes and laminae, and retracted with self-retaining retractors attached to a metal bar, which is itself fixed to the operating table. This system in conjunction with head fixation in a Mayfield-Kees head holder has been found to be very satisfactory. Thoracic and lumbar lesions are operated on in the prone position.

The posterior elements are removed in standard laminectomy fashion over the entire length of the tumor and associated varices, and the opening is extended bilaterally for better exposure. The Zeiss operating microscope is then brought into the field; the dura is carefully opened to avoid possible injury to the dorsal varices and is tacked up. The overlying varices and tumor are inspected and the arachnoid is opened. The tumor and varices are then explored. The main arterial feeding vessels are located, usually laterally, and are carefully dissected free over a short segment, coagulated with bipolar coagulation and divided. Following this, the numerous smaller feeding vessels and finally the draining veins are coagulated and sectioned. Abnormal vessels can usually be identified by their size, tortuosity, pulsation, and more reddish color. (Preoperative selective angiography is an invaluable aid here.) It is to be emphasized that this dissection would be extremely difficult without the operating microscope and bipolar coagulation. If the tumor is not on the surface, a careful midline longitudinal myelotomy is done. Hemangioblastomas are always sharply demarcated from the surrounding nervous tissue, which is protected with small cotton pledgelets during the procedure of freeing the tumor gently from the surrounding cord. Ventrally, there are usually one or more feeding vessels, often of significant size, coming from the anterior spinal artery. These are isolated, coagulated, and sectioned. Following this, it is usually possible to extirpate the entire tumor mass with its varices in one piece without injury to the cord. The cord is palpated and any cyst or syrinx is opened (this may be done prior to the actual excision of the tumor mass). Meticulous hemostasis is obtained and the dura is closed either primarily or with an exogenous graft of lyophilized dura. The fascia, musculature and skin are closed in layers and the wound is routinely drained for 24 hours.

Table 1. Twelve cases of intramedullary spinal hemangioblastomas at Kantonsspital Zürich 1967-1977

Case #	Patient	Age	Symptoms	Location	Operation	Date of Operation	Follow-up	Result	Additional Information
1.	HB	41	Headache x 3 years	Medulla + Cervical + Cerebellar	Posterior fossa expl. Laminectomy C1, 2, 3, Subtotal.	Nov. 1, 1967	11 months	Improved	Died due to unrelated cardiac causes Oct. 1968 Pancreas + renal cysts.
2.	HR	27	Headache + neck pain x 6 months	Medulla + Cervical	Posterior fossa expl. Laminectomy C1, 2. Total.	Feb. 6, 1973	4 years	Improved fair	Died 1 1/2 years later Bilateral IX-X-XII palsy
3.	RB	44	Headache x 5 years	Medulla + Cervical	Posterior fossa expl. Laminectomy C1, 2. Total.	Feb. 14, 1974	3 years	Improved	
4.	RS	38	Arm weakness x 8 months	Cervical + Cerebellar	Laminectomy C1 to C7. Total removal.	Apr. 23, 1970	6 1/2 years	Improved	Separate cerebellar expl. Pheochromocytoma. Retinal angioma. Post-op arm pain.
5.	PA	22	Arm weakness x 1 month	Cervical + Cerebellar	Laminectomy C2-C7. Apparently total.	July 9, 1974	2 1/2 years	Improved	Separate cerebellar expl. Pheochromocytoma. Positive family history.
6.	MM	49	Visual loss x 18 years	Cervical + Cerebellar	Posterior fossa expl. Laminectomy C1-C5. Total	Oct. 14, 1974	2 1/2 years	Improved fair	Multiple retinal angiomas. Positive family history.
7.	MI	30	Leg weakness x 3 years	Cervico-thoracic + Cerebellar	Posterior fossa expl. Laminectomy C1-T1. Total.	Mar. 13, 1974	3 years	Improved fair	Retinal angioma. Positive family history. Persistent post-op-arm pain.
8.	SB	62	Low back pain x 6 weeks	Thoracic + Cerebellar	Laminectomy T9-L1. Total removal.	Apr. 28, 1975	2 years	Improved No deficit	Cerebellar exploration is pending.
9.	HH	25	Neck pain x 11 months	Cervical	Laminectomy C2-C7. Total.	Feb. 26, 1973	4 years	Improved No deficit	Associated syrinx. Positive family history.
10.	MD	9	Thoracic pain x 6 mos.	Thoracic	Laminectomy T3-T8. Total.	Mar. 11, 1975	2 years	Improved No deficit	
11.	RM	23	Low back pain x 8 yrs.	Thoraco-lumbar	Laminectomy T11-L3. No removal	July 18, 1969	7 years	No change	
12.	RZ	59	Low back pain x 11 years.	Thoraco-lumbar	Laminectomy T11-L2. Total.	Feb. 14, 1973	4 years	Improved No deficit	

Results

In this series of 12 patients with spinal hemangioblastomas (Table 1) who were operated on using the microtechnique from 1969 to 1975, there were no surgical deaths. There were 11 total removals, and in 1 case the operation had to be terminated after laminectomy, when an inexperienced surgeon tried to extirpate the angioma from the center of the tumor, and hemostasis proved extremely difficult. Results are 11 improved, 1 unchanged. One of the patients (case number 2) had a large intramedullary angioma filling the dilated 4th ventricle and extending down to C2. This tumor also extended into the pons. Although it was not the intention of the surgeon to extirpate the intrapontine part, some bleeding occurred which required the removal of this part of the tumor. Postoperatively this patient had a bilateral palsy of the 9th, 10th and 12th cranial nerves. He died one and a half years later due to pulmonary difficulties. Two patients, cases 4 and 7, complain of persistent postoperative pain in the arm. In ten cases, multiple or single hemangioblastomas were radically removed.

The treatment of choice for intramedullary spinal hemangioblastomas is total extirpation utilizing microtechnique. It is imperative that the tumor be dissected sharply at its periphery. This can now be achieved with minimal mortality and, in view of the disease, a very reasonable morbidity.

The frequent association of these tumors with overlying pial varices, 6 out of 12 in our series, is to be noted. Selective angiography is of great value. The use of the operating microscope and bipolar cautery is absolutely essential.

Treatment of Spinal Angiomas by Embolization

René Djindjian

Embolization offers a new method of treatment for spinal angiomas. It is carried out with pieces of Gelfoam (Sterispon) and, more recently, by other emboligenic materials such as silicone or fragments of dura mater. Embolization should be planned according to the site of the angioma – retromedullary, intramedullary, or mixed. This stresses the importance of an accurate angiographic assessment in order to define clearly the feeding vessels – the posterior or the anterior spinal arteries. As a matter of fact, embolization of the posterior angiomas does not involve any risk of spinal cord ischemia, whereas embolization of the intramedullary angiomas may cause a paraplegia. We will, therefore, discuss the different forms of embolization which are available. Our statistics, based on 45 cases, are distributed as follows:

Intramedullary angiomas	14 cases
Mixed angiomas	15 cases
Posterior angiomas	16 cases

Embolization in the Retromedullary Angiomas

The emboli should block the intercostal, lumbar, or cervical arteries supplying the posterior spinal artery (Figs. 1, 2). It is useful to put in very small emboli to block the posterior spinal artery, but it is necessary previously to block the intercostal or lumbar artery, which requires a large number of emboli. A large embolus would block the intercostal artery at its origin, but the posterior spinal artery or an angioma which has not been embolized can be recanalized by intercostal arteries above and below or from the opposite side (Figs. 3 - 5).

In order to avoid these possible anastomoses, it is preferable straight away to embolize the intercostal arteries above, below, and on the opposite side, provided that one of them does not supply the anterior spinal artery. The use of a nonabsorbable material for the emboli constitutes a new advance; nevertheless, the ideal is to be able to embolize the angiomatous mass itself, in order to avoid revascularization by the neighboring intercostal arteries. The silicone material seems ideal for blocking of the angiomatous mass, but it can produce an ischemia of the posterior columns, as we have seen in two cases, although the situation actually improved at the end of a few months (Figs. 19, 20).

The contraindications to embolization are as follows. On the one hand, huge angiomas without any angiomatous barrier, because in these cases the emboli can block the draining veins with consequent congestion and increase in size of the angioma, with the risk of a massive hemorrhage; on the other hand, huge angiomas which are causing spinal cord compression. In these two instances, surgical removal remains the treatment of choice.

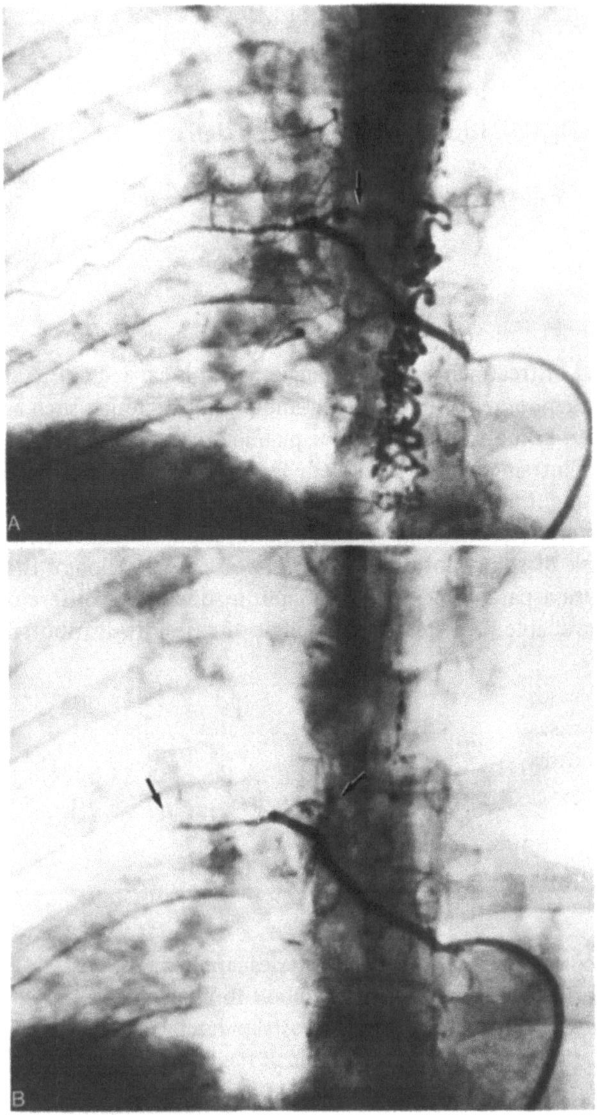

Fig. 1. Upper dorsal retromedullary angioma with one feeder/pedicle (D 5 R.) Films without subtraction. (A) Before embolization (feeding artery – arrow), (B) After embolization (arrows)

In retromedullary angiomas in an elderly subject, or one in poor general condition, embolization is the treatment of choice. In a young subject, if the routine follow-up films show that the angioma has revascularized, one may either repeat the embolization or else proceed to a surgical excision.

Embolization of the Mixed Angiomas

This involves the same treatment as the embolization of the retromedullary or intramedullary angiomas. However, embolization of a mixed angioma only allows one to embolize

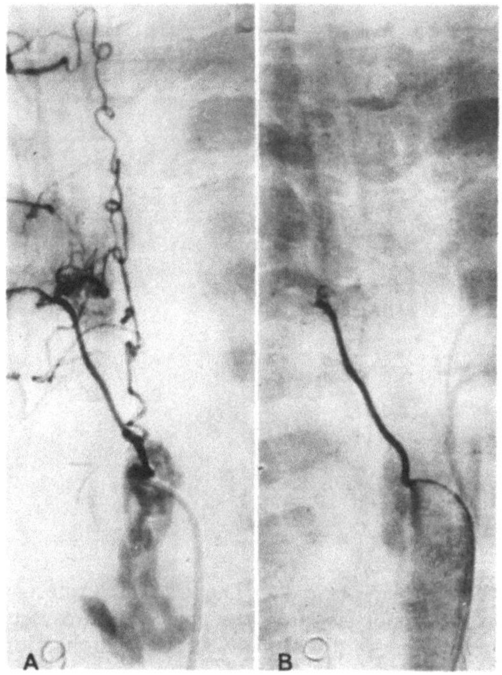

Fig. 2. Cervicodorsal retromedullary angioma with two feeders. (A) Posterior spinal arteries coming from the deep cervical and the fifth right intercostal arteries, (B) After embolization

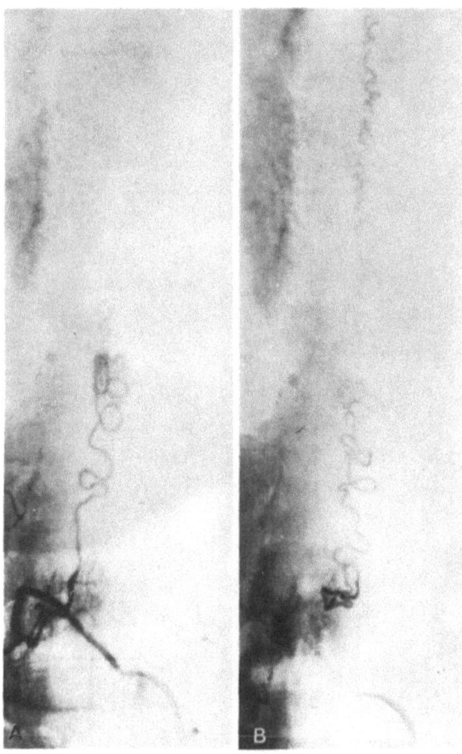

Fig. 3. (A) Dorsolumbar retromedullary angioma with one feeder (D 12 R.). (B) Posterior spinal artery feeder. Ascending draining vein

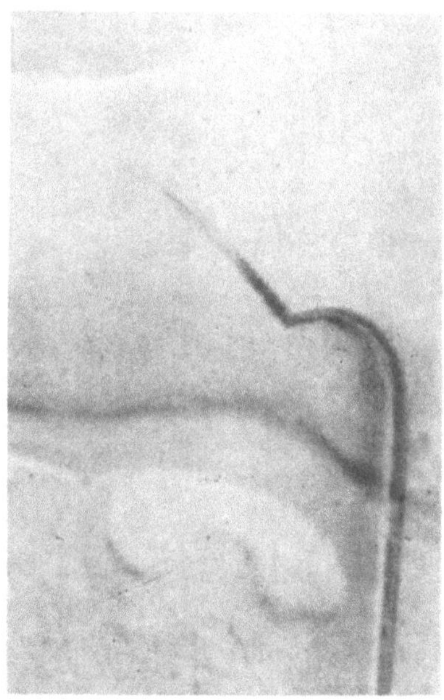

Fig. 4. Same case: Check angiogram several months after embolization. No filling of the angioma

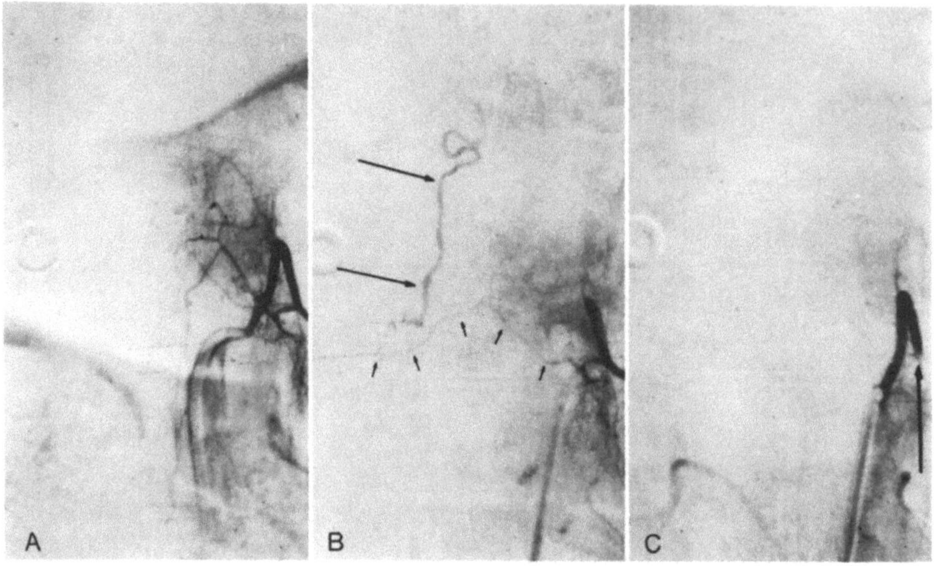

Fig. 5. Same case. (A) The same 12th intercostal artery (L) does not fill the angioma. (B) Several months later, the angioma is revascularized by the development of a retrocorporeal anastomosis (Arrows). (C) Embolization of the left 12th intercostal artery

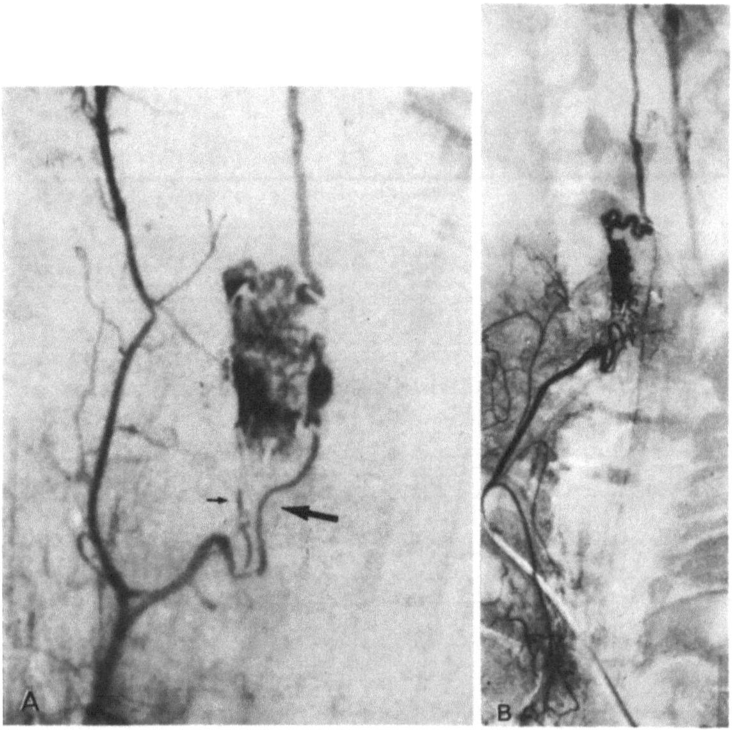

Fig. 6. Mixed cervical angioma with one pedicle. (A) Angioma fed by a common anterior spinal (large arrow) and posterior spinal (small arrow) trunk, coming from the right deep cervical artery. (B) Embolization of the ascending portion of the anterior spinal artery. The posterior spinal pedicle remains, opacifying the retromedullary portion of the angioma

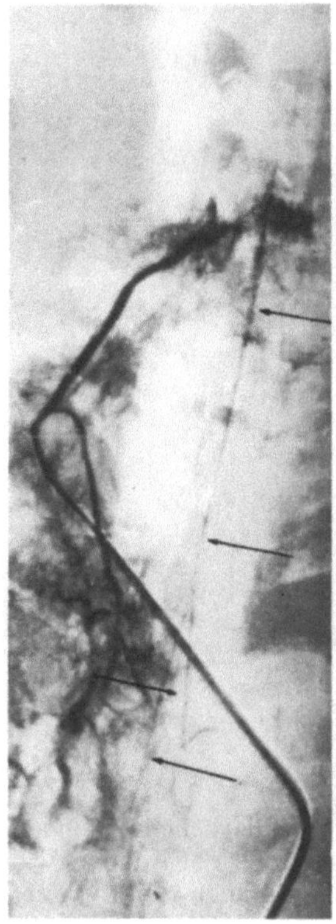

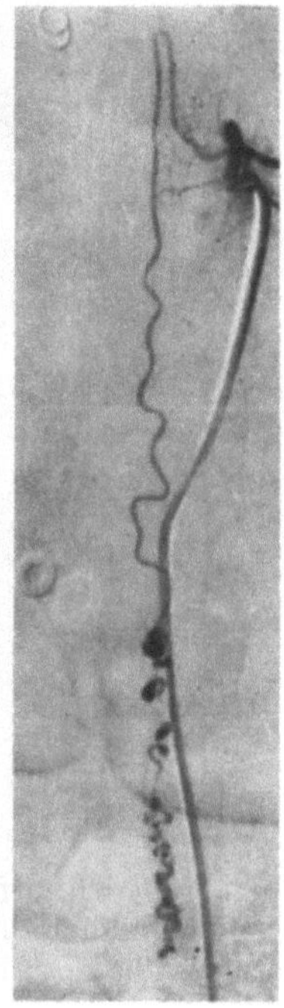

Fig. 7

Fig. 8

Fig. 7. Same case. Filling of the cervicodorsal portion of the anterior spinal trunk (arrow) with retrograde filling of an anterior spinal pedicle coming from the second intercostal artery on the *left*

Fig. 8. Dorsolumbar intramedullary angioma fed by the tenth intercostal artery (L). Tortuous descending branch, not dilated and not allowing the passage of emboli (risk of blockage by the emboli *at the level* of the descending branch)

one or more posterior feeders, while leaving the anterior spinal channel quite free. Indeed, the absence of embolization of an intramedullary angioma does not protect the patient from the complications inherent in the condition, but embolization of only the posterior pedicles leads to a reduction in the vascular "steal" produced by a retromedullary angioma, at the expense of the anterior spinal channels. This is especially more valuable if one has to deal with an elderly subject with a stenosed, atheromatous ostium of the intercostal artery which supplies the artery of Adamkiewicz.

This deliberately incomplete embolization can be carried out only if the artery of Adamkiewicz arises on its own from an intercostal artery different from the posterior spinal pedicles. In contrast, if there is a common trunk (artery of Lazorthes) to the anterior and posterior spinal arteries, it is very risky to attempt embolization of this common trunk, because it is difficult to estimate the size of these two arteries, and even more so to guide the emboli to their destination (Figs. 6, 7).

Embolization of the Intramedullary Angiomas

In these cases, embolization seems to be a treatment intermediate between doing nothing, with its many risks of complications, and undertaking radical surgical treatment, which is also not without risks to the anterior spinal trunk. The embolization should be terminal, blocking the malformation, and at the same time preserving the anterior spinal channel.

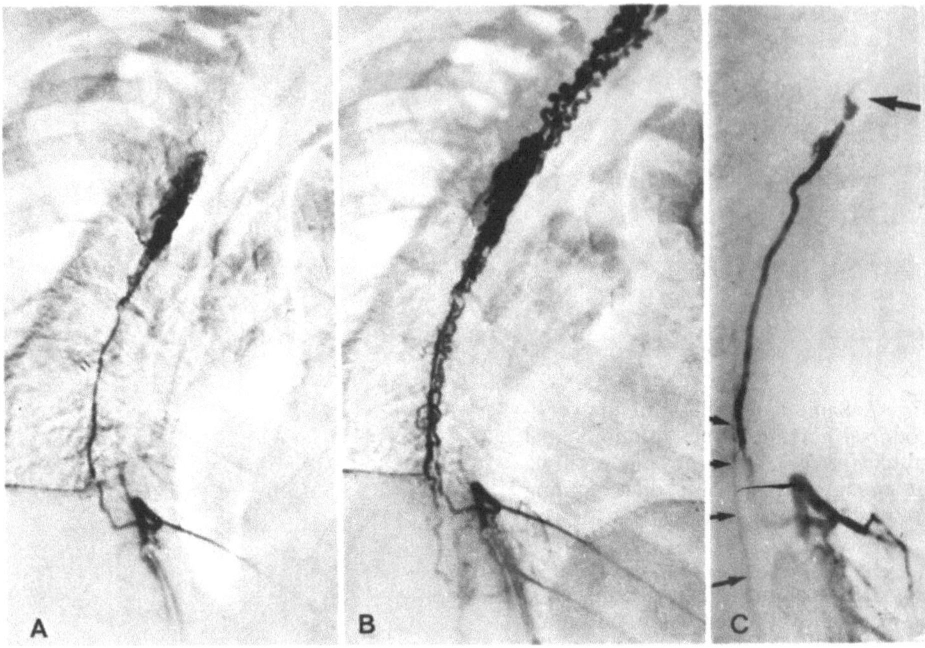

Fig. 9. Dorsal intramedullary angioma in a paraplegic patient. (A) Angioma fed by the ascending branch of the artery of Adamkiewicz which comes from the ninth *left* intercostal artery. The descending branch is not visible, (B) Late film showing the draining veins, (C) After embolization. The angioma is not filled. The feeding artery is dilated (ascending branch of the artery of Adamkiewicz). The descending branch is visible (arrows) confirming the disappearance of the "steal syndrome"

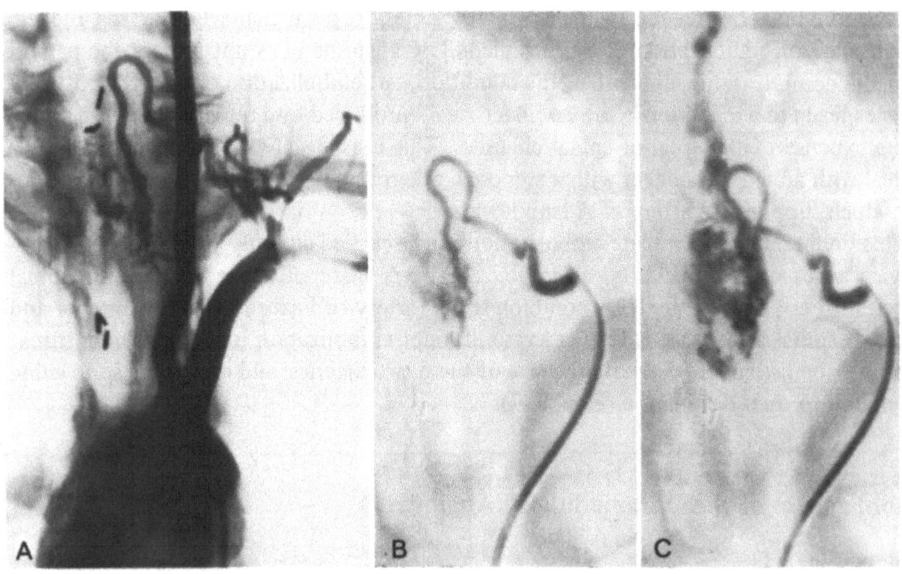

Fig. 10. Cervical intramedullary angioma in a paraplegic patient. (A) Intramedullary angioma fed by the artery of the cervical enlargement, from the deep cervical artery (L), (B) Selective arteriography of the artery of the cervical enlargement, (C) Late film. Ascending draining vein

Fig. 11

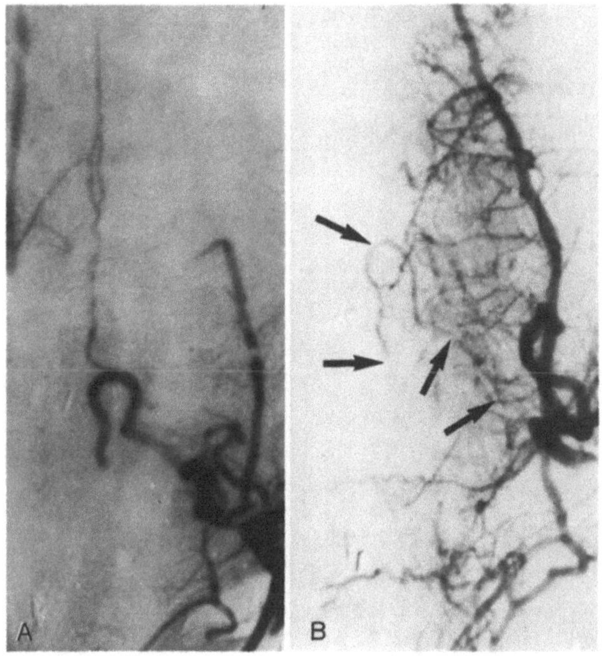

Fig. 11. (A) After embolization. No filling of the angioma. Filling of the ascending branch of the artery of the cervical enlargement (confirming the disappearance of the "steal syndrome") with an anterior radicular artery which fills the vertebral. (B) Check arteriography several months afterward. The angioma has remained embolized (arrow). The size of the artery of the cervical enlargement has returned to normal (arrows). The ascending branch of the anterior spinal artery is not filled. Clinically: disappearance of the root pains and relief of the spasticity allowing the wearing of prosthetic apparatus

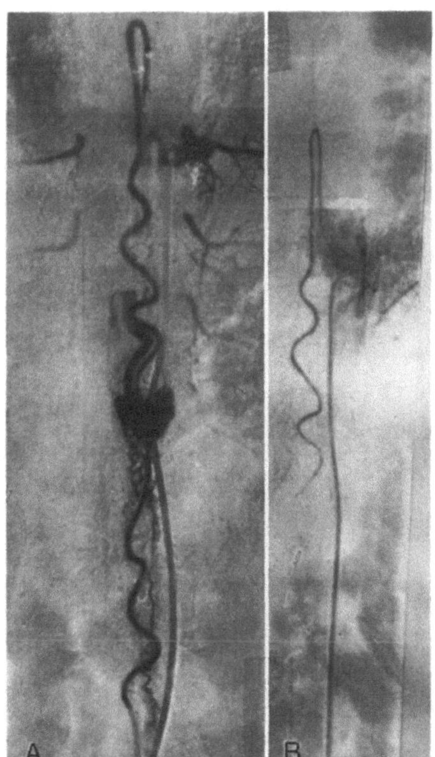

Fig. 12. Dorsolumbar intramedullary angioma in a paraparetic patient. (A) Dilated artery of Adamkiewicz coming off the tenth *left* intercostal artery. Angiomatous mass and descending draining vein. (B) Perfect embolization at the upper pole of the angioma, preserving all the underlying sulcocommissural arteries. The artery of Adamkiewicz has returned to a normal size with filling of its ascending branch

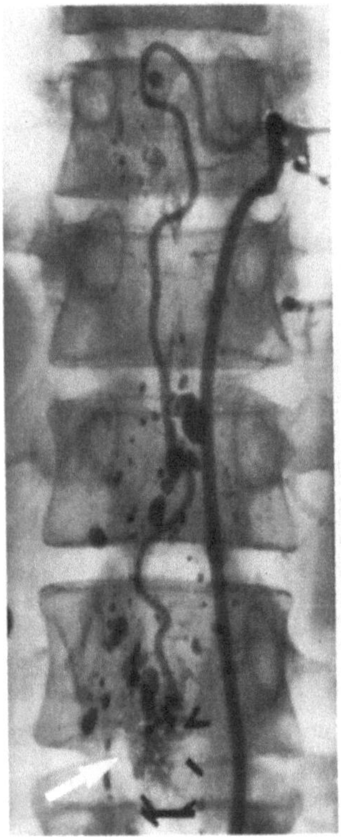

Fig. 13

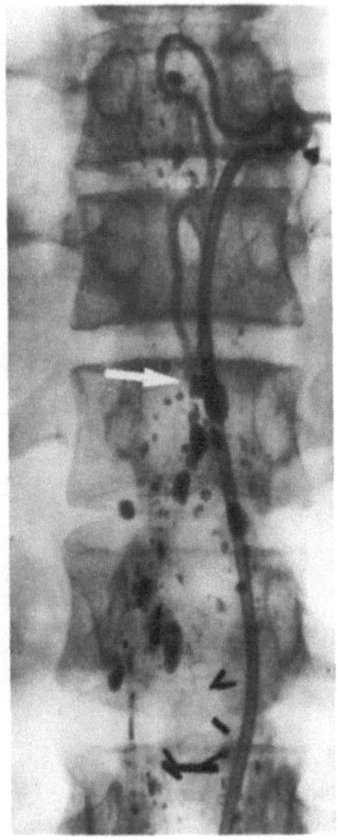

Fig. 14

Fig. 13. Dorsolumbar intramedullary angioma in a paraparetic patient. Angioma (arrow) fed by the dilated artery of Adamkiewicz, which is coming from the tenth intercostal artery (L)

Fig. 14. Same case. The embolus (very large) has remained impacted in the descending branch of the artery of Adamkiewicz at the upper border of the body of the 12th dorsal, producing a flaccid paraplegia. Partial recovery after several months (walking with two sticks)

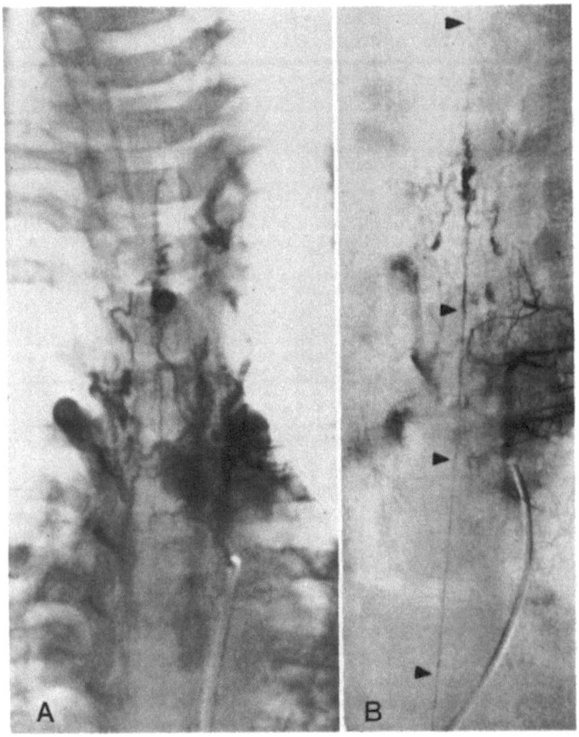

Fig. 15. Dorsal intramedullary angioma in a child, without paraplegia. (A) Pseudoaneurysmal angioma fed by an anterior spinal artery coming off the sixth intercostal artery (L). (B) Partial embolization

Fig. 16 and 17. Dorsolumbar intramedullary angioma (syndrome of Rendu-Osler-Weber). Angioma fed by the artery of Adamkiewicz coming from the tenth *right* intercostal artery. Huge vascular "lake" draining by a large vein in the right extradural spinal plexuses
Lateral views. Before and after embolization. Preservation of the sulcocommissural arteries. No filling of the vascular "lake"

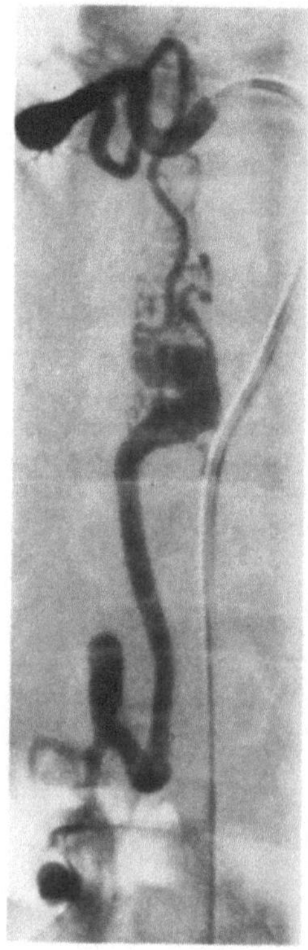

Fig. 16

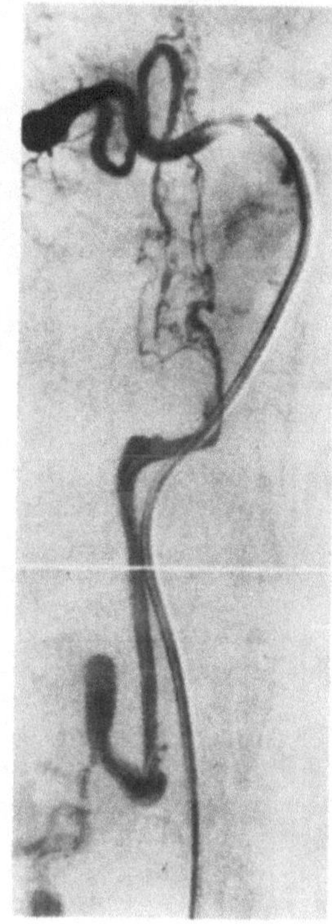

Fig. 17

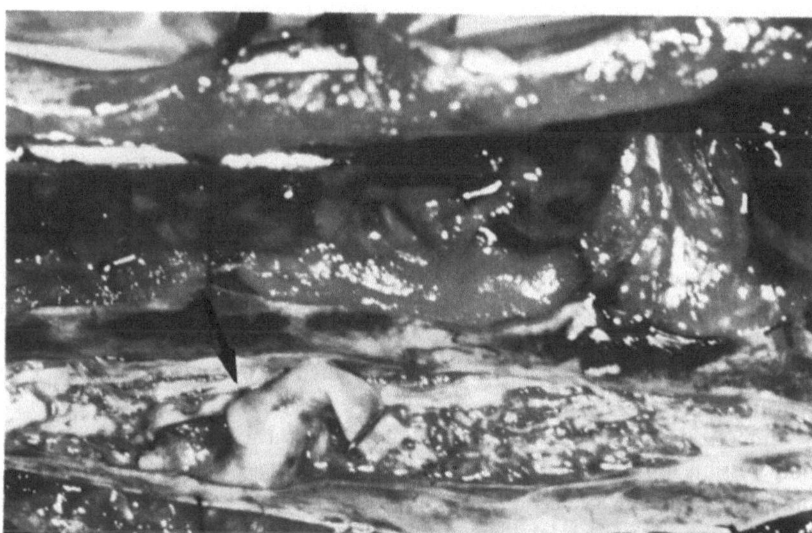

Fig. 18. Same case. At the operation (Prof. A. Hurth) there was spinal cord compression caused by the vascular "lake." This was partly thrombosed as a result of the embolization which facilitated the surgical procedure

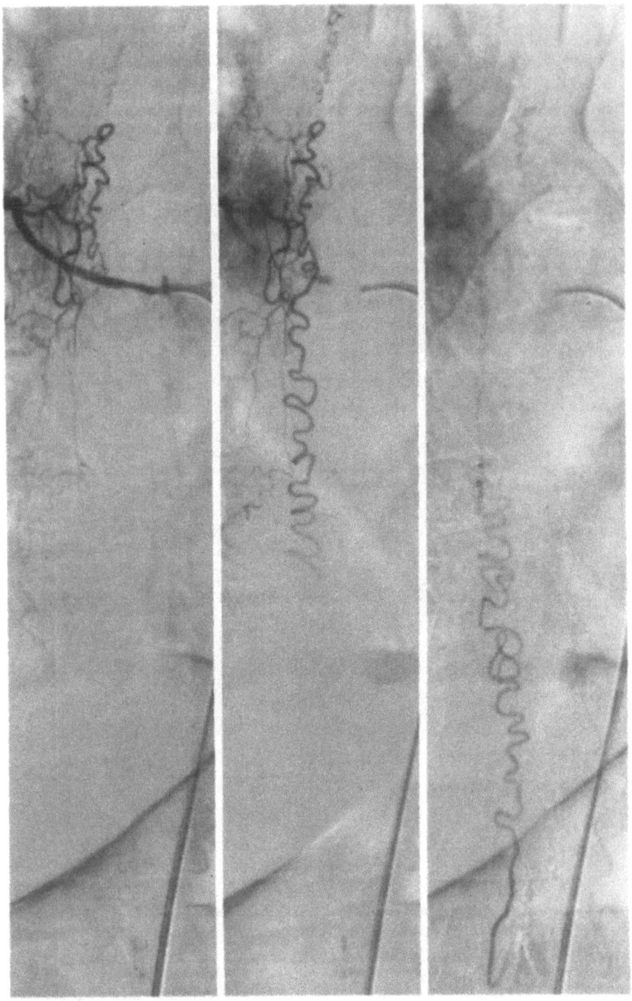

Fig. 19. Retromedullary angioma fed by one vessel from the fifth *right* intercostal artery. AP view

The obstruction ought to be done as close to the angioma as possible, as this reduces the risk of interruption of the important sulcocommissural arteries (Fig. 12). In this way, embolization offers a logical possibility of treating these progressive lesions, as opposed to radical excision which is sometimes unwise, when dealing with a cord made vulnerable by repeated ischemic attacks.

Embolization of the anterior spinal artery (cervical, upper dorsal, or Adamkiewicz) is only possible if this vessel is dilated, allowing the passage of microemboli capable of descending as far as the angioma (Fig. 8). In addition, it is necessary to consider the possibility of spasm of the artery of Adamkiewicz, in response to the passage of the embolus. If the embolus is very large, it will block the vessel at its origin or in its passage through the anterior spinal artery and will precipitate a paraplegia or a tetraplegia.

The indications for embolization are dependent on the neurologic state of the patient and the clinical progress of the lesion. Paraplegic patients (Figs. 9 - 11) can benefit from

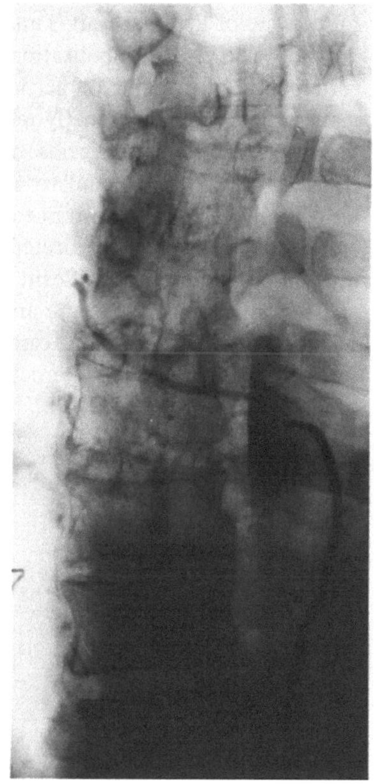

Fig. 20. Same case. Embolization with opaque silicone beads. Check films by aortography

embolization just as much as from surgical excision. In cases where there has been a recent acute episode, it is reasonable to wait for a few weeks in order that the patient may benefit from a possible natural improvement. The situation is quite different in patients with an established chronic paraplegia. In these cases, embolization can abolish root pains, suppress further subarachnoid hemorrhages, and reduce the spasticity which, because of repeated attacks of clonus, hinders the use of prosthetic apparatus. In the cases without paraplegia (Figs. 12 - 15), embolization ought to be discussed and carried out with the greatest circumspection, particularly in the dorsal region and in the artery of Adamkiewicz, in order to avoid a subsequent massive deficit. In the cervical region, the multiplicity of anterior afferents is able to compensate for the obstruction of one of those feeding the angioma. In the intramedullary angiomas composed of large efferent vascular lakes which can produce cord compression, embolization allows one to block these vascular lakes, thus allowing a later surgical excision without any risks of severe hemorrhage (Figs. 16 - 18).

Conclusions

1. Embolization appears to be one of the available methods of treatment for spinal vascular malformations. Because of its technical ease and its elegance, it offers great satisfaction. We have described the indications and the risks in dealing with the retromedullary and intra-

medullary angiomas. If it is carried out in a specialized department with a medical team fully aware of its hazards, it is undoubtedly a technique of the future.

2. The weakness of embolization is that one is not able to assess in advance the anatomic certainty of treatment, on account of the absorption of the Gelfoam. A nonabsorbable material for embolization (lyophilized dura, silicone, Isobutylmethylacrylate) which is being studied at present, seems to have resolved this problem (Fig. 19, 20).

3. Recent progress in medullary arteriography (directional photography coupled with rapid seriography) now allows intramedullary angiomas (both intra- and retroependymal, median and lateral) to be precisely located, thus permitting surgical excision (posterior commissural myelotomy) without significant postoperative risk (A. Rey, M. Djindjian, R. Houdart, and R. Djindjian). Systematic arteriographic reexamination has confirmed the success of such operations; in only one case has embolization been necessary. Surgery might in such cases be preferable to the alternatives.

Embolization of Spinal Arteriovenous Malformations

John L. Doppman

Operative embolization techniques were pioneered by neurosurgeons (Brooks, 1930; Luessenhop and Spence, 1960) and were directed principally at carotid-cavernous fistulas and cerebral arteriovenous malformations. Embolization through percutaneously placed catheters, a logical progression from the more cumbersome surgical approach, was developed by radiologists seeking a more controlled method for achieving intravascular occlusion. In fact, the first successful *transcatheter* embolization was directed at spinal arteriovenous malformations (Doppman et al., 1968; Newton and Adams, 1968). We embolized our first spinal arteriovenous malformation in October, 1967 and have since embolized 17 more lesions. Current embolizing materials are not ideal, and in most instances the technique is not curative, at least in the same sense as a complete surgical excision. But as a preoperative measure to reduce vascularity and facilitate resection or as a palliative measure in unresectable lesions, transcatheter embolization substantially contributes to the care of these patients.

Techniques

Our technique for embolizing spinal arteriovenous malformations has remained essentially unchanged since its introduction in 1967. The goal is to occlude all arterial feeders and the malformation without jeopardizing blood flow to the normal cord. Metallic or opaque silicone pellets are used initially to obstruct each arterial feeder within the spinal canal. This is the most important technical point since proximal obstruction of intercostal or lumbar arteries merely encourages collateral inflow from adjacent lumbar or intercostal vessels. The point of arrest of pellets can be approximately predicted by comparing pellet diameters with the diameter of downstream vessels. Spinal arteries frequently narrow as they pass through the dura, and this is a common site of pellet impaction (Fig. 1). Pellets too small in diameter usually lodge within the malformation rather than embolizing in the venous system. Obstruction of the venous side of a malformation, as may occur with some of the injectable plastics, is potentially dangerous and must be avoided at all costs.

When an arterial feeder has been occluded within the spinal canal by an appropriate sized pellet, Gelfoam is embolized proximal to the obstructing pellet to occlude the lumbar or intercostal artery and to stimulate thrombosis. However, the use of Gelfoam as the only embolizing agent (Djindjian, 1975) although technically less demanding since smaller catheters can be used, is unsatisfactory in our opinion for several reasons.

1. Gelfoam occlusion is not permanent. Several laboratory studies (Gold and Grace, 1975) and a growing clinical experience (Fig. 2 A-C) have demonstrated recanalization

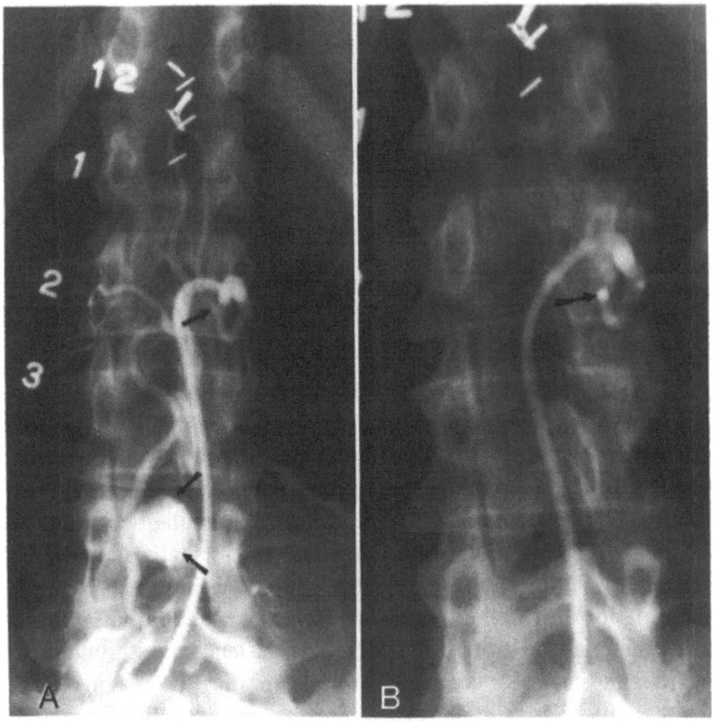

Fig. 1. (A) Note narrowing of artery of Adamkiewicz (upper arrow) as it passes through dura to supply AVM. Lower arrows identify aneurysm of enlarged anterior spinal artery. (B) Pellet of appropriate size impacted at site of transdural narrowing (arrow). Objective in this patient was to reduce risk of bleeding from the aneurysm without obstructing anterior spinal artery

within 3-4 months of vessels occluded with Gelfoam. For the control of bleeding or for tumor infarction, a 2-3 month occlusion is adequate, but for congenital lesions of blood vessels, a more permanent obturation is desired. Occlusion of the feeding vessel with metallic or silicone pellet is permanent. We recently restudied our first embolized case: the position of the pellet and occlusion of the feeding artery remain unchanged after 10 years. We have never seen pellet migration in any of our cases on follow-up radiographs can 3 months - 10 years. Since plain films provide no evidence about the fate of Gelfoam, a long term study with follow-up angiograms would be required to demonstrate the permanence of these occlusions. To our knowledge, such a study has not yet been published. Recent demonstration of the ability to visualize spinal arteriovenous malformations (AVM) by computerized tomography after bolus injections of contrast media (Di Chiro et al., 1977) will facilitate serial studies of such lesions although arteriography will still be necessary to identify individual feeders.

Fig. 2. (A) Large spinal AVM supplied by right tenth intercostal feeder. Vessel was progressively occluded with small, followed by large Gelfoam emboli. No pellets were used, (B) Arrow indicates complete obstruction at conclusion of embolization, (C) Arteriogram 3 years later demonstrates recanalization of feeding artery and malformation, (D) Paraplegic male with large intramedullary AVM and severe lumbar radicular pain. Anterior spinal artery obstructed (arrow) with good relief of pain ▶

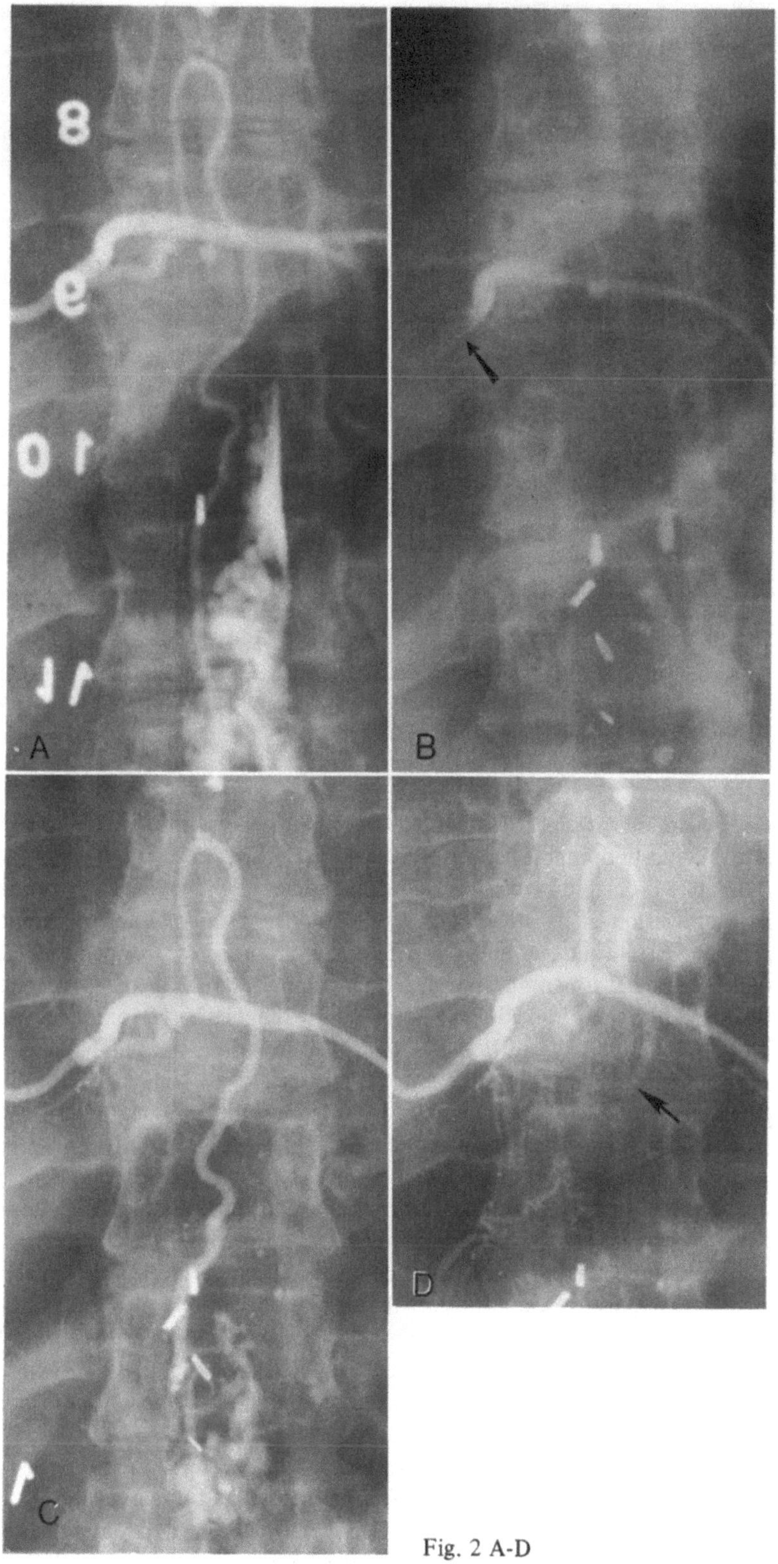

Fig. 2 A-D

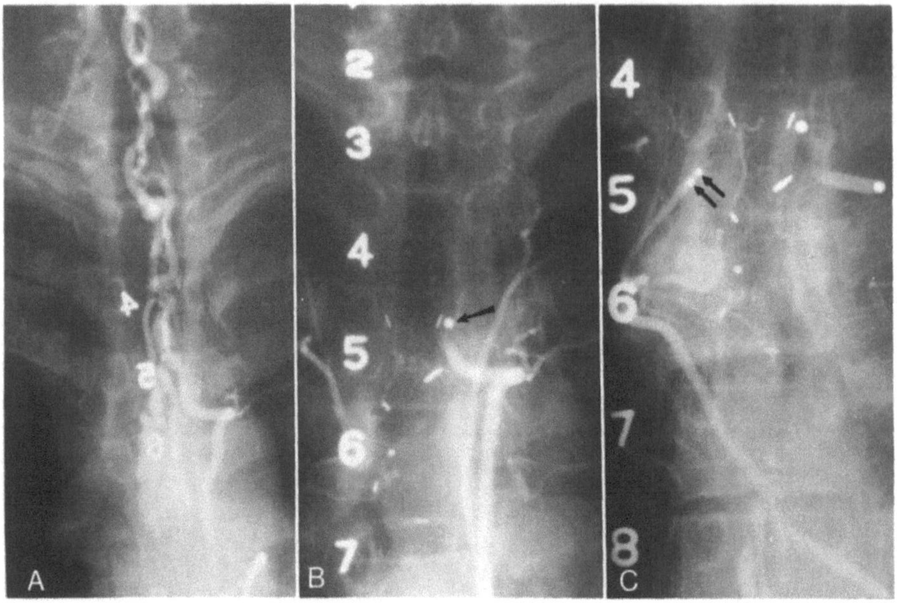

Fig. 3. Large cervicothoracic malformation. (A-B) Demonstration of intraspinal obstruction of left highest intercostal feeder by pellet (arrow). (C) Demonstration of obstruction of smaller feeder from right highest intercostal artery by 2 pellets (arrows). Two more feeding arteries were obstructed at same session

2. Gelfoam embolization is less controllable than pellet embolization. As originally theorized by Luessenhop and Spence (1960), the downstream distribution of pellets can be approximately predicted by comparing pellet and vessel diameters. Gelfoam, regardless of the pseudoprecision of its preparation (e.g., 2 x 2 mm squares), forms an amorphous, poorly coherent mass when wet and is capable under arterial pressure of considerable compression and plastic deformation. To use Gelfoam emboli to pass through the anterior spinal artery (ASA) into an intramedullary or mixed angioma is to risk proximal ASA obstruction. In spite of the possibility of flow in either direction in the ASA and also its ready reversibility, obstruction just below the entry of the artery of Adamkiewicz will produce paraplegia as demonstrated experimentally by Fried et al. (1969). In addition, Gelfoam may embolize normal sulcocommissural branches which are end arteries. When embolization was first undertaken, our philosophy was to provide palliation only if it could be reasonably accomplished without jeopardizing remaining cord function (Doppmann et al., 1971). None of our patients has deteriorated as a result of embolization. We have refused to embolize anterior spinal arteries (intramedullary and most mixed angiomas) because with current techniques, we cannot direct the embolus accurately into the malformation. Certain AVMs, in our opinion, cannot be embolized without *considerable* risk to the cord and must await the development of more precise embolization techniques. However, when no significant spinal cord function remains, we have embolized the anterior spinal artery (Fig. 2D) to control pain or decrease spasticity.

Multiple feeding arteries can be embolized at the same sitting without increased morbidity. We have embolized up to five separate feeding arteries at a single session (Fig. 3 A-C). The limiting factor is usually the volume of contrast material (a catheter in the urinary bladder is essential to prevent overdistension), and we have consistently used 400 - 500 cc

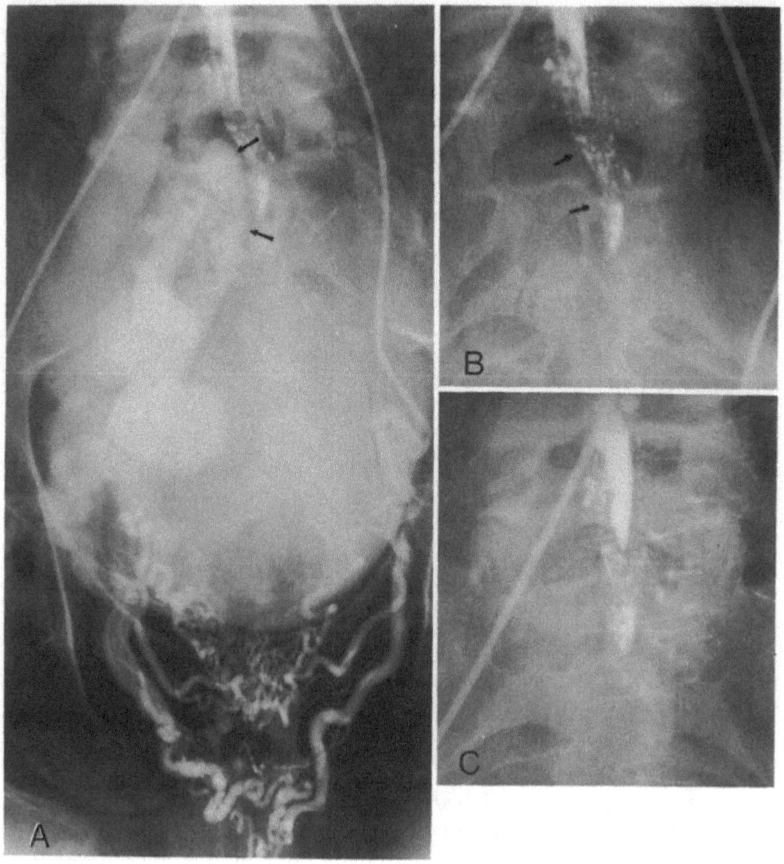

Fig. 4. Large pelvic arteriovenous fistula resulting from a bullet wound. Note in A drainage into enlarged epidural veins (arrows) compressing the caudal sac. Pelvic fistula was occluded with IBCA. Caudal sac returned to midline; compare B (preembolization) with C (2 weeks postembolization). Patient recovered ability to walk without assistance

meglumine iothalmate (Conray 60) over 2 - 3 hours without significant toxicity. We also feel that embolization should be performed under local rather than general anesthesia, since the reaction of the patient to the initial embolus may modify the subsequent handling of the procedure.

Arterial or venous aneurysms within AVMs are occasionally observed, especially in patients with a history of recurrent subarachnoid bleeding (Herdt et al., 1971). We have successfully employed embolization to lessen the risk of recurrent hemorrhage from such lesions, as illustrated in Figure 1.

Neurosurgeons and neuroradiologists must keep in mind that rarely extraspinal vascular lesions may present with neurologic symptoms and myelographic findings which resemble those found in spinal AVMs. Aortic coarctation is the best known example (Doppmann et al., 1968) and produces an ischemic myelopathy by stealing blood from the cervicothoracic cord segment as a result of collateral circulation through this portion of the anterior spinal artery. This phenomenon, which we call "spinal steal," may be associated with aortic obstructive lesions or large AV fistulas of the trunk. Less common than "spinal steal" has been spinal compression caused by greatly dilated extradural veins draining an extraspinal

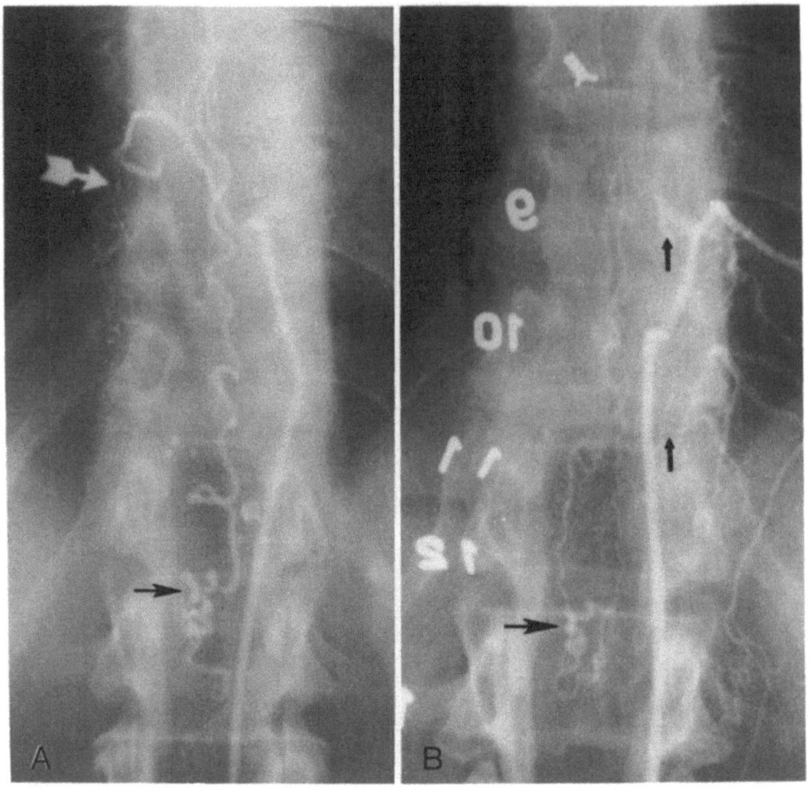

Fig. 5. Thoracolumbar spinal AVM with point of AV shunting (nidus) at black arrow. Major feeder (white arrow) (A) was surgically occluded (clip). (B) Two years later, posterolateral spinal arteries supply same nidus (compare horizontal arrows A and B). Ninth and tenth left intercostal feeders (vertical arrows, B) did not supply malformation at time of initial arteriographic study

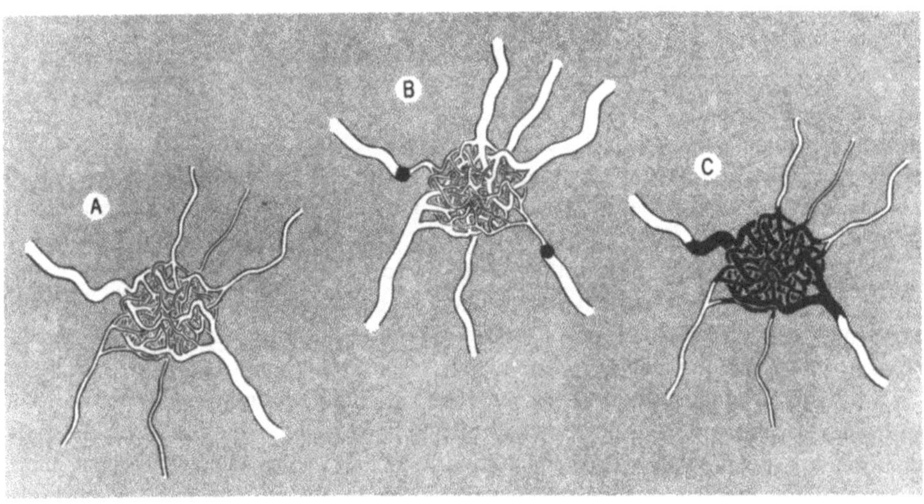

Fig. 6. (A) AVM with two large, i.e., angiographically demonstrable, and multiple small feeders, (B) Occlusion of major feeders results in temporary palliation only until new collaterals develop. (C) Complete obturation of nidus prevents development of collaterals and permanently obliterates arteriovenous shunt. (Reproduced with permission of the publisher, Doppman et al., 1971)

AVM. Figure 4 illustrates abnormal subarachnoid vessels and compression of the caudal sac in a young man with a posttraumatic arteriovenous fistula in the right pelvis. Surgical excision of the fistula had been attempted four times over a 10-year period but had always failed. Progressive paraplegia had developed in the course of 1 year, confining the patient to a wheelchair. Embolic obliteration of the pelvic fistula led to disappearance of the abnormal intraspinal vessels and neurologic recovery. It must be kept in mind that extraspinal vascular lesions may present with predominantly spinal syndromes and myelographically may show abnormal intraspinal vessels. Embolization of the extraspinal lesions is often free of risk and dramatically effective in reversing the neurologic syndrome.

If embolization is to compete with surgery as a therapeutic alternative for spinal cord AVMs, it must do more than simply obstruct feeding arteries. Since most spinal angiomas are abnormal arteriovenous connections, the obstruction of multiple feeding arteries results in only temporary improvement until additional feeders develop (Fig. 5). If the site of arteriovenous shunting, the so-called "nidus," could be identified and filled with a material injected as a liquid but polymerizing to form a solid mass, potential collaterals could not develop. Figure 6 illustrates this concept of "vascular casting" (Doppman et al., 1971). The nidus of an AVM can usually be identified by careful, thorough angiography (Doppman, 1971); its recognition should also simplify surgical excision. The following points help in its identification: 1) it is the point of convergence of multiple arterial feeders, 2) it is the point of divergence of venous flow, 3) it is sometimes associated with an abrupt increase in vessel diameter (Fig. 7). The ideal embolizing technique would obturate the

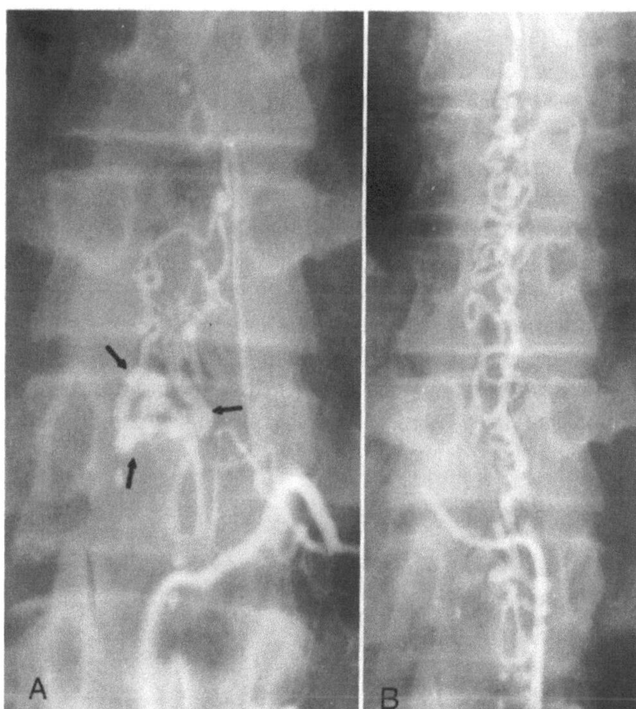

Fig. 7. Nidus (arrows, A) is the point of convergence of right 11th and left 12th intercostal feeding arteries. Common venous drainage from either injection (B) represents enlarged posterior veins which should regress when AV shunt or "nidus" is obliterated

Table 1. Embolizing Plastics

Silicone Rubber	IBCA
Opaque	± Opaque
Variable viscosity	Nonviscous
Requires catalyst	Instantaneous polymerization in body fluids
Inert	Fibrosing
Balloon catheters	Coaxial catheters
Low flow lesions	High flow lesions

nidus without compromising normal spinal arteries or veins. Such a technique obviously would apply only to posterior malformations, but these are the most common adult lesions. Two plastics are currently being investigated as possible embolizing agents. Table 1 summarizes the physical properties and potential applications of silicone rubber (Doppman et al., 1971) and isobutyl cyanoacrylate (IBCA) (Kerber, 1975a, b; Zanetti and Sherman, 1972). Silicone rubber requires the addition of a catalyst for polymerization, is biologically inert and nonreactive, but is rather viscous for delivery through tiny balloon catheters. IBCA polymerizes rapidly on contact with body fluid, is biologically more reactive, but viscosity is not a problem. Both plastics may be rendered opaque by the addition of tantalum powder. The ability to float tiny balloon catheters through tortuous feeding arteries has already been demonstrated by Serbinenko (1974) and Pevsner et al. (1976). This promises to be the ideal technique for embolizing plastics, and clinical examples have already been presented by Kerber (1975a, b), Hilal and Michelsen (1975), and Hilal et al. (1975). Efforts to improve both the delivery techniques and the embolizing agent are under way in many laboratories.

The development of microsurgical techniques has dramatically improved the results of surgical therapy for spinal AVMs. Yasargil et al. (1975) have recently reported complete excision of 11 intramedullary angiomas of the cervical cord with excellent results. In the light of such emerging surgical prowess, one must wonder about the current role of embolization techniques in this disease. Preoperative embolization, in our experience, significantly reduces the vascularity of AVMs and simplifies excision. It should be routinely performed preoperatively in all cases when only posterior spinal arteries are involved. In addition, embolization can provide palliation for patients who are unsuitable for operation because of extensive arachnoiditis, long-standing paraplegia, or serious associated diseases. But until embolization techniques are refined to the point of permitting precise placing of more suitable embolizing agents, surgical excision will remain the treatment of choice for resectable spinal cord AVMs.

References

Adotti, F., Chelloul, N., Ponchon, Y., Roujeau, J.: Les anévrysmes artério-veineux médullaires. Sem Hôp. Paris **47**, 1971 553-558.

Agnoli, A. L., Bauer, B.L., Kirchhoff, D.: Neuroradiologische Untersuchungsmethode zur Differentialdiagnose spino-caudaler Fehlbildungen. In: Spinale raumfordernde Prozesse (Hrsg. W. Schiefer und H.H. Wieck), 211-214. Straube 1976. Perimet Verlag Dr. Straube 1976.

Agnoli, A.L., Popovic, H., Popovic, M., Schönmayr, R., Schepelmann, F.: Differential diagnosis of sciatica. – Analysis of 3000 disc prolapse operations. Presented Ann. Meeting German Soc. Neurosurgery, Berlin 1976.

Aminoff, M.J.: Spinal Angiomas. Oxford–London–Edinburgh–Melbourne: Blackwell 1976.

Aminoff, M.J., Barnard, R.O., Logue, V.: The pathophysiology of spinal vascular malformations. J. Neurol. Sci. **23**, 255-263 (1974).

Aminoff, M.J., Logue, V.: Clinical features of spinal vascular malformations. Brain (1974) **97**, 197-210.

Aminoff, M.J., Logue, V.: The prognosis of patients with spinal vascular malformations. Brain. (1974) **97**, 211-218.

Ansari, F.: Hämatomyelie bei arteriovenösem Hämangiom des Rückenmarks. Ein Beitrag zur Pathogenese der Foix-Alajouaninschen Krankheit. Beitr. path. Anat. **131**, 137-161 (1965).

Antoni, N.: Spinal vascular malformations (angiomas) and myelomalacia. Neurology (Minneap.) **12**, 795-804 (1962).

Arseni, C., Samitca, D.: Vascular malformations of the spinal cord. Acta psychiat. Scand. **34**, 10-17 (1959).

Arseni, C., Simionescu, M.D.: Vertebral hemangioma. Acta psychiat. scand. **34**, 1958 1-9.

Bailey, W.L., Sperl, M.P.: Angiomas of the cervical spinal cord. J. Neurosurg. **30**, 560-568 (1969).

Baker, H.L., Love, J.G., Layton, D.D.: Angiographic surgical aspects of spinal cord vascular anomalies. Radiology. **88**. 1078-1085 (1967).

Balck, C.A.: A case of angioma of the spinal cord with recurrent haemorrhages. Brit. med. J. (1900) **II**, 1707-1708.

Baló, J.: Über ein Aneurysma der Rückenmarksarterien, welches Tabes-dorsalis-artige Symptome vortäuschte. Dtsch. Z. Nervenheilk. **85**, (1925) 86-95.

Bannerjee, T., Hunt, W.: A Case of Spinal Cord Hemangioblastoma and Review of the Literature. Surg. **38**, 460 (1972).

Bardal. D., Heilbronn, Y.D., Schiffer, J.M.: Microneurosurgical Excision of an Intra- and Extramedullary Cervical Angioma. Israel J. med. Sci. **9** 92-97 (1973).

Bassett, R.C., Peet, M.M., Holt, J.F.,: Pial medullary angiomas. Clinicopathologic features and treatment. Arch. Neurol. Psychiat. (Chic.) **61**, 558-568 (1949).

Battifora, H.: Hemangiopericytoma: Ultrastructural study of five cases. Cancer (Philad.) **31**, 1418-1432 (1973).

Bednar, B.: Foixova-Alajouaninova angiohypertroficka myelomalacie. Cs. Patol. **6**, 11-16 (1970).

Béraud, R. Meloche, B.R.: A propos des malformations vasculaires médullaires. Description de deux cas et revue de littérature. U. méd. Can. **94**, 176-188 (1965).

Béraud, R.: Vascular malformations of the spinal cord. In: Handbook of Clinical Neurology (P.J. Vinchen and G.W. Bruyn, eds.), Vol. 12, pp. 548-555. Amsterdam: North Holland 1972.
Berenbruch, K.: Ein Fall von multiplen Angiolipomen, kombiniert mit einem Angiom des Rückenmarks. Inaug.-Diss. Tübingen, 1890.
Berger, G., Patricot, L.M., Boucheron, Mlle, Boissen, D.: La myélite nécrotique subaiguë de Foix et Alajouanine. Conception actuelle, à propos d'un cas anatomo-clinique. Lyon méd. **230**, 41-45 (1973).
Bergstrand, A., Möök, O., Lidvall, H.: Vascular malformations of the spinal cord. Acta neurol. scand. **40**, 169-183 (1964).
Bergstrand, H., Olivecrona, H., Tönnis, W.: Gefäßmißbildungen und Gefäßgeschwülste des Gehirns. Leipzig: Thieme 1936.
Bettaieb A.: Les tumeurs primitives intramédullaires extirpables de la région cervicale et dorsale. Thèse de Paris, 1960. (Quoted Guidetti, 1964).
Bischof, W., Schettler, G.: Zur Klinik und Therapie der arteriovenösen Angiome und Varikosen des Rückenmarks. Dtsch. Z. Nervenheilk. **192**, 46-68 (1967).
Black and Farber (Quoted Wyburn-Mason, 1943).
Blahd, M.E.: Hemangioma of the spinal cord. J. Amer. med. Ass. **80**, 1452-1453 (1923).
Bodechtel, G., Erbslöh, F.: Die Foix-Alajouaninesche Krankheit ("Myélite nécrotique subaiguë"-Angiodysgenetische Myelomalacie). In: Hdb. spez. path. Anat. Histol. Vol. XIII/1 B, pp. 1576-1599. Berlin-Göttingen-Heidelberg: Springer 1957.
Bogaert, L. van: Pathologie des angiomatoses. Acta neurol. belg. **50**, 525-610 (1950).
Bräutigam, M.W.: Über eine spontane Hämatomyelie durch Ruptur eines durch angeborene Gefäßschwäche entstandenen Aneurysmas der Arteria spinalis dorsalis. Dtsch. Z. Nervenheilk. **181**, 119-129 (1960).
Brasch, F.: Über einen schweren spinalen Symptomencomplex, bedingt durch eine aneurysma-serpentinum-artige Veränderung eines Teiles der Rückenmarksgefässe. Berl. klin. Wschr. **37**, 1210-1213, 1239-1241 (1900).
Brion, S., Netzky, M.G., Zimmermann, H.M.: Vascular malformations of the spinal cord. Arch. Neurol. Psychiat. (Chic.) **68**, 339-361 (1952).
Brooks, B.: The treatment of traumatic arteriovenous fistula. Sth. med. J. (Bgham, Ala.) **23**, 100-106, (1930).
Browne, T.R., Adams, R.D., Robertson, G.H.: Hemangioblastoma of the spinal cord. Arch. Neurol. (Chic.) **33**, 435-441 (1976).
Buckley, A.C.: Hematomyelia secondary to hemangioma. J. nerv. ment. Dis. **83**, 422-429 (1936).
Carpenter, G., Schwartz, H., Walker, A.E.: Neurogenic polycythaemia, Ann. intern. Med. **19**, 470 (1943).
Cassinari, V., Bernasconi, V.: Tumours and malformations of spinal blood vessels. Acta neurochir. (Wien) **9**, 612 (1961).
Casteigne, P., David, M., Pertuiset, B., Escourolle, R., Poirrier, J.: L'ultrastructure des hémangioblastomes du système nerveux central. Rev. neurol. **118**, 5 (1968).
Chatterjee, R.N.: Spinal vascular malformations. Their classification, pathogenesis, and the rationale of treatment by excision of the draining veins. 46 Exc.Med.(1969)I.C.S. Nr.193
Christian, P., Noder, W.: Akute Rückenmarkssymptome bei Isthmusstenose der Aorta als Folge eines pathologischen Kollateral-Kreislaufes über die Arteria spinalis anterior. Z. Kreisl. Forsch. **43**, 125-131 (1954).
Christoferson, L.A., Gustafson, M.B., Peterson, A.G.: Von Hippel-Lindau's Disease. **178**, 280 (1961).
Cobb, S.: Hemangioma of the spinal cord, associated with skin naevi of the same metamere. Ann. Surg. **62**, 641-649 (1915).
Collins E.T.: Intraocular Growths. Trans. Ophthal. Soc. U.K. **14**, 141 (1894).
Corbin, J.L.: Anatomie et pathologie artérielle de la moëlle. Paris: Masson 1961.
Cramer, F., Kinsey, W.H.: The Cerebellar Hemangioblastoma: a review of 53 cases. Arch. Neurol. Psychiat. (Chic.) **67**, 237 (1952).
Craig, W. McK., Horrax, G.: The occurrence of hemangioblastomas (two cerebellar and one spinal) in 3 members of a family. J. Neurosurg. **6**, 518 (1949).
Craig, W. McK., Wagener, H.P., Kernohan, J.W.: Lindau-von Hippel Disease. Arch. Neurol. Psychiat. (Chic.) **46**, 36 (1941).

Cross, G.O.: Subarachnoid cervical angioma with cutaneous hemangioma of a corresponding metamere. Arch. Neurol. Psychiat. (Chic.) **58**, 359-366 (1947).
Cube, H.M.: Spinal extradural hemorrhage. J. Neurosurg. **19**, 171-172 (1962).
Cushing, H., Bailey, P.: Tumors arising from the blood vessels of the brain. Angiomatous malformations and hemangioblastomas. Springfield/Ill.: C.G. Thomas 1928.
Dalloz, J.C., Queileau, P., Canlorbe, P., Rubin, S.: Modifications de la statique rachidienne au cours des compressions médullaires par tumeur chez l'enfant. Arch. franç. Pédiat. **20**, 309-319 (1963).
David, E., Müller, D., Schulze, H.A.F., Unger, R.R.: Angiodysgenesis cerebrospinalis. Schweiz. Arch. Neurol. **96**, 318-336 (1965).
David, E., Schulze, H.A.F., Busch, G.: Zur Abgrenzung der angiodysgenetischen nekrotisierenden Myelopathie (Foix-Alajauanine). Wien. Z. Nervenheilk. **19**, 44-58 (1962).
David, M., Garcin R., Sachs M., Metzger J.: Maladie de von Hippel-Lindau à localisations multiples. Neurochirurgia (Stuttg.) **9**, 12 (1966).
David, M., Messimy, R., Sachs, M., Chedru, F.: Hemangioblastomes cérébelleux et compression médullaire. Presse méd. **76**, 2413 (1968).
Dawson, B.H.: Paraplegia due to spinal epidural haematoma. J. Neurol. Neurosurg. Psychiat. **26**, 171-173 (1963).
Decker, R., Stein, H., Epstein, J.: Complete embolization of artery of Adamkiewicz to obliterate an intra-medullary arterio-venous aneurysm. Case report. J. Neurosurg. **43**, 486-489 (1975).
Deeb, Z.L., Rosenbaum, A.E., Bensky, J.J., Scarff, T.B.: Calcified intramedullary aneurysm in spinal angioma. Neuroradiology **14**, 1-4 (1977).
Di Chiro, G.,: Combined retino-cerebellar angiomatosis and deep cervical angiomas: Case report. J. Neurosurg. **14**, 685-687 (1957).
Di Chiro, G.: Spinal cord angiography. Proc. roy. Soc. Med. **63**, 184 (1970).
Di Chiro, G., Doppman, J.G.: Differential angiographic features of hemangioblastomas and arteriovenous malformations of the spinal cord. Radiology **93**, 25-30 (1969).
Di Chiro, G., Doppman, J.L.: Endocranial drainage of spinal cord veins. Radiology. **95**, 555-560. (1970).
Di Chiro, G., Doppman, J., Ommaya, A.K.: Selective arteriography of arteriovenous aneurysms of spinal cord. Radiology **88**, 1065-1077 (1967).
Di Chiro, G., Doppman, J.L., Ommaya, A.K.: Radiology of spinal cord arterio-venous malformations. Progr. Neurol. Surg. **4**, 329-354 (1971).
Di Chiro, G., Doppman, J.L., Wener, L: Computed tomography of spinal cord arteriovenous malformations. Submitted for publication.
Di Chiro, G., Jones, A.E., Johnston, G.S.: Radioisotope angiography of the spinal cord. Preliminary note. J. Nucl. Med. **13**, 567-569 (1972).
Di Chiro, G., Wener, L.: Angiography of the spinal cord. J. Neurosurg. **39**, 1-29 (1973).
Dilenge, D., Héon, M., Metzger, J.: Selective spinal angiography in multiple CNS lesions. J. Canad. Ass. Radiol. 24, 178-183 (1973).
Djindjian, M.: Le traitement chirurgical des angiomas intra-médullaires, Thèse, Paris 1976.
Djindjian, R.: Vascularisation médullaires par phlébographie et artériographie. Rev. neurol. **106**, 707-717 (1962).
Djindjian, R.: Arteriography of the spinal cord. Roentgenology **107**, 461-478 (1969).
Djindjian, R.: Angiography of the spinal cord. Baltimore: University Park, 1970.
Djindjian, R.: Spinal cord hemangioblastomas and von Hippel-Lindau's disease, Rev. neurol. **124**, 495 (1971).
Djindjian, R.: Neuro-radiological examination of spinal cord angiomas. Handbook of clinical neurology, Vol. **12**, 631-643 (1972).
Djindjain, R.: Vascular malformations. In: Myelography (ed. by R. Shapiro). Yearbook medical **14**, 249-278 (1975).
Djindjian, R.: Embolization of angiomas of the spinal cord. Surg. Neurol. **4**, 411-420 (1975).
Djindjian, R., Cophignon, J., Rey, A., Theron, J., Merland, J.J., Houdart, R.: Super-selective arteriography; embolization by the femoral route in neuroradiology. Neuro-radiology **6**, 132-142. (1973).
Djindjian, R., Cophignon, J., Theron, J., Merland, J.J., Houdart, R.: L'embolisation en neuro-radiologie vasculaire. A propos de 30 cas. Nouv. Presse méd. **1**, 2153-2158 (1972).

Djindjian, R., Dumesnil, M., Fauré, C., Lefebre, J., Leveque, P.: Étude angiographique d'un angiome intra-rachidien. Rev. neurol. **106**, 278-285 (1962).
Djindjian, R., Dumesnil, M., Fauré, C., Tavernier, J.B.: Angiome médullaire dorsal. Rev. neurol **108**, 432-434 (1963).
Djindjian, R., Fauré, C.: Investigations neuro-radiologiques dans les malformations vasculaires médullaires. Neuro-radio Roentgen Europ. **6-7**, 171-183 (1963).
Djindjian, R., Fauré, C.: L'aortographie dans les angiomes médullaires dorsaux. J. Radiol. Électrol. **46**, 680-682 (1965).
Djindjian, R., Fauré, C., Houdart, R., Lefebre, J.: Artériographie des angiomes médullaires. La radiographie des formations intra-rachidiennes. Paris: Masson, 1965.
Djindjian, R., Fauré, C., Houdart, R., Lefevre, J.: Exploration angiographique des malformations vasculaires de la moëlle épinière. Acta radiol. diagn. **5**, 145-162 (1966).
Djindjian, R., Fauré, C., Hurth, M.: Les angiomes de la moëlle dorso-lombaire. J. Radiol. Électrol. **46**, 168-170 (1965).
Djindjian, R., Houdart, R., Cophighon, J., Hurth, M.: Premiers essais d'embolisation par voie fémorale dans un cas d'angiome médullaire et dans un cas d'angiome alimenté par la carotide externe. Rev. neurol. **125**, 119-130 (1971).
Djindjian, R., Houdart, R., Fauré, C., Lefevre, J., Lebesnerais, Y., Hurth, M.: L'artériographie des angiomes de la moëlle. Rev. neurol. **109**, 640-645 (1963).
Djindjian, R., Houdart, R., Hurth, M.: Les angiomes de la moëlle épinière. Paris: Sandoz, 1969.
Djindjian, R., Houdart, R., Hurth, M., Cophignon, J., Rey, A., Thurel, C.: Embolisation dans les angiomes de la moëlle. J. Neuroradiologie **2**, 73-172 (1975).
Djindjian, R., Hurth, M.: Angiomas médullaires. Traité de Radiodiagnostic. Paris: Masson, Paris. 1971.
Djindjian, R., Hurth, M., Djindjian, M., Houdart, R.: Où en est l'angiographie médullaire en 1973 ? Nouv. Presse méd **2**, 22-29 (1973).
Djindjian, R., Hurth, M., Fauré, C.: Artériographie des angiomes médullaires. Expansion scientifique, 1966.
Djindjian, R., Hurth, M., Houdart, R.: Artériographie de la moëlle épinière dorsale et dorso-lombaire par aortographie sélective. **49**, 289-294 (1968).
Djindjian, R., Hurth, M., Houdart, R.: Les angiomes médullaires. Paris: Sandoz 1969.
Djindjian, R., Hurth, M., Houdart, R.: L'angiographie de la moëlle épinière. Paris: Masson 1970.
Djindjian, R., Hurth, M., Houdart, R.: Angiomas médullaires, dysplasies vasculaires segmentaires ou généralisées et phacomatoses. Rev. neurol. **124**, 121-142 (1971).
Djindjian R., Hurth, M., Houdart, R.: Hemangioblastomes médullaires et maladie de von Hippel-Lindau. Rev. neurol. **124**, 495 (1971).
Djindjian, R., Hurth, M., Mamo, H., Houdart, R.: L'embolisation de la voie artérielle spinale antérieure. Rev. neurol. **128**, 385-400 (1973).
Djindjian, R., Hurth, M., Rey, A., Houdart, R.: Angiomas médullaires dans la maladie de Rendu-Osler. J. Neuroradiol. **1**, 289-350 (1974).
Djindjian, R., Hurth, M., Thurel, Cl.: Cervico-cranial phlebography of angiomas of the spinal cord. Neuroradiology **1**, 42-46 (1970).
Doppman, J.L.: The nidus concept of spinal cord arteriovenous malformations. A surgical recommendation based upon angiographic observations. Brit. J. Radiol. **44**, 758-763 (1971).
Doppman, J., Di Chiro, G.: Subtraction angiography of spinal cord vascular malformations. Report of a case. J. Neurosurg. **23**, 440-443 (1965).
Doppman, J.L., Di Chiro, G., Glancy, D.L.: Collateral circulation through dilated spinal cord arteries in aortic coarctation and extraspinal arteriovenous shunts. An arteriographic study. Clin. Radiol. **20**, 192-197 (1968).
Doppman, J.L., Di Chiro, G., Ommaya, A.K.: Obliteration of spinal cord arteriovenous malformations by percutaneous embolization. Lancet 1968, 477.
Doppman, J.L., Di Chiro, G., Ommaya, A.K.: Selective arteriography of the spinal cord. St. Louis: Warren H. Green 1969.
Doppman, J.L., Di Chiro, G., Ommaya, A.K.: Percutaneous embolization of spinal cord arteriovenous malformations. J. Neurosurg. **34**, 48-55 (1971).
Doppman, J.L., Wirth, F.P., DiChiro, G., Ommaya, A.K.: Value of cutaneous angiomas in

the arteriographic localization of spinal-cord arteriovenous malformations. N. Engl. J. Med. **281**, 1440-1444 (1969).
Doppman, J.L., Zapol, W., Pierce, J: Transcatheter embolization with a silicone rubber preparation: Experimental observations. Invest. Radiol. **6**, 304-309 (1971).
Dorndorf, W., Gänshirt, H.: Die Klinik der arteriellen zerebralen Gefäßverschlüsse. In: Der Hirnkreislauf (Gd. H. Gänshirt), pp. 512-650 Stuttgart: Thieme 1972.
Dynes, J.B., Smedal, M.J.: Radiation Myelitis: Amer. J. Roentgenol. **83**, 78 (1960).
Echols, D.D. and Holcombe, R.G.: Extramedullary aneurysm of spinal cord. New Orleans med. Surg. J. 93, 582-583 (1941).
Elsberg, Ch. A.: The surgical significance and operative treatment of enlarged and varicose veins of the spinal cord. Amer. J. med. Sci. **151**, 642-652 (1916).
Engelhardt, F., Gruß, P.: Über ein spinales Angiom der Leptomeninx mit raumforderndem mikroangiomatösem Gebilde. Z.Neurol. **205**, 275-286 (1973).
Epstein, B.S., Govoni, A.F.: Aspetti mielografici delle aracnoiditi. Radiol. med. (Torino) **45**, 113-122 (1959).
Epstein, J.A., Beller, A.J., Cohen, I.: Arterial anomalies of the spinal cord. J. Neurosurg. **6**, 45-56 (1949).
Fischgold, H., Clement, J.C., Talairach, J., Ecoiffier, J.: Opacification des systèmes veineux rachidiens et craniens par osseuse voie. Presse méd. **60**, 599-601 (1952).
Flament, J., Nune Vicente, A., Coers, C., Guazzi, G.C.: La myélomalacie angiodysgénétique (Foix-Alajouanine) et sa differentiation des nécroses spinales sur angiomatose intramédullaire. Rev. neurol. **103**, 12-29 (1960).
Foerster, Ch., Kazner, E.: Spinales Angiom mit Querschnittslähmung bei Klippel-Trenaunay Syndrom. Neuropädiatrie **4**, 180-186 (1973).
Foix, Ch., Alajouanine, Th.: La myélite nécrotique subaiguë. Myélite centrale angio-hypertrophique à évolution progressive. Paraplégie amyotrophique lentement ascendante, d'abord spasmodique, puis flasque, s'accompagnant de dissociation albumino-cytologique. Rev. neurol. **33**, 1-42 (1926).
Fried, L.C., Di Chiro, G., Doppman, J.L.: Ligation of major thoracolumbar spinal cord arteries in monkeys. J. Neurosurg. **31**, 608-614 (1969).
Fuchs, E.: Aneurysma arterio-venosum retinae. Arch. Augenheilk. **11**, 440 (1882).
Gagel, O., Mészaros, A.: Zur Frage der Myelitis necroticans. Arch. Psychiat. **179**, 423-429 (1948).
Garcin, R., Kipfer, M., Gruner, J., Van Reeth, P.Ch.: Angiomatose disséminée du névraxe avec foyer hémorrhagique médullaire. Etude anatomo-clinique. Rev. neurol. **85**, 1-4 (1951).
Garcin, R., Lapresle, J.: Télangiectasies de la moëlle dorsale révélées à l'âge de 75 ans par une myélopathie transverse, avec une discussion sur l'atrophie spinale segmentaire. Ideggyóg. Szle. **21**, 34-40 (1968).
Garcin, R., Zülch, K.J., Lazorthes, G., Gruner, J.: Pathologie vasculaire de la moëlle. Rev. neurol. **106**, 531-645 (1962).
Gaupp, J.: Casuistische Beiträge zur pathologischen Anatomie des Rückenmarks und seiner Häute. Beitr. path. Anat. **2**, 510-524 (1888).
Giampalmo, V.: Zur Frage der "nekrotisierenden Myelopathie" ("Myelitis necroticans" Foix-Alajouanine). Nervenarzt **16**, 168-172 (1943).
Ginsbourg, M.: Contribution à l'étude des formations vasculaires pathologiques vertébro-médullaires. Thèse, Paris 1961.
Globus, J.H., Strauss, I.: Intraspinal iodolography. Subarachnoid injection of iodized oil as an aid in the detection and localisation of lesions compressing the spinal cord. Arch. Neurol. Psychiat. (Chicago) **21**, 1331-1386 (1929).
Globus, O.H., Doshay, L.J.: Venous dilatations and other spinal alterations, including true angiomata, with signs of cord compression. Surg. Gynec. Obstet. **48**, 345-366 (1929).
Gloor, P., Woringer, E., Schneider, J., Brogly, G.: Lombo-sciatiques par anomalies vasculaires épidurales. Schweiz. med. Wschr. **82**, 537-542 (1952).
Gold, R.R., Grace, D.M.: Gelfoam embolization of the left gastric artery for bleeding ulcer. Experimental considerations. Radiology **116**, 575-580 (1975).
Goran, A., Carlson, D.J., Fischer, R.G.: Successful treatment of intramedullary angioma of the cord. J. Neurosurg. **21**, 311-314 (1964).

Goulon, M., Escourolle, R., Grosbuis, S., Lougovoy-Visconti, J., Lefebvre, Y.: Paraplégie, puis troubles psychiques et dysarthrie en rapport avec des télangiéctasies diffuses du système nerveux central. Rev. neurol. **125**, 425-434 (1971).

Greenfield, J.G., Turner, J.W.: Acute and subacute necrotic myelitis. Brain **62**, 227-252 (1959).

Greitz, T., Liliequist, E., Mueller, R.: Cervical vertebral phlebography. Acta radiol. (Stockh.) **57**, 353-365 (1962).

Grode, M.L.: Hemangiopericytoma of the central nervous system. N.Y. St. J. Med. **72**, 2557-2561 (1972).

Gümbel, U., Pia, H.W., Vogelsang, H.: Lumbosacrale Gefäßanomalien als Ursache von Ischialgien. Acta neurochir. (Wien.) **20**, 131-151 (1969).

Guidetti, B.: Surgical treatment of vascular tumors and vascular malformations of the spinal cord. Vasc. Surg. **4**, 179-185 (1970).

Guidetti, B., Fortuna, A.: Surgical treatment of intramedullary hemangioblastoma of the spinal cord. Report of six cases. J. Neurosurg. **27**, 530-540 (1967).

Guidetti B., Fortuna, A., Moscatelli, G., Riccio, A.: I Tumori Intramidollari. Lavo neuropsichiat. **35**, 1-379 (1964).

Guidetti, B. and Silipo, P.: Considerazioni sul trattamento chirugico della anomalia vascolani del midollo. Minerva Neurochirurgica 5, 118-123 (1961).

Guillain, G., Alajouanine, Th.: Paraplégie par compression due à un volumineux angiocèle de la pie-mère spinale. J. Neurol. (Brux.) **11**, 69 (1925).

Guillain, G., Alajouanine, T.: Paraplégie par compression due à un volumineux angiocèle de la pie-mère spinale. Contribution à l'étude des compressions médullaires dues à des formations vasculaires pathologiques. J. Neurol. (Brux.) **25** 689-698 (1925).

Guillain, G., Bertrand, I., Lereboullet, J.: Hémangioblastomes du système nerveux central à localizations multiples. Rev. neurol. **47**, 432-441 (1932).

Guizzetti, P., Cordero, A.: Aneurisma dell'arteria centrale del midollo spinale con ematomielia secondaria. Rif. med. **19**, 761-767 (1903).

Gullota, U., Heller, H. Hämangioperizytome der Hirnhäute aus der Sicht des Radiologen. Fortschr. Röntgenstr. **120**, 561-566 (1974).

Guthkelch, A.N.: Haemangiomas involving spinal epidural space. J. Neurol. Neurosurg. Psychiat. **11**, 199-210 (1948).

Haberer, H.: Ein Fall von seltenem Collateralkreislauf bei angeborener Obliteration der Aorta und dessen Folgen. Z. Heilk. **24**, 26-38 (1903).

Hackel, W.: Über die Ectasie der Vena spinalis externa posterior mit der Querschnittskompressionsläsion des Rückenmarks. Z. Ges. Neurol. Psychiat 122, 550-559 (1929).

Hadlich, R.: Ein Fall von Tumor cavernosus des Rückenmarks mit besonderer Berücksichtigung der neueren Theorien über die Genese des Kavernoms. Virchows Arch. path. Anat. **172**, 429-441 (1930).

Hash, C.J.: Concurrent intracranial and spinal cord arteriovenous malformations. J. Neurosurg. **43**, 104-107 (1975).

Hebold, O.: Aneurysmen der kleinsten Rückenmarksgefäße. Arch. Psychiat. Nervenkr. **16**, 813-823 (1885).

Heidrich, R.: Die subarachnoidale Blutung. Leipzig: Thieme 1970.

Heindel, C., Dugger, G., Guinto, G.: Spinal arteriovenous malformation with hypogastric blood supply. J. Neurosurg. **42**, 462-464 1975.

Henson, R.A., Croft, P.B.: Spontaneous spinal subarachnoid haemorrhage. Quart. J. Med. **25**, 53-66 (1956).

Herdt, J.R., Di Chiro, G., Doppman, J.L.: Combined arterial and arteriovenous aneurysms of the spinal cord. Radiology **99**, 589-593 (1971).

Herdt, J.R., Shimkin, P.M., Ommaya, A.K., Di Chiro, G.: Angiography of vascular intraspinal tumors. Amer. J. Roentgenol. **115**, 165-170 (1972).

Herrmann, E., Lorenz, R., Vogelsang, H.: Zur Diagnostik der spinalen epiduralen Hämatome und Abszesse. Radiologe **5**, 504-508 (1965).

Hetzel, H.: Ein Fall von "Myélite nécrotique subaiguë" (Foix-Alajouaninesche Krankheit) mit Syringobulbie und Syringomyelie. Schweiz. Arch. Neurol. **86**, 70-81 (1960).

Hiecke, L.: Über Hämatomyelie bei intramedullären Telangiektasien. Beitr. path. Anat. 433-440 (1949).

Hilal, S.K., Michelsen, J.W.: Therapeutic percutaneous embolization for extra-axial vascular lesions of the head, neck and spine. J. Neurosurg. **43**, 275-287 (1975).
Hilal, S.K., Michelsen, J., Sane, P.H.: Intravascular adhesive for the treatment of vascular lesions of the spinal cord. Presented at 61st Annual Meeting of the RSNA, Nov. 30-Dec. 5, 1975, Chicago Ill.
Hindmarsch, T.: Myelography with a non-ionic water-soluble contrast medium (Metrizamide). Stockholm: 1974.
Hippel, E., von: Über eine sehr seltene Erkrankung der Netzhaut. Klinische Beobachtungen. Albrecht v. Graefes Arch. Ophthal. **59**, 83 (1904).
Hippel, E., von: Die anatomische Grundlage der von mir beschriebenen "sehr seltenen Erkrankung der Netzhaut" Albrecht von Graefes Arch. Ophthal. **79**, 350 (1911).
Höök, O., Lidvall, H.: Arteriovenous aneurysms of the spinal cord. A report of two cases investigated by vertebral angiography. J. Neurosurg. **15**, 84-91 (1958).
Hoffman, H.B., Bagan, M.: Cervical epidural arteriovenous malformation occurring with a spinal neurofibroma. Case report. J. Neurosurg. **26**, 346-351 (1967).
Hopkins, C.A., Wilkie, F.L., Voris, D.C.: Extramedullary aneurysm of the spinal cord. Case report. J. Neurosurg. **24**, 1021-1023 (1966).
Horten, B.C., Urich, H., Rubinstein, L.J., Montague, S.R.: The angioblastic meningioma: a reappraisal of a nosological problem. J. Neurol. Sci. **31**, 387-410 (1977).
Houdart, R.: Contribution à l'étude des angiomes de la moëlle, angiomes intra-duraux extra-médullaires. Thèse, Paris 1944.
Houdart, R.: Chirurgie des angiomes de la moëlle. Neurochirurgie **15**, Suppl. 1 (1969).
Houdart, R.: Les angiomes de la moëlle et leur traitement chirurgical. Nouv. Presse méd. **79**, 1533-1537 (1971).
Houdart, R., Djindjian, R.: Hémangioblastomes du cervelet, de la moëlle, du tronc cérébral et maladie de von Hippel-Lindau. J. méd. Leysin. **55**, 773 (1974).
Houdart, R., Djindjian, R., Hurth, M.: L'artériographie des angiomes de la moëlle. Étude anatomique et perspectives thérapeutiques. Presse méd. **73**, 525-530 (1965).
Houdart, R., Djindjian, R., Hurth, M.: Vascular malformations of the spinal cord: the anatomic and therapeutic significance of arteriography. J. Neurosurg. **24**, 583-594 (1966).
Houdart, R., Djindjian, R., Hurth, M.: Les angiomes de la moëlle. Étude clinique. Mécanisme de l'atteinte médullaire. Possibilités thérapeutiques. A propos de 32 cas. Rev. neurol. **118**, 97-110 (1968).
Houdart, R., Djindjian, R., Hurth, M.: Chirurgie des angiomes de la moëlle. Rapport 19e Congrès de Neurochirurgie. Neurochirurgie **15**, n°1. (1969).
Houdart, R., Djindjian, R., Hurth, M., Rey, A.: Treatment of angiomas of the spinal cord. Surg. Neurol. **2**, 3 (1974).
Hughes, J.T.: Pathology of the spinal cord. London: Lloyd-Duke 1966.
Huk, W., Klinger, M.: The diagnosis of cervical spinal angioblastomas. Neuroradiol. **5**, 174 (1973).
Hurth, M.: Les anévrysmes artério-veineux de la moëlle épinière. Considérations anatomo-cliniques et thérapeutiques à propos de 11 cas. Thèse, Paris: Foulon 1964.
Hurth, M., André, J.M., Djindjian, R., Escourolle, R., Houdart, R., Poirier, J., Rey, A.: Les hémangioblastomes intrarachidiens. Neuro-chirurgie. **21**, Suppl. 1 (1975).
Hurth, M., Djindjian, R., Houdart, R.: L'exérèse complète des anévrysmes artério-veineux de la moëlle épinière. Intérêt de l'artériographie médullaire sélective à propos de 11 cas. Neurochirurgie **14**, 499-514 (1968).
Hurth, M., Djindjian, R., Houdart, R.: Angiome médullaire cervical inextirpable pseudo-tumoral chez un malade porteur d'une maladie de Rendu-Osler. Neurochirurgie **16**, 287-295 (1970).
Hurth, M., Djindjian, B., Houdart, D., Ray, A., Djindjian, M.: Les angiomes de la moëlle. Progr. Neurol. Surg. 1976.
Hurth, M., Julian, H., Djindjian, R., Houdart, R.: Le traitement chirurgical des anévrysmes artério-veineux de le moëlle épinière à la lumière de l'artériographie médullaire. Neurochirurgie **12**, 437-450 (1966).
Iizuka, J.: Differential diagnosis of intraspinal hemangioblastomas. Minerva neurochir. **14**, 100-105 (1970).
Illingworth, R.D.: Phaeochromocytoma and cerebellar haemangioblastoma. J. Neurol. Neurosurg. Psychiat. **30**, 443-445 (1967).

Jackson, H.: A series of cases illustrative of cerebral pathology. Med. Times (Lond.) **2**, 541 (1872).
Jacob, M.: Angiome du cône médullaire avec stase papillaire. Neurochirurgie **15**, 586-590 (1969).
Jakesz, R.: Meningiales Hämangioperizytom mit zweizeitigen Spätmetastasen in Lunge und Thoraxwand. Thoraxchirurgie **24**, 23-29 (1976).
Jantz, H.: Zur Differentialdiagnose zwischen Arachnoiditis spinalis und Tumor spinalis im Myelogramm. Nervenarzt **18**, 175-179 (1947).
Jeffreys, R.V.: Supratentorial haemangioblastoma. Acta neurochir. (Wien) **31**, 55-65 (1974).
Jellinger, K.: Zur Orthologie und Pathologie der Rückenmarksdurchblutung. Berlin–Heidelberg–New York: Springer 1966.
Jellinger, K: The morphology of centrally situated angiomas. In: Cerebral Angiomas (ed. H.W. Pia, J.R.W. Gleave, E. Grote, J. Zierski), pp. 9-18. Berlin-Heidelberg-New York: Springer 1975.
Jellinger, K., Minauf, M., Garzuly, F., Neumayer, E.: Angiodysgenetische nekrotisierende Myelopathie. Arch. Psychiat. Nervenkr. **211**, 377-404 (1968).
Jellinger, K., Slowik, P.: Histological subtypes and prognostic problems in meningiomas. J. Neurol. **208**, 279-298 (1975).
Jellinger, K., Sturm, K.W.: Delayed radiation myelopathy in man. J. neurol. Sci. **14**, 389-408 (1971).
Kaplan, H.A., Aronson, S.M., Browder, E.J.: Vascular malformations of the brain. An anatomical study. J. Neurosurg. **18**, 630-635 (1961).
Kaplan, P., Hollenberg, R.D., Fraser, F.C.: Spinal arteriovenous malformation with hereditary cutaneous hemangiomas. Am. J. Dis. Child. **130**, 1329-1334 (1976).
Kastendieck, H., Klöppel, G., Altenähr, E.: Morphologie und klinische Bedeutung des meningealen Hämangiopericytoms. Z. Krebsforsch. **85**, 287-297 (1976).
Kaufman, H.H., Ommaya, A.K., Di Chiro, G., Doppman, J.L.: Compression av "steal". The pathogenesis of symptoms in arteriovenous malformations of the spinal cord. Arch. Neurol. **23**, 173-178 (1970).
Kendall, B.E., Logue, V.: Spinal epidural angiomatous malformation draining into intrathecal veins. Neuroradiology **13**, 181-190 (1977).
Kendall, B., Russell, J.: Haemangioblastomas of the spinal cord. Brit. J. Radiol. **39**, 817-823 (1966).
Kerber, C.: Intracranial cyanoacrylate. A new catheter therapy for arteriovenous malformations. Invest. Radiol. **10**, 536-538 (1975).
Kerber, C.: Experimental arteriovenous fistulas. Creation and percutaneous catheter obstruction with cyanoacrylate. Invest. Radiol. **10**, 10-17 (1975).
Kinney, T.D., Fitzgerald, P.J.: Lindau-von Hippel disease with hemangioblastoma of the spinal cord and syringomyelia. Arch. Path. **43**, 439 (1947).
Klug, W.: Die Angiome der Wirbelsäule und ihres Inhalts. Zbl. Neurochir. **18**, 279-291 (1948).
Koeppen, A.H., Barron, K.D., Cox, J.F.: Foix-Alajouanine syndrome. Acta neuropath. (Berl.) **29**, 187-197 (1974).
Koos, W.T., Böck, F.: Spontaneous multiple intramedullary hemorrhage. Case report. J. Neurosurg. **32**, 581-584 (1970).
Kothe, H.: Über Angiodysgenesia spinalis. Dtsch. Z. Nervenheilk. **169**, 409-420 (1953).
Kourbage, A.: Angiomes épiduraux intra-rachidiens. Thèse, Lyon 1972.
Krause, F.: Chirurgie des Gehirns und Rückenmarks. Berlin: Urban und Schwarzenberg 1911.
Krayenbühl, H., Benini, A., Bollinger, A., Wellauer, J., Senning, A.: Ein Fall von Klippel-Trénaunay-Weber-Syndrom mit arteriovenöser Fistel im Bereich der Brustwirbelsäule. Neurochirurgia (Stuttg.) **13**, 228-232 (1970).
Krayenbühl, H., Yasargil, M.G.: Die Varicosis spinalis und ihre Behandlung. Schweiz. Arch. Neurol. Psychiat. **92**, 74-92 (1963).
Krayenbühl, H., Yasargil, M.G.: Klinik der Gefäßmibildungen und Gefäßfisteln. In: Der Hirnkreislauf (Hrsz. H. Gänshirt), pp. 465-511. Stuttgart: Thieme 1972.
Krayenbühl, H., Yasargil, M.G., McClintock, H.G.: Treatment of spinal cord vascular malformations by surgical excision. J. Neurosurg. **30**, 427-435 (1969).
Krieger, A.J.: A vascular malformation of the spinal cord in association with a cauda equina ependymoma. Vasc. Surg. **6**, 167-172 (1972).
Krishnan, K.R., Smith, W.T.: Intramedullary haemangioblastoma of spinal cord associated

with pial varicosities simulating intradural angioma. J. Neurol. Neurosurg. Psychiat. **24**, 350-352 (1961).
Kunc, Z., Bret, J.: Diagnosis and treatment of vascular malformations of the spinal cord. J. Neurosurg. **30**, 436-445 (1969).
Labauge, R., Péguret, C., Torrès, F.: Les résaux cervicaux de suppléance au cours des obstructions athéromateuses de l'artère vertébrale. Rev. neurol. **121**, 467-481 (1969).
Langlois, M., Darlegug, P., Arron-Vignod, J.L., Toga, M., Vigoroux, R.: Maladie de von Hippel-Lindau avec hémangioblastome kystique de la moëlle dorsale opéré. Rev. neurol. **110**, 145-152 (1964).
Langmaid, C.: Personal communication. In: Observations on intradural spinal angiomas (Sheppard, R.H.). Neurochirurgia (Stuttg.) **6**, 58-74 (1963).
Lazorthes, G.: La vascularisation artérielle de la moëlle. Recherches anatomiques et application à la pathologie médullaire et aortique. Neurochirurgie **4**, 3-19 (1958).
Lazorthes, G., Gouazé, A., Zadeh, J.D., Santin, J.J., Lazortes, Y., Burdin, P.: Arterial vascularization of the spinal cord: Recent studies of the anastomotic substitution pathways. J. Neurosurg. **35**, 253-262. (1971).
Lazorthes, S., Gouazé, A., Djindjian, R.: Vascularisation et pathologie vasculaire de la moëlle épinière. Paris: Masson 1973.
Ledinsky, Q., Vrbik, J., Dura, J.: Aneurysm of arteria spinalis dorsalis. Plzenský lék. Sborn. **22**, 145-148 (1963).
Leech, P.J.: Unruptured aneurysm of the anterior spinal artery presenting as paraparesis. J. Neurosurg. **45**, 331-333 (1976).
Lepage, M., Djindjian, R., Hurth, M., Houdart, R.: Étude clinique et artériographique d'un angiome médullaire à pédicules multiples. Exérèse chirurgicale. Rev. neurol. **118**, 82-87 (1968).
Lepoire, J., Tridon, P., Montant, J., Hepner, H., Picard, L., Weber, M: Angioréticulome récidivant au cours d'une maladie de von Hippel-Lindau. Neurochriurgie **15**, 529-534 (1969).
Leu, H.J., Rüttner, J.R.: Angioretikulome des Zentralnervensystems. Acta neurochir. (Wien) **29**, 73-82 (1972).
Levin P.: Multiple hereditary hemangiomas of the nervous system. Arch. Neurol. Psychiat. (Chic.) **36**, 384-391 (1936).
Ley, A.: A-v. malformations of spinal cord: angiographic diagnosis and microsurgical techniques. Presented 25. Ann. Meeting Span. Society of Neurosurgery, April 1973, Malaga.
Lhermitte, J., Fribourg, B., Kyriaco, N.: La gliose angio-hypertrophique de la moëlle épinière (Myélite nécrotique de Foix-Alajouanine). Rev. neurol. **38**, 37-53 (1931).
Liebeskind, A.L., Schwartz, K.S., Coffey, E.L., Beresford, H.R.: Spinal epidural hematoma with delayed appearence of neurological symptoms. Neuroradiology **8**, 191-193 (1975).
Liliequist, B.: Spinal cord angiomas diagnosed by gas myelography. Neuroradiology **12**, 15-19 (1976).
Lindau, A.: Studien über Kleinhirncysten: Bau, Pathogenese und Beziehungen zur Angiomatosis Retinae. Acta Path. microbiol. Scand. Suppl. **1**, 1-128 (1926).
Lindau, A.: Discussion on vascular tumours of the brain and spinal cord. Proc roy. Soc. Med. **24**, 363-370 (1931).
Lindau, A.: Capillary angiomatosis of the central nervous system. Acta. genet: (Basel) **7**, 338 (1957).
Lindemann, A.: Varicenbildung der Gefäße der Pia mater spinalis und des Rückenmarks als Ursache einer totalen Querschnittsläsion. Z. ges. Neurol. Psychiat. **12**, 522-529 (1912).
Lindgren (1950): Quoted in Olsson, O.: Vertebral Angiography. Acta radiol. (Stockh.) **40**, 9 (1953).
Linoli, O.: Das histologisch-anatomische Bild und die Pathogenese der angiodysgenetischen Myelomalacie der Foix und Alajouanineschen Krankheit. Frankfurt. Z. Path. **69**, 247-267 (1958).
Logue, V., Aminoff, M.B., Kendall, S.: Results of surgical treatment for patients with a spinal angioma. J. Neurol. Neurosurg. Psychiat. **37**, 1074-1081 (1974).
Lombardi, G., Migliavacca, F.: Angiomas of the spinal cord. Brit. J. Radiol. **32**, 810-814 (1959).
Lorenz, O.: Cavernöses Angiom des Rückenmarks. Inaug.-Diss., Jena 1901.

Losacco, G.: Zur Frage der Lokalisation der angiodysgenetischen nekrotisierenden Myelopathie (Foix-Alajouaninesche Krankheit). Arch. Psychiat. Nervenkr. **208**, 360-370 (1966).
Lougheed, W.M., Hoffman, H.J.: Spontaneous spinal epidural hematoma. Neurology (Minneap.) **10**, 1059-1063 (1960).
Luessenhop, A.J., Dela Cruz, T.D.: The surgical excision of spinal intradural vascular malformations. J. Neurosurg. **30**, 552-539 (1969).
Luessenhop, A.J., Spence, W.T.: Artificial embolization of cerebral arteries: Report of use in case of arteriovenous malformation. J. Amer. med. Ass. **172**, 1153-1155 (1960).
Mair, W.G.P., Folkert S.J.E.: Necrosis of the spinal cord due to thrombophlebitis (subacute necrotic myelitis). Brain **76**, 563-575 (1953).
Manelfe, C., Djindjian, R.: Exploration artériographique des angiomes vertébraux. IX Symposium neuroradiologicum. Göteborg. Acta radiol. (Stockh.) **13**, 818-828 (1972).
Marc, J.A., Takei, Y., Schechter, M.M., Hoffman, J.C.: Intracranial hemangiopericytomas. Angiography, pathology and differential diagnosis. Amer. J. Roentgenol. **125**, 823-832 (1975).
Mares, A., Dumitrasco, I., Ionesco, M.: Accidents médullaires au cours de la coarctation de l'aorte. Hémorrhagie médullaire et subarachnoidienne par rupture d'anévrysme de l'artère spinale antérieure. Rev. roum. Neurol. **4**, 197-204 (1967).
Marty, L.: Contribution à l'étude de l'hématomyélie. Thèse, Bordeaux 1899.
McAllister, V.L., Kendall, B.E., Bull, J.W.D.: Symptomatic vertebral haemangioma. Brain **98**, 71-80 (1975).
McCormick, W.F.: The pathology of vascular ("arteriovenous") malformations. J. Neurosurg. **24**, 807-816 (1966).
Melmon, K.L., Rosen, S.W.: Lindau's Disease. Review of the literature and study of a large kindred. Amer. J. Med. **36**, 595 (1964).
Merry, G.S., D.B.: Spinal arterial malformation in a child with hereditary hemorrhagic telangiectasia. J. Neurosurg. **44**, 613-616 (1976).
Meyer, O., Köhler, B.: Über eine auf kongenitaler Basis entstandene cavernomähnliche Bildung des Rückenmarks. Frankfurt. Z. Path. **20**, 37-56 (1917).
Minckler, J. (ed.): Pathology of the Nervous System. New York: McGraw Hill 1971.
Möller, H.V.: Familial Angiomatosis Retinae et Cerebelli–Lindau's Disease. Acta opthal. (Kbh) **7**, 244 (1929).
Morris, L: Angioma of the cervical spinal cord. Case report. Radiology **75**, 785-787 (1960).
Muller, J., Mealey, J.Jr.: The use of tissue culture in differentiation between angioblastic meningioma and hemangiopericytoma. J. Neurosurg. **34**, 341-348 (1971).
Nadjmi, M., Engelhardt, F., Jensen, H.P., Gruß, P., Müller, H.A.: Zur Diagnose der Lindau-Tumoren bei retrogradem Brachialisangiogramm. Fortschr. Röntgenstr. **116**, 190 (1972).
Newman, M.J.D.: Racemose angioma of the spinal cord. Quart. J. Med. **28**, 97-108 (1959).
Newton, Th., Adams, J.: Angiographic demonstration and non-surgical embolization of a spinal cord angioma. Radiology **91**, 873-876 (1968).
Nibbelink, D.W., Peters, B.H., McCormick, W.F.: On the association of pheochromocytoma and cerebellar hemangioblastoma. Neurology (Minneap.) **19**, 455-460 (1969).
Nittner, K., Tönnis, W.: Symptomatologie, Diagnostik und Behandlungsergebnisse der Rückenmarks- und Wirbelangiome. Zbl. Neurochir. **10**, 317-333 (1950).
Odom, G.L.: Vascular lesions of the spinal cord. Clin. Neurosurg. **8**, 196-236 (1962).
Odom, G.L., Woodhall, B., Margolis, G.: Spontaneous hematomyelia and angiomas of the spinal cord. J. Neurosurg. **14**, 192-202 (1957).
Ohlmacher, J.: Multiple cavernous angioma, fibroendothelioma, osteoma and hematomyelia of the central nervous system. J. nerv. ment. Dis. **26**, 395-412 (1899).
Olivecrona, H., Tönnis, W.: Handbuch der Neurochirurgie, Vol. **7** II. Berlin–Heidelberg–New York: Springer 1971.
Oliver, A.D., Wilson, C.B., Boldrey, E.B.: Transient postprandial paresis associated with arteriovenous malformations of the spinal cord. Report of two cases. J. Neurosurg. **39**, 652-655 (1973).
Ommaya, A.K., Di Chiro, G., Doppman, J.L.: Ligation of arterial supply in the treatment of spinal cord arteriovenous malformations. J. Neurosurg. **30**, 679-692 (1969).
Ortner, W.D., Kubin, H., Pilz, P.: Ein zervikales kavernöses Angiom. Fortschr. Röntgenstr. **18**, 475-476 (1973).

Osterland, G.: Ein morphologischer Beitrag zur Kenntnis der Foix-Alajouanineschen Krankheit (Phlebodysgenetische Myelomalacie). Arch. Psychiat. Nervenkr. **800**, 123-145 (1960).
Otenasek, F., Silver, M.: Spinal hemangioma (Hemangioblastoma) in Lindau's Disease. Report of six cases in a single family. J. Neurosurg. **18**, 295-300 (1961).
Padget, D.H.: The development of the cranial arteries in the human embryo. Contr. Embryol. Carneg. Inst. **32**, 205-261 (1948).
Paillas, J.E., Bordouresgues Combalkert, A., Bérard, M., Salomon, G.: Angioréticulomes de la moëlle cervicale. Rev. Neurol. **117**, 416-417 (1967).
Palmer, J.J.: Haemangioblastomas: A review of 81 cases. Acta neurochir. (Wien) **27**, 125-148 (1972).
Panas, F., Rémy, D.A.: Anatomie pathologique de l'oeil. Paris: Delahaye 1879.
Papo, I., Salvolini, U., Vecchi, A.: Extradural spinal hemangioblastomas. J. neurosurg. Sci. **17**, 184-192 (1973).
Pecker, J.: Lindau's Disease. Presse méd. **79**, 635 (1971).
Pena, C.E.: Intracranial hemangiopericytoma. Acta neuropath. (Berl.) **33**, 279-284 (1975).
Perlmutter, I., Horrax, G., Poppen, J.: Cystic hemangioblastomas of the cerebellum. Surg. Gynec. Obstet. **91**, 88 (1950).
Perret, G., Nishioka, H.: Arteriovenous malformations. J. Neurosurg. **25**, 467-490 (1966).
Perthes, G.: Über das Rankenangiom der weichen Häute des Gehirns und Rückenmarks. Dtsch. Z. Chir. **203**, 93-103 (1927).
Pevsner, P.H., Strash, A., Kunz, R., Stinnett, R.: The computerized scan and experimental stroke in a new primate model. Presented at the International Symposium and Course on Computerized Tomography, Apr. 5-9, 1976, San Juan, Puerto Rico.
Pia, H.W.: Angiolipomatöse Dysplasien als Ursache von Ischialgien. Zbl. Chir. **85**, 1026-1033 (1960).
Pia, H.W.: Klinische Problematik der spinalen Angiome. In: Wirbelsäule und Nervensystem (Hrsg. E. Trostdorf und H. St. Stender), p. 90-96. Stuttgart: Thieme 1970.
Pia, H.W.: Diagnosis and treatment of spinal angiomas. J. Neurol. Neurosurg. Psychiat. **33**, 715 (1970).
Pia, H.W.: Diagnosis and treatment of spinal angiomas. Neurol. med. chir. (Tokyo) **11**, 11-16 (1971).
Pia, H.W.: The operative treatment of spinal arteriovenous malformations. Proc. 4th Europ. Congr. Neurosurgery, Avicenum Czechoslov. Med. Press, p. 385-387. Prague, 1972.
Pia, H.W.: Die operative Behandlung der Rückenmarkangiome. Dtsch. med. J. **23**, 186-189 (1972).
Pia, H.W.: The operative treatment of spinal angiomas. Phronesis 211-221 (1973).
Pia, H.W.: Diagnosis and treatment of spinal angiomas. Acta neurochir. (Wien) **28**, 1-12 (1973).
Pia, H.W.: Die Rückenmarkangiome. Dtsch. Ärztebl. **72** 727-734 (1975).
Pia, H.W.: Diagnose und Behandlung spinaler Angiome. In: Spinale raumfordernde Prozesse (Hrsg. W. Schiefer und H.H. Wieck), p. 345-356. Erlangen: Perimed 1976.
Pia, H.W., Vogelsang, H.: Diagnose und Therapie spinaler Angiome. Dtsch. Z. Nervenheilkd: **187**, 74-96 (1965).
Picard, L., Renard, M., Hepner, H., Lepoire,: Aspects radio-anatomiques des angiomes médullaires. A propos de deux observations. Neurochirurgie **15**, 519-528 (1969).
Pitkethly, D., Hardman, J.M., Kempe, L.G., Earle, K.N.: Angioblastic meningiomas. J. Neurosurg. **32**, 539-544 (1970).
Pool, J.L.: Arteriovenous malformations of the brain. In: Handbook of Clinical Neurology (P.J. Vinken and G.W. Bruyn, eds.), Vol. 12, pp. 227-266. Amsterdam: North Holland 1972.
Poole, G.J., Larsen, J.L.: Spinal arteriovenous malformation diagnosed by gas myelography. Neuroradiology **2**, 119-121 (1971).
Popoff, N.A., Malinin, T.I., Rosomoff, H.L.: Fine structure of intracranial hemangiopericytoma and angiomatous meningioma. Cancer (Philad.) **34**, 1187-1197 (1974).
Poser, C.M.: The relationship between syringomyelia and neuroplasm. Springfield Ill: Chas. Thomas 1953.
Pouyanne, L., Bergnouignan, M., Caillon, F.: Angiomes racémeux de la moëlle. Rev. neurol. **83**, 494-497 (1950).

Prieto, A., Cantu, R.C.: Spinal subarachnoid hemorrhage associated with neurofibroma of the cauda equina. J. Neurosurg. **27**, 63-69 (1967).
Profeta, G., Guarnieri, L., de Rosa, G., Ambrosio, A., Petrone, G., Calabro, A.: Arterio-venous aneurysms of the spinal cord. J. neurosurg. Sci. **18**, 98-108 (1974).
Puusepp, L: Zur Frage der Varices spinales und ihrer operativen Therapie. Zbl. Neurochir. **3**, 158-168 (1938).
Rand, R.M., Rand. D.W.: Intraspinal tumors of childhood. Vascular anomalies of the spinal cord, pp. 281-284. Springfield Ill: C.C. Thomas 1970.
Rasmussen, T., Kernohan, J., Adson, A.: Pathologic classification with surgical consideration of intraspinal tumors. Ann. Surg. **111**, 513-530 (1940).
Raynor, R.B., Kingman, A.F., Jr.: Hemangioblastoma and vascular malformations as one lesion. Arch. Neurol. **12**, 39-48 (1965).
Reeth, P.C. van: Contribution à l'étude de l'angiomatose médullaire. Acta neurol. belg. **52**, 354-366 (1952).
Reichman, O.H., Sorenson, B.F.: Excision of spinal cord arteriovenous malformation. Rocky Mtn. med. J. **68**, 21-24 (1971).
Reinisch, H.: Über das Wesen der Foix-Alajouanineschen Krankheit. Virchows Arch. path. Anat. **336**, 570-579 (1963).
Resche, F., Lefrane, G., Pradal, G., Lajat, Y., Collet, M., Descuns, P.: Les hémangioblastomes du névraxe. Rev. Oto-neuro-ophtal. **46**, 1-20 (1974).
Rey, A., Djindjian, R., Djindjian, M., Houdart, R.: Les angiomes antérieures de la moëlle et leur traitement chirurgical Rev. neurol. **132**, 364 (1976).
Reznik, M.: Le ramollissement médullaire. Acta neurol. belg. **65**, 294-317 (1965).
Ribadeu-Dumas, Ch., Djindjian, R.: Angiome médullaire cervical. Étude clinique et artériographique. Rev. neurol. **108**, 54-56 (1963).
Richardson, J.C.: Spontaneous haematomyelia. Brain **61**, 17-36 (1938).
Roman, B.: Ein Fall von Hämangiom des Rückenmarks. Zbl. allg. path. Anat. **24**, 993 (1913).
Roussy, G., Oberling, C.: Presse méd. **38**, 179 (1930).
Rubinstein, L.J.: Tumors of the central nervous system. Atlas of tumor pathology, 2nd series, Fasc. 8. Washington: Armed Forces Inst. of Pathology, 1972.
Russell, D.S.: Capillary haemangioma of spinal cord associated with syringomyelia. J. Path. Bact. **35**, 103-112 (1932).
Russell, D.S., Rubinstein, L.J.: Pathology of tumours of the nervous system. 3rd ed. London: Arnold 1972.
Sadka, M., Merrit, A.A.: Vascular anomaly of the spinal cord illustrated by three case reports. Aust. Ann. Med. **5**, 136-140 (1956).
Sahs, A.L. Perret, G.E., Locksley, H.B., et al.: Intracranial aneurysms and subarachnoid hemorrhage. A cooperative study. Philadelphia: Lippincott 1969.
Saito, I.: Total removal of hemangioblastoma of the spinal cord. Brain Nerve (Tokyo) **23**, 13 (1971).
Sakhai, H.: Hemangioblastoma of the Spinal Cord with Paraplegia: Recovery following surgical removal. Proc. Third Inter. Cong. Neurol. Surg. in Excerpta. med. (Amst.) 806, (1966).
Sargent, P.: Haemangioma of the pia mater causing compression paraplegia. Brain **48**, 259-267 (1925).
Schirger, A., Uilhein, A.L., Parker, H.L., Kernohan, J.W.: Hemangiopericytoma recurring after 26 years. Mayo Clin. Proc. **33**, 347-352 (1958).
Schmorl, G., Junghanns, H.: Die gesunde und kranke Wirbelsäule im Röntgenbild. Leipzig: Thieme 1932.
Scholz, W., Manuelidis, E.E.: Angiodysgenetische Myelopathie. Dtsch. Z. Nervenheilk. **165**, 56-71 (1951).
Scholz, W., Wechsler, W.: Ein weiterer Beitrag zur angiodysgenetischen nekrotisierenden Myelopathie (Foix-Alajouaninesche Krankheit). Arch. Psychiat. Nervenkr. **199**, 609-629 (1959).
Schröder, J.M., Brunngraber, C.V.: Über ein intramedulläres cavernöses Angiom. Acta neurochir. (Wien) **12**, 632-641 (1964).
Schultze, F.: Weiterer Beitrag zur Diagnose und operativen Behandlung von Geschwülsten des Rückenmarks. Dtsch. med. Wschr. **38**, 1767-1679 (1912).

Scoville, W.B.: Intramedullary arteriovenous aneurysm of the spinal cord. Case Report with operative removal from the conus medullaris. J. Neurosurg. 5. 307-312 (1948).
Seiler, R.: Rückenmarkskompression durch Wirbelhämangiome. Schweiz. Arch. Neurol. Neurochir. Psychiat. **108**, 4-22 (1971).
Serbinenko, F.A.: Balloon catheterization and occlusion of major cerebral vessels. J. Neurosurg. **41**, 125-145 (1974).
Seze, S., Hurth, M., Djindjian, R., Kahn, M.F., Hubault, A., Dryll, A.: A propos d'un cas d'angiomatose métamérique cutanéo-vertébro-médullaire. Rev. Rheum. **9**, 455-460 (1966).
Shenkin, H.A., Jenkins, F., Kim, K.: Arteriovenous anomaly of the brain associated with cerebral aneuryms. J. Neurosurg. **34**, 225-228 (1971).
Shephard, R.H.: Observations on intradural spinal angiomas. Neurochirurgia (Stuttg) **6**, 58-74 (1963).
Silver, M.L.: Hereditary vascular tumors of the nervous system. J. Amer. med. Ass. **156**, 1053-1056 (1954).
Sloof, J.L., Kernohan, J.W., MacCarty, C.S.: Primary intramedullary tumors of the spinal cord and filum terminale. Philadelphia: Saunders 1964.
Spence, A.M., Rubinstein, L.J.: Cerebellar capillary hemangioblastoma: its histogenesis studied by organ culture and electron microscopy. Cancer (Philad.) **35**, 326-341 (1975).
Steimle, R., Lecomte, R., Weill, F., Hanhart, P., Jacquet, G., Bonneville, J.-F.: Angiome para-médullaire avec compression de la moëlle cervicale. Sem. Hôp. Paris **47**, 1242-1247 (1971).
Stein, S.C., Ommaya, A.K., Doppman, J.L.: Arteriovenous malformation of the cauda equina with arterial supply from branches of the internal iliac arteries. Case report. J. Neurosurg. **36**, 649-651 (1972).
Stochdorph, O.: Pathologie des Rückenmarks. In: Handbuch der Neurochirurgie (ed. H. Olivecrona, W. Tönnis), Vol. **7**, Part 1, pp. 238-304. Berlin-Heidelberg-New York: Springer 1969.
Stout, A.P., Murray, M.R.: Hemangiopericytoma. A vascular tumor featuring Zimmermann's pericyte. Ann. Surg. **116**, 26-33 (1942).
Streeter, G.L.,: The developmental alterations in the vascular system of the brain of the human embryo. Contr. Embryol. Carneg. Instn **8**, 5-38 (1918).
Suh, T.H., Alexander, L.: Vascular System of the Human Spinal Cord. Arch. Neurol. Psychiat. 41, 659-677 (1939).
Suter-Lochmatter, H.: Die spinale Varikose. Acta neurochir. (Wien) **1**, 154-195 (1950).
Svien, H.J., Baker, H.L., Jr.: Roentgenographic and surgical aspects of vascular anomalies of the spinal cord. Surg. Gynec. Obstet. **112**, 729-735 (1961).
Tarlov, I.M.: Spinal extradural hemangioblastomas roentgenographically visualized with diodrast at operation and successfully removed. Radiology **49**, 717 (1947).
Taylor, A.R.: Surgical treatment of spinal arteriovenous malformations. J. Neurol. Neurosurg. Psychiat. **27**, 578-579 (1964).
Taylor, J.R., Van Allen, M.W.: Vascular malformation of the cord with transient ischemic attacks. J. Neurosurg. **31**, 576-578 (1969).
Teng, P., Papatheodorou, G.: Myelographic appearance of vascular anomalies of the spinal cord. Brit. J. Radiol. **37**, 358-366 (1964).
Teng, P., Shapiro, M.J.: Arterial anomalies of the spinal cord. Myelographic diagnosis and treatment by section of dentate ligaments. Arch. Neurol. Psychiat. **80**, 577-586 (1958).
Thomas, M., Burnside, R.M.: Von Hippel-Lindau's Disease. Amer. J. Ophthal. **51**, 140 (1961).
Töpfer, D.: Zur Kenntnis der Wirbelangiome. Frankfurt. Z. Path. **36**, 337-345 (1928).
Toga, M., Bérard-Badier, M., Chrestian, M.-A., Choux, R., Gambarelli, D., Hassoun, J., Pellissier, J.-F., Tripier, M.-F.: Tumeurs du système nerveux. Ultrastructure. Marseille: Diff. Gen. Libr. 1976.
Torr, J.B.D.: The embryological development of the anterior spinal artery in man. J. Anat. (London) **91**, 587 (1957).
Trupp, M. and Sachs, E.: Vascular tumors of brain and spinal cord and their treatment. J. Neurosurg. 5. 354-371 (1948).
Turnbull, I.M.: Blood supply of the spinal cord. In: Handbook of Clinical Neurology (P.J. Vinken and G.W. Bruyn, eds.), Vol. **12**, pp. 478-491. Amsterdam: North Holland 1972.

Turner, O.A., Kernohan, J.W.: Vascular malformations and vascular tumors involving the spinal cord. A pathologic study of forty-six cases. Arch. Neurol. Psychiatry (Chicago) **46**, 444-463 (1941).
Ule, G., Kolkmann, F.-W.: Pathologische Anatomie. In: Der Hirnkreislauf (ed. H. Gänshirt), pp. 47-160. Stuttgart: Thieme 1972.
Umbach, H.: Klinik und Verlauf bei 192 spinalen Prozessen mit besonderer Berücksichtigung der Gefäßtumoren. Acta neurochir. (Wien) **10**, 167-193 (1962).
Vanderkelen, B., Brihaye, J., Flament-Durand, J., Retif, J., Sadeghi, B.: Angiomes de l'espace épidural. Acta neurol. helg. **75**, 99-106 (1975).
Verbiest, H. et Calliauw, L.: Les angiomes racémeux intraduraux de la moëlle épinière. Rev. Neorol. 102, 230-243 (1960).
Virchow, R.: Die krankhaften Geschwülste. Berlin: Hirschfeld 1863.
Vogelsang, H.: Intraosseous spinal venography. Excerpta med. (Amst.) 1970.
Vogelsang, H.: Intraosseous spinal venography. Baltimore: Williams and Wilkins 1970.
Vogelsang, H.: Neuroradiological diagnosis of intradural spinal angiomas in children and infants. Neuropädiatrie **4**, 414-426, (1973).
Vogelsang, H.: Die selective spinale Arteriographie und ihre Bedeutung für die Diagnostik spinaler Angiome. Fortschr. Röntgenstr. **119**, 692-702 (1973).
Vogelsang, H.: Neuroradiological diagnosis of intradural spinal angiomas in children and infants. Neuropaed. **4**, 414-426 (1973).
Vogelsang, H.: Angiography. In: Handbook of Clinical Neurology (P.J. Vinken and G.W. Bruyn, eds.). Vol. **19** / Part I. Amsterdam: North Holland 1975.
Vogelsang, H.: Angiographische Untersuchungen von Wirbelsäule, Spinalkanal und Rückenmark. In: Handbuch der medizinischen Radiologie (L. Diethelm und S. Wende, Edt.), Band XIV/1. Berlin–Heidelberg–NewYork: Springer 1978, submitted for publication.
Vogelsang, H., Dietz, H.: Cervical spinal angioma combined with arterial aneurysm. Neuroradiology **8**, 223-228 (1975).
Voigt, K., Yasargil, M.G.: Cerebral cavernous haemangiomas or cavernomas. Neurochirurgia (Stuttg.) **19**, 59-68 (1976).
Vollmar, J., Diezel, P.B., Georg, H.: Das sogenannte Rankenangiom des Kopfes (Angioma racemosum Virchow). Langenbecks Arch. Klin. Chir. **307**, 8-14 (1964).
Vraa-Jensen G.: Angioma of the spinal cord. Acta psychiat. scand. **24**, 709-721 (1949).
Waldman, T.A. et. al., Amer. J. Med. **31**, 318 (1961) (Quoted Minckler, 1971).
Walker, A.E.: Dilatation of the vertebral canal associated with congenital anomalies of the spinal cord. Amer. J. Roentgenol. **52**, 571-582 (1944).
Ward, A.A. Jr., Foltz, E.L., Knopp, L.M.: "Polycythemia" associated with cerebellar hemangioblastoma. J. Neurosurg. **13**, 248-258 (1956).
Weenink H.L. Smilde, J.: Spinal cord lesions due to coarctatio aortae. Psychiat. Neurol. Neurochir. (Amst.) **67**, 259-269 (1964).
West, H.H.: Arterio-venous malformations as a cause of progressive myelopathy. Neurology (Minneap. **22**, 403. (1972).
Wirth, P.P., Post, R.P., DiChiro, G., Doppman, J.L., Ommaya. A.K.: Foix Alajouanine disease. Spontaneous thrombosis of a spinal cord malformation. Neurology (Minneap.) **20**, 114-118 (1970).
Woltman, H.W., Kernohan, J.W., Adson, A.W., Craig, W.McK.: Intramedullary tumors of spinal cord and gliomas of intradural part of filum terminale. Arch. Neurol. Psychiat. **65**, 378-395 (1951).
Wright, R.L.: Familial von Hippel-Lindau's Disease (Case Report). J. Neurosurg. **30**, 281-285 (1969).
Wyburn-Mason, R.: The vascular abnormalities and tumours of the spinal cord and its membranes. London: Kimpton 1943.
Yasargil, M.G.: Surgery of vascular lesions of the spinal cord with the microsurgical technique. Clin. Neurosurg. **17**, 257-265. (1969).
Yasargil, M.G.: Diagnosis and treatment of spinal cord arteriovenous malformations. Progr. Neurol. Surg. **4**, 355-428 (1971).
Yasargil, M.G., Antic, J., Laciga de Preux, Fideler, R.W., Boone, S.C.: The microsurgical removal of intramedullary spinal hemangioblastomas – Report of twelve cases and a review of the literature. Surg. Neurol. **6**, 141-148 (1976).
Yarsargil, M.G., De Long, W.B., Guarnaschelli, J.J.: Complete microsurgical excision of

cervical extramedullary and intramedullary malformations. Surg. Neurol. **4**, 211-224 (1975).
Zakov, S.B.: Vertebral hemangiona. Vestn. Rentgenol. Radiol. **6**, 54-59 (1953).
Zanetti, P.H., Sherman, F.E.: Experimental evaluation of a tissue adhesive as an agent for the treatment of aneurysms and arteriovenous malformations. J. Neurosurg. **36**, 72-79 (1972).
Zülch, K.J.: Angioblastome (Lindau-Zystem). In: Handbuch der Neurochirurgie (Ed. W. Krenkel, H. Olivecrona and W. Tönnis), Vol. **3**. Berlin–Göttingen–Heidelberg: Springer 1956.
Zülch, K.J.: Biologie und Pathologie der Hirngeschwülste. V. Gefäßgeschwülste, Gefäßmißbildungen und raumbeengende Gefäßveränderungen (Angiome und Aneurysmen). In: Handbuch der Neurochirurgie III, S. 555-573. Berlin–Göttingen–Heidelberg: Springer 1956.

Subject Index

MIX
Papier aus verantwortungsvollen Quellen
Paper from responsible sources
FSC® C105338

If you have any concerns about our products,
you can contact us on
ProductSafety@springernature.com

In case Publisher is established outside the EU,
the EU authorized representative is:
Springer Nature Customer Service Center GmbH
Europaplatz 3, 69115 Heidelberg, Germany

Printed by Libri Plureos GmbH
in Hamburg, Germany